# Quality Cancer Care

Peter Hopewood · Mary J. Milroy
Editors

# Quality Cancer Care

## Survivorship Before, During and After Treatment

Springer

*Editors*
Peter Hopewood
Cape Cod Healthcare
Falmouth, MA
USA

Mary J. Milroy
University of South Dakota Sanford
School of Medicine
Vermillion, SD
USA

ISBN 978-3-319-78648-3 ISBN 978-3-319-78649-0 (eBook)
https://doi.org/10.1007/978-3-319-78649-0

Library of Congress Control Number: 2018944116



Printed on acid-free paper

This Springer imprint is published by the registered company Springer International Publishing AG part of Springer Nature
The registered company address is: Gewerbestrasse 11, 6330 Cham, Switzerland

*This book is dedicated to cancer care providers and their patients.*

*We also dedicate this book to Mary's husband Dr. Dan Johnson and four daughters Carrie, Laura, Leslie, and Amy, and Peter's wife Lindsay and three sons Andrew, Ian, and Gavin.*

Mary J. Milroy
Peter Hopewood

# Preface

When we began training as residents in general surgery during the 1980s, cancer was primarily a surgical disease. The majority of cancer patients did not see other specialists. They had surgery, received routine postoperative care, and then were discharged home to face an uncertain future. The following decades, however, have seen a transformation in the prevention, diagnosis, treatment, and survivorship of cancer. Cancer is now a very multidisciplinary disease and not only involves dedicated professionals from many specialties but also encourages active patient engagement. These dramatic changes have resulted in improvements in both treatment and survival but have also created, at times, the seemingly overwhelming task of providing the highest quality, accessible, affordable cancer care to an increasing number of diverse patients. For this book, respected experts were asked to contribute information that would help cancer care providers "in the trenches" meet this challenge. We believe this book will be an invaluable resource and thank our authors for their willingness to share their expertise with our readers. Thanks also to Stephanie Frost for her work on this project.

Vermillion, SD Mary J. Milroy
Falmouth, MA Peter Hopewood

# Contents

# Contributors

**Domna Antoniadis** New York Legal Assistance Group, New York, NY, USA

**Allison J. Applebaum** Department of Psychiatry and Behavioral Sciences, Caregivers Clinic, Memorial Sloan Kettering Cancer Center, New York, NY, USA

**Tomas Bednar** Philadelphia, PA, USA

**James G. Brueggemann** Emeritus Physician, Essentia Health, Duluth, MN, USA

**Geoffrey P. Dunn** Department of Surgery, Palliative Care Consultation Service, UPMC Hamot, Erie, PA, USA

**Matthew A. Facktor** Department of Thoracic Surgery, Geisinger Health System, Danville, PA, USA

**Frederick L. Greene** Cancer Data Services, Levine Cancer Institute, Charlotte, NC, USA

**John D. Halporn** DFCI – POPC, Adult Palliative Care Clinic, Dana-Farber Cancer Institute, Harvard Medical School, Boston, MA, USA

Harvard Medical School Center for Palliative Care, Harvard Medical School, Boston, MA, USA

**Susan Hedlund** Department of Patient and Family Support Services, Knight Cancer Institute, School of Medicine, Oregon Health and Science University, Portland, OR, USA

**Carl E. Heltne** Emeritus Physician, Essentia Health, Duluth, MN, USA

**Peter Hopewood** American College of Surgeons Commission on Cancer, Falmouth, MA, USA

**Vicki A. Jackson** Division of Palliative Care and Geriatrics, Department of Medicine, Massachusetts General Hospital, Boston, MA, USA

Harvard Medical School Center for Palliative Care, Harvard Medical School, Boston, MA, USA

**Ted A. James** Department of Breast Surgical Oncology, Beth Israel Deaconess Medical Center, Harvard Medical School, Boston, MA, USA

**Wendy G. Lichtenthal** Department of Psychiatry and Behavioral Sciences, Bereavement Clinic, Memorial Sloan Kettering Cancer Center, New York, NY, USA

**Neil Maniar** Bouvé College of Health Sciences, Northeastern University, Boston, MA, USA

**Allison Marziliano** Department of Psychiatry and Behavioral Sciences, Memorial Sloan Kettering Cancer Center, New York, NY, USA

**Kimberly A. Maurer** BreastCare Center, Beth Israel Deaconess Medical Center, Harvard Medical School, Boston, MA, USA

**Mary J. Milroy** Department of Surgery, Sanford School of Medicine, University of South Dakota, Vermillion, SD, USA

**Aliza A. Panjwani** Department of Psychology, The Graduate Center, City University of New York, New York, NY, USA

**Jennifer Pruskowski** Department of Pharmacy and Therapeutics, University of Pittsburgh Medical Center, Palliative Supportive Institute (PSI), Pittsburgh, PA, USA

**Vishwa S. Raj** Section of Rehabilitation, Department of Supportive Care, The Levine Cancer Institute, Charlotte, NC, USA

Department of PM&R, Carolinas Rehabilitation, Carolinas Medical Center, Carolinas Healthcare System, Charlotte, NC, USA

**Simone P. Rinaldi** Division of Palliative Care and Geriatrics, Department of Medicine, Massachusetts General Hospital, Boston, MA, USA

Harvard Medical School Center for Palliative Care, Harvard Medical School, Boston, MA, USA

**Kailey E. Roberts** The New School for Social Research, New York, NY, USA

Department of Psychiatry and Behavioral Sciences, Memorial Sloan Kettering Cancer Center, New York, NY, USA

**Julie K. Silver** Department of Physical Medicine and Rehabilitation, Harvard Medical School, Boston, MA, USA

Spaulding Rehabilitation, Massachusetts General and Brigham and Women's Hospitals, Charlestown, MA, USA

**Lisa K. Simonian** Palliative Care Consultation Service, UPMC Hamot, Erie, PA, USA

**Paula M. Termuhlen** University of Minnesota Medical School, Duluth Campus, Duluth, MN, USA

**Richard Wender** American Cancer Society, Atlanta, GA, USA

**Ruth E. Westra** Department of Family Medicine and Community Health, University of Minnesota Medical School, Duluth Campus, Duluth, MN, USA

**Tracy Wiedt** American Cancer Society, Atlanta, GA, USA

**Eric M. Wisotzky** Rehabilitation Medicine, Georgetown University School of Medicine, Washington, DC, USA

Division of Rehabilitation Medicine, Cancer Rehabilitation, MedStar National Rehabilitation Network, Washington, DC, USA

The original version of this book was revised: Affiliation of Tomas Bednar was incorrectly listed in the contributor's list. This is corrected and updated in the contributor's list.

# Chapter 1
# Outlining the Crisis in Cancer Care

Mary J. Milroy

## Outlining the Crisis in Cancer Care

Cancer care teams are charged with the task of providing accessible, affordable, high-quality care to an increasing number of diverse patients. Unfortunately many stressors are present that make these goals increasingly difficult to achieve. Chief among the stressors are:

- Overall increasing numbers of cancer patients
- The increasing age and needs of cancer patients
- The increasing numbers of cancer survivors
- The projected shortages of adequately trained cancer care providers
- The increasing complexity of cancer diagnosis and treatment
- Increased demand for better communication and coordination between patients and providers and among providers
- The need for informed and engaged patients
- The difficulty in identifying and measuring quality parameters
- The unsustainable increasing cost of care
- The changing and unpredictable political climate
- Adopting quality cancer care into diverse local cancer programs

This literature review provides an overview of these stressors in order to assist cancer care teams in their strategic planning as they prepare to meet these challenges.

The United States Census Bureau December 2016 [1] estimated the US population at 323,127,513. This represented a 0.07% population increase (2.2 million persons) from July 2015 to July 2016. Of greater interest is the projected dramatic

M. J. Milroy
Department of Surgery, Sanford School of Medicine,
University of South Dakota, Vermillion, SD, USA



P. Hopewood, M. J. Milroy (eds.), *Quality Cancer Care*,
https://doi.org/10.1007/978-3-319-78649-0_1

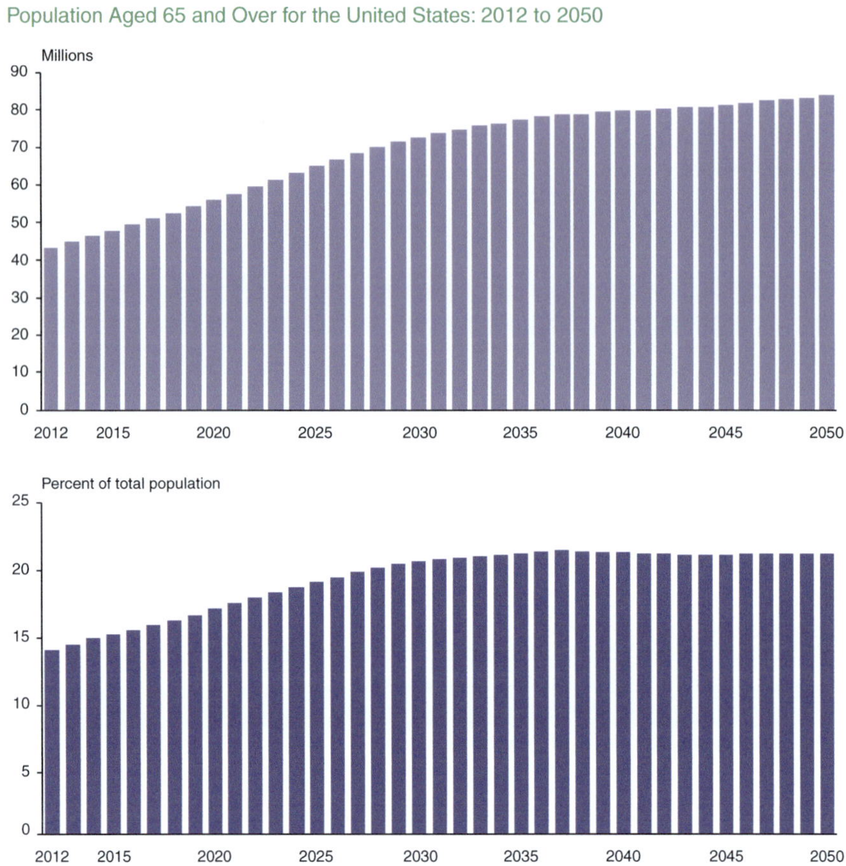


**Fig. 1.1** Population aged 65 and over for the United States: 2012–2050 [2]. Reprinted from US Census Bureau, 2012 Population Estimates and 2012 National Projections. An Aging Nation: The Older Population in the United States. Population Estimates and Projections. Current Population Reports. Ortman JM, Velkoff VA, Hogan H. May 2014; P25–1140. U.S. Department of Commerce Economics and Statistics Administration. https://www.census.gov/content/dam/Census/library/publications/2014/demo/p25-1140.pdf

increase in the percent of persons 65 years of age and older. In 2050 the US population over 65 is projected to be 82.7 million—almost double the estimated population of 43.1 million older persons in 2012 (Fig. 1.1).

## Increased Diversity of Population

In addition, the US Census Bureau notes that the population will be more racially and ethnically diverse [1]. The Pew Research Center also projects that the United States will continue to become more diverse and that by 2055 the United States will not have a single racial or ethnic majority [3]. Much of the increase in diversity is due to immigration. The populations with greatest increase are Hispanic and Asian-Americans [3].

Cancer is recognized as the second overall leading cause of death in the United States. In addition, the American Cancer Society (ACS) Facts and Figures 2017 [4] note that cancer is the leading cause of death in 22 states and in Hispanic and Asian-Americans. This will impact cancer services as the proportion of Hispanic and Asian-Americans grows. Cancer is also the leading cause of death in women aged 40–79 years and among men aged 45–79 years. The ACS projects 1,688,780 new cancer cases and 600,920 cancer deaths in the United States in 2017 [4]. SEER data estimates the lifetime risk of a male developing invasive cancer at 42.05% or one in two, and the lifetime risk of dying of cancer at 22.62% or one in four. For females, the risk of developing invasive cancer is 37.58% or one in three, and the risk of dying is 19.13% or one in five [5, 6].

## Aging Population

Increased age is recognized as the leading risk factor for the development of cancer. The incidence of cancer is increased 11-fold after the age of 65 and nearly 80% of all cancers are diagnosed in persons over age 55 [7–9]. This increasing proportion of older American at risk for developing cancer has been called the "silver tsunami" [10]. The challenges associated with treating older persons with cancer are multifactorial. Older individuals have traditionally been excluded from clinical trials [11] which makes evidence-based treatment guidelines scarce. Older individuals experience physiologic changes associated with aging [9] and are more likely to present with comorbidities, defined as "coexistence of disorders in addition to a primary disease of interest" [12]. Data from Medicare indicates that four of ten patients with cancer have at least one other chronic condition and 15% have two or more. The most common chronic conditions include cardiovascular disease, obesity, metabolic illness, mental health problems, and musculoskeletal conditions [13]. This affects both treatment choices and outcomes. Most treatment guidelines are not designed to consider the interaction between cancer and comorbidity and many providers do not have experience with managing patients with a wide variety of comorbidities [13]. Comorbidity may impact the timing of diagnosis both positively and negatively. Increased contact with health providers may lead to more screening opportunities and an earlier diagnosis or on the other hand the comorbidities may distract the patient and provider leading to a delayed diagnosis [13]. Patients with existing comorbidities may be less likely to receive curative treatment and are less likely to receive treatment that is concordant with clinical guidelines [13]. Comorbidity and cancer outcomes have been difficult to evaluate but have been found to adversely affect survival and lead to poorer quality of life [13]. In addition, older cancer patients often present with greater needs for social support [14] during treatment and in survivorship [14, 15].

## Impact of Cancer on the Population

Cancer statistics follow incidence, mortality, years of life lost, years lived with disability (YLD), and disability-adjusted life years (DALY) to determine the full impact of cancer on a population [16]. Survivorship is defined as people living with and beyond cancer and can also include those caring for them [17]. Increased survivorship represents a great success in cancer treatment and one of the biggest changes in the field of cancer care. An estimate of survivors rose from 3 million in 1971 to more than 15.5 million in 2016 and is estimated to reach 20.3 million by 2026 [17]. Survivors are currently estimated to account for 5% of the US population. Survivors are a diverse population and experience varying ongoing physical, psychological, and social needs associated with their cancer treatment [17–19].

### *Workforce Shortages*

The workforce that will be required to deal with the increased number of cancer patients is noted to be in crisis [20, 21]. The Institute of Medicine National Cancer Policy Forum Workshop convened in 2010 to address this challenge [20]. The workshop noted "there is a crisis in the oncology workforce. Health professionals involved in prevention, early detection, diagnosis, treatment, survivorship, palliative care, and research are experiencing significant workforce shortages that are expected to worsen. This is because of the rapidly growing population of Americans requiring cancer care, an aging oncology workforce, and inadequate numbers of newly trained workers. This mismatch between supply and demand for cancer care could threaten patient care, safety and quality" [20]. The increased demand was noted to be due to an aging population with higher rates of cancer and with changes in cancer treatments that were less toxic but require more frequent administration and increased patient visits. The critical workforce shortage was predicted to involve oncologists, nurses, allied health providers, public health workers, social workers, pharmacists, and primary care providers adequately trained to care for cancer patients. The age of the current workforce was noted as a principal factor as more members are approaching retirement age than are currently in training to replace them and far less than what will be required to meet the increasing needs. ASCO State of Cancer 2016 [21] noted that 1/5 of practicing oncologists are of age 64 or older. There continues to be underrepresentation of racial and ethnic minorities in the oncology workforce and there is uneven distribution of oncologist in the United States with 19% of American living in a rural area while only 6% of oncologists practice in rural areas. ASCO State of Cancer 2017 continued to identify a looming critical workforce shortage in oncology [22]. This shortage will make traditional methods of providing cancer care unsustainable and urgently calls for innovative new methods of providing quality care.

## Complexity of Cancer Care

The increasing complexity of cancer care is affecting both the diagnosis and treatment of cancer. ASCO's State of Cancer 2016 [21] noted that complexity of cancer care involves screening recommendations, implementation of precision medicine treatments, and aging of the US population. Implementation of screening programs is challenging in the face of conflicting and changing screening guidelines. The importance of weighing the risks and benefits of screening in order to avoid over- as well as under-screening and incorporating the individual patient's desires in order to make individualized screening recommendations creates challenges for cancer programs attempting to implement cancer screening programs. Precision medicine expands treatment options and improves survivals but both providers and patients are now faced with overwhelming amounts of complex and evolving information. This is often difficult to process and utilize in making treatment decisions. This complexity must be taken into account as programs plan for the future.

## Importance of Good Communication

The increasing complexity of treatment and the increasing number of diverse providers involved in a patient's care create the need for good communication among providers and with patients. Survivors identify poor communication and lack of coordination as barriers to care [17]. Survivors express desire that their needs be addressed by their oncology team and also request involvement of their primary care providers. This coordination of care is important during all aspects of treatment and aftercare. Patients who experienced communication gaps experienced confusion, insecurity, a sense of vulnerability, and abandonment. There is increasing need for models of health care that promote effective coordination and communication especially during times of transition.

## Patient-Reported Cancer Care Experience

Patient-reported outcomes are now playing an increasingly important role in the care of cancer patients. The following study from Cancer Care provides an example of the types of information that can be obtained from patient-reported outcomes. If problems are identified, cancer care providers can then design and implement quality improvement actions In order to assess the patient experience with cancer diagnosis, treatment, and survivorship, Cancer Care [23] designed six online surveys. Each survey included at least 500 patients diverse in age, gender, ethnicity, education, income, geography, cancer type, and stage. In all, over 3000 patient results were analyzed. Their 2016 report provides patient insight into their cancer experience. Highlights from their survey are as follows.

- Survey 1 assessed the patient's understanding of the diagnosis of cancer. Most patients reported following their physician's recommendation for diagnostic testing and understood the risks and benefits. Nearly all were able to access testing and expressed confidence in their doctor. However ¼ of patients aged 25–54 disagreed with some of the recommendations and did not follow them. Less than ½ discussed the cost of follow-up testing.
- Survey 2 assessed treatment planning, including communication and shared decision-making. Only two-thirds of patients felt that they were provided adequate information regarding treatment options. Only 13% felt that they received adequate information regarding clinical trials. Less than half said that they had adequate information on matters such as their ability to continue to work during treatment, how much home care they would need, the emotional impact of cancer and treatment, and how much of the cost of care they were personally responsible for. Half sought a second opinion and the majority felt that they had gotten the best care. Only half reported their care team regularly inquiring about their level of distress. Patient satisfaction was low regarding access to clinical trials and new treatments.
- Survey 3 looked at communication. Most patients were satisfied and felt that their care was coordinated; they understood the discussions and could connect with members of the team in a reasonable time. However 20% of African-American patients reported serious communication problems and experienced discomfort talking about cultural, religious, and personal values and their effect on treatment. Only half of patients reported being asked about their distress and very few were referred to counseling.
- Survey 4 looked at financial and insurance concerns. Half felt that they understood their insurance completely or very well. Twenty-five percent reported stopping work completely and 13% switched from full- to part-time work. Only one-third were able to continue working full time. Fifty-eight percent reported distress about finances. Twenty-five percent felt that financial concerns were never considered in treatment planning and 34% said that finances were only sometimes considered. Many patients reported using care-altering strategies to reduce cost. Many cut back on daily living costs such as groceries and transportation and borrowed money. Twenty-one percent missed paying a utility bill and 17% missed a rent or mortgage payment. Forty-four percent of patients aged 25–64 experienced the fear that if they could not continue to work they would lose their insurance.
- Survey 5 looked at symptoms, side effects, and quality of life. The majority reported moderate-to-severe fatigue. One-quarter to one-third felt that their ability to perform day-to-day activities was dramatically compromised.
- Survey 6 looked at survivorship. The survey noted that profound physical, emotional, financial, social, and spiritual changes occurred as a result of cancer diagnosis and treatment. A significant stress was the concern for the impact their cancer diagnosis and treatment had on family members. Most had end-of-life discussions with their family. There, however, was widespread misconception regarding hospice and palliative care.

## Measuring Quality of Cancer Care

Parameters for identifying and measuring quality of cancer care are essential but have not been widely determined and adopted. Organizations such as the National Quality Forum, the National Comprehensive Cancer Network, the American Medical Association Physician Consortium for Performance Improvement, the National Committee for Quality Assurance, the Center for Medicare and Medicaid, and the Agency for HealthCare Research Quality all work to promote healthcare quality through measurement and reporting. Unfortunately there are many diverse measures without consensus agreement on meaningfulness. Often measures have been collected based on the ease of obtaining the information without regard to clinical relevance. The time involved and the cost of obtaining meaningful data remain a challenge. Comparative effectiveness research (CER) is beneficial in guiding research, clinical oncology practice, and national healthcare policy. CER evaluates the benefits and harms of available diagnostic and therapeutic strategies in order to determine the most effective, safe, and cost-effective treatments [24]. Measure development includes not just survival but other measures such as quality of life and patient-reported outcomes. However, measures are often determined from large population databases and not from individual oncology practices. Measures are often cancer type specific. The Quality Oncology Practice Initiative (QOPI) [25] allowed individual practitioners to evaluate their practice's quality of care compared to published practice guideline and consensus-derived indicators of quality of care with the goal of improving quality in individual practitioners' offices. The challenge of developing and measuring quality parameters remains a work in progress.

## Cost of Health Care

The cost of health care in the United States has been steadily rising. Serious concerns have been raised that the high cost of care especially for diseases such as cancer with fast diffusions of expensive new technologies could jeopardize the quality of care [26]. This has been largely due to a fee-for-service payment system that reimbursed quantity but not quality and resulted in unsustainable healthcare spending that grew by 5.8% in 2015 to $3.2 trillion and represented 17.8% of the US GDP, the highest in the world [27]. Cost of cancer care is of vital interest to both patients and payers.

The increased cost of cancer care has led to increased cost shifting to patients. "Average out-of-pocket (OOP) spending by cancer patients is estimated at $1730 to $4727 per year depending on insurance status" [28, 29]. Financial burden can affect outcomes with patients delaying or forgoing care, avoiding filling prescriptions, and experiencing increased financial stress and lower satisfaction with care [28, 29]. Individual costs of oncology care present a burden for patients. Insured patients report high deductibles and high drug prices. 24% of Americans reported having a hard time paying for prescription drugs and 72% felt that drug prices were unreasonable. 31 million underinsured had difficulty with out-of-pocket costs [21, 28]. ASCO State of Cancer 2017 states that "even among patients with health insurance, a cancer diagnosis can be financially catastrophic" [22]. Many patients struggle financially during and after cancer treatment [30] and economic recovery has been proposed as a measure of the quality of cancer treatment and survivorship [31].

## Health Insurance Status

Health insurance status impacts patient outcomes [32]. Reports of patients with various tumors from germ cell tumor to breast cancer to glioblastoma note that patients who are either uninsured or have Medicaid coverage present at later stage with larger tumors and increased likelihood of metastatic disease. The type of insurance also affects the treatment received. Significant differences are observed in patients receiving optimal care with insurance status affecting the likelihood of lymph node dissection, radiation therapy, surgical therapy, and referral to specialists. Less than optimal care is felt to result in poorer outcomes for uninsured and Medicaid patients.

The American Society of Clinical Oncology established a Cost of Care Task Force in 2007 and published guidelines that encouraged cost communication as a key component of high-quality care [33]. A literature search conducted at MD Anderson noted that while the majority of patients desired cost communication with their providers, less than 33% actually had such discussions. Over 75% of physicians felt that these discussions were their responsibility; however, the majority were uncomfortable with these discussions and expressed the need for accurate cost information [33].

### *Affordable Care Act*

The Affordable Care Act consisted of the Patient Protection and Affordable Care Act (P.L. 111–148) and the Health Care and Education Reconciliation Act of 2010 (P.L. 111–152) and was intended to expand coverage, hold insurance companies accountable, lower healthcare costs, guarantee more choice, and enhance the quality of care for all Americans. The law was enacted in March 2010 and the most significant changes took effect in January 2014. At the end of 2015 there remained 28.5 million uninsured people but represented a decrease of 13 million uninsured people. The majority of people who remained uninsured cited high cost as the reason for not obtaining insurance. Economic evaluation defined as "the comparative analysis of alterative courses of action in terms of both their costs and consequences" may assist in priority setting and allocation efficiency [26]. The passage of the Medicare Access and CHIP Reauthorization Act of 2015 (MACRA) was adopted to attempt to address this crisis. This law created the Merit-based Payment System (MIPS) and the Advanced Alternative Payment Models (APMs). MACRA attempts to replace a volume-based system with a quality-based system [34]. In addition, MACRA section 102 established the Quality Measure Development Plan (MDP) to build a framework to build and improve quality measures for clinicians. These measures were to support MIPS and advanced APMS. Unfortunately the rules were not finalized until November 2016 when MACRA was due to take effect in January 2017. This limited time frame burdened providers and healthcare systems to scramble towards implementation. Recent data show that the uninsured rate in the United States continues to fall. Gallup and Healthways reported in July 2017 that the uninsured rate in the United States was 11.7% which was slightly increased from the previous quarter but significantly lower than the 18% peak in 2013 before the Affordable Care Act's individual mandate which took effect in 2014 [35].

## *National Health Policy*

However, uncertainty regarding the future of healthcare spending occurred with the change in federal administration in January 2017 and "the United States has never experienced a sea change in national health policy like that which occurred in early 2017" with the "First steps of Repeal, Replace, and Repair" [36]. The Affordable Care Act has come under fierce debate in both the US House and Senate and the question of continued coverage for the millions of Americans that obtained coverage under the ACA is undetermined at this time. This leaves the future of health care uncertain and creates challenges to programs attempting to plan for the future.

## *Care at the Local Level*

Improving care at the local level is essential. The Institute of Medicine's report Best Care at Lower Cost: The Path to Continuously Learning Health Care in America [37] identified significant gaps in quality care and recommended new strategies to align science and informatics, patient-clinician partnerships, incentives, and a culture of continuous improvement to produce the best care at lower cost. The Commission on Cancer (CoC) is a consortium of professional organizations dedicated to survival and quality of life for cancer patients through standard-setting prevention, research, education, and monitoring of quality care. In 2012, the CoC released their new patient-centered standards. Programs of all sizes can adopt these standards, measure compliance, and undergo survey to check adherence to these standards and receive accreditation. Even small local programs can show that they are adhering to high national standards. The Institute of Medicine's detailed report Delivering High-quality Cancer Care: Charting a New Course for a System in Crisis [38, 39] can be a helpful resource for programs working to incorporate quality improvement at the local level.

## Summary

Cancer care programs are charged with the task of providing accessible, high-quality, patient-based care. Knowledge of the stressors facing cancer programs from increasing numbers of patients, increasing age and ethnic and racial diversity of patients, increasing numbers of survivors, workforce shortages, increasing complexity of cancer care, increasing need for improved communication and patient engagement, development and measuring of quality parameters, providing accessible and affordable care in a climate of increasing cost, uncertain political climate, as well as incorporating quality care at a local level can assist cancer programs in the successful achievement of that goal.

## References

1. United States Census Bureau. Tuesday December 20, 2016. Release number: CB16-214.
2. Ortman JM, Velkoff VA, Hogan H. An aging nation: the older population in the United States. Population Estimates and Projections. Current Population Reports. US Department of Commerce, Economics and Statistics Administration, US Census Bureau. 2014. p. 25–1140. https://www.census.gov/prod/2014pubs/p25-1140.pdf.
3. Pew Research Center. The changing face of America 1965–2065. www.pewresearch.org/ft_16-01-25_nextamerica_fig.2_1_495px/.
4. American Cancer Society. Cancer Facts and Figures 2017. https://www.cancer.org/research/cancer-facts-statistics/all-cancer-facts-figures/cancer-facts-figures-2017.html.
5. Lifetime risk (percent) of being diagnosed with cancer by site and race/ethnicity:males, 18 SEER Areas, 2010–2012 (Table 1.16). http://seer.cancer.gov/csr/1975_2012/browse_csr.php?sectionSEL=1&pageSEL=sect_01_table.16.html and females, 18 SEER Areas, 2010–2012 (Table 1.17) http://seer.cancer.gov/csr/1975_2012/browse_csr.php?sectionSEL=1&pageSEL=sect_01_table.17.html.2014.
6. Lifetime risk (percent) of dying from cancer by site and race/ethnicity:males, Total US, 2010–2012 (Table 1.19) http://seer.cancer.gov/csr/1975_2012/browse_csr.php?sectopmSEL=1&pageSEL=sect_01_table.19.html and females, total US, 2010–2012 (Table 1.20) http://seer.cancer.gov/csr/1975_2012/browse_csr.php?sectionSEL=1&pageSEL=set_01_table.20.html.2014.
7. Serrano M. Unraveling the links between cancer and aging. Carcinogenesis. 2016;37(2):107.
8. Li D, de Glas NA, Hurria A. Cancer and aging: general principles, biology, and geriatric assessment. Clin Geriatr Med. 2016;32(1):1–15.
9. Marosi C, Koller M. Challenge of cancer in the elderly. ESMO Open. 2016;1(3):e000020. eCollection 2016.
10. Bluethmann SM, Mariotto AB, Rowland JH. Anticipating the "Silver Tsunami": prevalence trajectories and comorbidity burden among older cancer survivors in the United States. Cancer Epidemiol Biomark Prev. 2016;25(7):1029–36.

11. Hutchins L, Unger J, Crowley J, Coltman C, Albain K. Underrepresentation of patients 65 years of age or older in cancer-treatment trials. N Engl J Med. 1999;341:2061–7.
12. Feinstein A. The pre-therapeutic classification of co-morbidity in chronic disease. J Chronic Dis. 1970;23:45–469.
13. Sarfati D, Koczwara B, Jackson C. The impact of comorbidity on cancer and its treatment. CA Cancer J Clin. 2016;66:337–50.
14. Mohile S, Hurria A, Cohen H, Rowland J, Leach C, Arora N, et al. Improving the quality of survivorship for older adults with cancer. Cancer. 2016;122:2459–68.
15. Rowland J, Bellizzi K. Cancer survivorship issues: life after treatment and implications for an aging population. J Clin Oncol. 2014;32(24):2662–8.
16. Global Burden of Disease Cancer Collaboration. Global, Regional, and National Cancer Incidence, Mortality, years of life lost, years lived with disability, and disability-adjusted life-years for 32 cancer groups, 1990 to 2015: a systematic analysis for the global burden of disease study. JAMA Oncol. 2017;3(4):524–48.
17. Mayer D, Nasso S, Earp J. Defining cancer survivors, their needs, and perspectives on survivorship health care in the USA. Lancet Oncol. 2017;18:e11–8.
18. Snyder C, Frick K, Herbert R, Blackford A, Neville B, Lemke K, et al. Comorbid condition care quality in cancer survivors: role of primary care and specialty providers and care coordination. J Cancer Surviv. 2015;9:641–9.
19. Mayer D, Shapiro C, Jacobson P, McCabe M. Assuring quality cancer survivorship care: we've only just begun. Am Soc Clin Oncol Educ Book. 2015:e583–91.
20. Levit L, Smith A, Benz E, Ferrell B. Ensuring quality cancer care through the oncology workforce. J Oncol Pract. 2010;6(1):7–11.
21. ASCO State of Cancer 2016. American Society of Clinical Oncology. 2016. doi:101200/JOP2015.010462.
22. ASCO. The State of cancer care in America 2017. Proc Am Soc Clin Oncol. 2017;13(4):e353–94. https://doi.org/10.1200/JOP.2016.020743.
23. CancerCare. CancerCare patient access and engagement report. New York: CancerCare; 2016.
24. Lyman G, Levine M. Comparative effectiveness research in oncology: an overview. J Clin Oncol. 2012;30(34):4181–4.
25. Neuss M, Desch C, McNiff K, Eisenberg P, Gesme D, Jacobson J. A process for measuring the quality of cancer care: the quality oncology process initiative. J Clin Oncol. 2005;23(25):6233–9.
26. Tina Shih YC, Mullins Daniel C, Drummond M. The role of economic evaluation in meeting IOM's recommendations on delivering high-quality cancer care. Value Health. 2014;17(5):497–500.
27. Martin A, Hartman M, Washington B, Catlin A, The National Health Expenditures Accounts Team. National health spending: faster growth in 2015 as coverage expands and utilization increases. Health Aff (Millwood). 2017;36(1):166–76.
28. Collins S, Rasmussen P, Beulet S, Doty M. The problem of underinsurance and how rising deductibles will make it worse: findings from the common wealth fund biennial health insurance survey, 2014. Issue Brief (Commonw Fund). 2015;13:1–20.
29. Kale H, Carroll N. Self-reported financial burden of cancer care and its effect on physical and mental health-related quality of life among US cancer survivors. Cancer. 2016;122:1283–9.
30. Pisu M, Azuero A, Benz R, McNees P, Meneses K. Out-of-pocket costs and burden among rural breast cancer survivors. Cancer Med. 2017;6(3):572–81.
31. Bradley C. Economic recovery: a measure of the quality of cancer treatment and survivorship. Cancer. 2015;121:4282–5.
32. Halpern M, Brawley O. Insurance status, health equity, and the cancer care continuum. Cancer. 2016;122:3106–9.
33. Shih Y, Chien C. A review of cost communication in oncology: patient attitude provider acceptance, and outcome assessment. Cancer. 2017;123:928–39.
34. Kaiser Family Foundation. "Key facts about the uninsured population" KFF.org. 2016. http://www.kff.org/uninsured/fact=sheet/key-facts-about-the-uninsured-population/.

35. Auter Z. U.S. Uninsured rate rises to 11.7%. www.news.gallup. July 10, 2017. Gallup and Healthways U.S. Uninsured Rate Rises to 11.7%. Healthcare. 2017. http://news.gallup.com/poll/213665/uninsured-rate-rises.aspx.
36. Jost T. First steps of repeal, replace, and repair. Health Aff. 2017;36(3):398–9.
37. Institute of Medicine. Best care at lower cost: the path to continuously learning health care in America. 2012. http://www.nationalacademies.org/hmd/Reports/2012/Best-Care-at-Lower-Cost-The-Path-to-Continuously-Learning-Health-Care-in-America.aspx.
38. The National Academy of Sciences, Engineering and Medicine: Delivering high-quality cancer care: charting a new course for a system. 2013. http//nationalacademes.org/hmd/reports/2013/delivering-high-quality-cancer-care-charting-a-new-course-for-a-system-in-crisis.aspx.
39. Nekhlyudov L, Levit L, Hurria A, Ganz P. Patient-centered, evidence-based, and cost-conscious cancer care across the continuum: translating the Institute of Medicine report into clinical practice. CA Cancer J Clin. 2014;64:408–21.

# Chapter 2
# Public Reporting of Institution and Provider-Level Outcomes

**Frederick L. Greene**

## Introduction

The development of quality benchmarks in cancer care, although imperative for comparison and opportunities for patient selection, is ultimately destined for use by agencies to reward or penalize institutions and individual practitioners when benchmarks are, respectively, exceeded or unmet. This strategy is particularly evident in many aspects of cancer management and is destined to play a major role both in accreditation of providers and institutions and reimbursement for cancer care.

The Accreditation Program of the Commission on Cancer (CoC) is a prime example of the Donabedian concept of structure, process, and outcome that may be used for assessment and reporting [1]. In more than 1500 institutions in the United States that are currently accredited under this program, the information relating to diagnosis and treatment is already available on a public website maintained by the CoC. These examples of Level I data are provided by institutions in the Survey Application Record (SAR) and are available to patients who desire to choose a facility for their cancer care. The specific indicators in the Level I data refer to types of diagnostic radiology techniques available, specialties of physicians who treat cancer, specific surgical approaches available, and other diagnostic and treatment modalities that would be of importance to patients seeking cancer treatment.

The next level of data (Level II) is also publically reported, but is dependent on the institution's agreement to release information relating to volume of cancers treated and the various stages of malignancy seen at the institution. The frequency of treating certain cancers may be a benchmark of improved quality, both at the physician and institutional level, and, thus, is important to patients seeking treatment locations. The stage (American Joint Committee on Cancer TNM staging system) of various cancers treated is an indication of the institution's experience with

F. L. Greene
Cancer Data Services, Levine Cancer Institute, Charlotte, NC, USA
e-mail: fgreene@med.unc.edu

 
P. Hopewood, M. J. Milroy (eds.), *Quality Cancer Care*,
https://doi.org/10.1007/978-3-319-78649-0_2

early- and late-stage cancer. Once released by the hospital cancer committee and administration, these data are also available to the public through the CoC website.

The ultimate benchmarks of care—cancer survival statistics—are available to the individual CoC-accredited institutions, but are not released for public scrutiny. Until now, the survival statistics generated by the National Cancer Data Base (NCDB), developed by the CoC and the American Cancer Society, have not been risk adjusted and have not been appropriate for public reporting. These Level III data and the ultimate use of these by patients, insurers, accrediting agencies, and federal reimbursement systems are the subject of this chapter.

## The Mission of Public Reporting

Public reporting is a strategy to address quality and cost in the healthcare system by providing consumers, payers, and healthcare providers, such as treating physicians and hospitals, with information about the performance of these providers and patient outcomes. It can include such tools as "report cards" on hospital performance, including the information found on Medicare's Hospital Compare website. Public reports can allow for the comparison of costs, quality (such as rates of hospital-acquired infections), and satisfaction levels of patients with healthcare services. Advocates of public reporting believe that release of this information helps consumers make informed decisions when choosing among physicians, hospitals, and health plans; guides employers and other purchasers when selecting insurance plans; and aids providers when making referrals to specialists. Providers and health plans, in turn, are motivated to improve their performance to protect their reputations and the demand for their services. Publicly reported information may also be useful to policy makers when assessing system performance and value.

Modern efforts to promote public reporting date back to the 1980s, when the Health Care Financing Administration (the predecessor to today's Centers for Medicare and Medicaid Services) began publishing death rates at the nation's hospitals [2]. The effort was highly controversial among hospitals; many complained that the data were not "risk adjusted," failing to take into account that their particular population of patients may have been older or sicker and at greater risk of mortality than patients at other institutions. Although the effort was ultimately abandoned, it paved the way for growing use of public reporting in the decades that followed. Over the last several years public reporting has advanced considerably in depth and scope. Various measures have been developed to capture information about the quality of health care. Some of these measures provide performance while other benchmarks focus on healthcare outcomes—for example, how likely are patients to die after receiving emergency cardiac procedures at one hospital versus another.

Public reports increasingly are being developed and used by a range of stakeholders including federal, state, and local governments; hospitals and other healthcare institutions; professional associations; health insurance plans; employers; and consumers. The enactment of the Affordable Care Act (ACA) of 2010 created a new context for these initiatives by framing a national strategy for quality improvement which also incorporated public reporting [3]. Two federal agencies within the Department of Health and Human Services (HHS) share primary responsibility for these activities: the Agency for Healthcare Research and Quality (AHRQ) and the Centers for Medicare and Medicaid Services (CMS) [4]. AHRQ supports research and works with public and private stakeholders to develop quality measures, report aggregate national- and state-level data, and conduct research on the science of public reporting. It does not, however, report measures at the provider level. CMS collects data on performance measures from providers participating in the Medicare, Medicaid, and the Children's Health Insurance Program. CMS posts comparative provider-specific information about hospitals, doctors, nursing homes, home health agencies, and kidney dialysis facilities [5]. The amount of information CMS provides varies by type of provider. The most information reported at the national level is for general hospitals and is available at www.hospitalcompare.hhs.gov [6]. Since 2005 this site has reported on quality measures focusing on myocardial infarction, heart failure, pneumonia, and surgical care for all US acute care hospitals. The Hospital Compare website also includes measures developed from patient surveys in such areas as communication with doctors and nurses, responsiveness of hospital staff, pain management, cleanliness and quietness, and instructions about medications and discharge. CMS) also maintains www.medicare.gov, which provides information allowing consumers to compare the Medicare Advantage and Part D drug plans available in their area [7].

The ACA directed the secretary of HHS to establish a national strategy for quality improvement that includes public reporting of performance information through healthcare quality websites. CMS and AHRQ were required under the law to convene multiple stakeholder groups and develop performance measures tailored to the needs of "hospitals and other institutional health care providers, physicians and other clinicians, patients, consumers, researchers, policy makers, states, and other stakeholders" [3]. The resulting performance measures were to include clinical conditions, be provider specific, and be detailed enough to meet the needs of patients with different clinical conditions. The ACA also called for public reporting of performance measures on quality, cost, and other metrics and mandated that reports be prepared on hospitals, physicians, and other healthcare providers who participate in Medicare's "value-based purchasing" program, which will base hospital payment in part on whether providers achieve targets for delivering higher quality care [8]. These performance data are also to be posted at www.healthcare.gov. For Medicaid, the law required HHS to adopt an initial core set of quality measures; develop a standardized format for reporting by states; and make the information publicly available annually.

A majority of states currently have public reporting programs in place. The information collected varies considerably from state to state by health condition, process, and outcome measures reported. Some of these activities are publicly sponsored and funded; others are carried out in conjunction with nonprofit organizations or regional or community collaboratives in which provider systems, large purchasers of health care, and other stakeholders work together to advocate for quality improvement. As executive and legislative assaults continue to transform the ACA, the final impact of this law on outcome reporting, especially relating to cancer, is questionable.

## The Setting for Public Reporting

Cancer is the second leading cause of death in the United States: one in four deaths is the result of cancer. It is estimated that more than 1.6 million new cancer cases were diagnosed in the United States in 2017 [9]. The continuous decline in cancer death rates over the last two decades has resulted in an overall drop of 25% resulting in 2.1 million fewer cancer deaths during this time period. Conversely, 5-year relative survival rates for cancer have improved, rising from 50% in the 1970s to 68% in the early twenty-first century, owing to earlier detection and more effective therapies [9].

As a result of improved survival rates, more people are living longer with a cancer diagnosis. This has effectively transformed cancer into a chronic disease for many patients. The aging of the US population will increase the numbers of people diagnosed and living with cancer over the next 20 years. In a fee-for-service environment, where compensation is based on the volume and intensity of services provided, these factors will lead to increased costs of cancer treatment. Cornerstones of quality improvement in health care are the definition and application of meaningful measures. The fundamental challenge of defining quality measures is that the precise definition of "meaningful" is subjective and differs among providers, patients, caregivers, and payers. Meaningful measures may be defined as "quantifiable factors that influence the decision making of patients, caregivers, providers, payers, and policy makers" [10]. Meaningful measures for cancer may encompass objective criteria, such as whether a patient can speak following treatment for oropharyngeal cancer. These may also encompass subjective criteria, such as whether a breast cancer patient is satisfied with her appearance following therapeutic and reconstructive surgery.

Minimal progress has been made in developing meaningful measures for cancer care, in part because of the complexity of the disease. Cancer represents a set of diseases with some common traits, but tremendous variability, unlike more homogeneous conditions such as diabetes. Cancers vary greatly depending on location, type, stage, and molecular and genetic characteristics. Treatment may involve multiple specialists including medical, surgical, and radiation oncologists, which presents a unique challenge for attributing patient outcomes to a particular provider. Similarly, most cancer treatment is delivered as outpatient care, which has been underrepresented in efforts to develop measures. These factors underlie the formidable challenge of representing a disparate set of diseases with a uniform set of quality measures and reportable outcomes.

Generic quality measures that are not disease specific, such as length of stay and hospital readmission rates, are relatively simple to report, although these measures provide limited insight into the quality of cancer care because they cannot assess long-term outcomes. However, when general quality measures are paired with cancer-specific measures—such as long-term survival rates—and are publicly reported, identification of opportunities for immediate and long-term improvements in cancer care will be possible.

## Cancer Care Quality Measurement

In the publication "Crossing the Quality Chasm: A New Health System for the Twenty-First Century," the Institute of Medicine (IOM) recommended the establishment of a monitoring system to evaluate the healthcare system's accomplishments with regard to six aims for improvement—safety, effectiveness, patient-centeredness, timeliness, efficiency, and equity—and to report these results annually to Congress [11].

Subsequently, the IOM published ten recommendations to improve the quality of cancer care [12] (Table 2.1). They included a core set of quality measures that were applicable to all aspects of cancer care—from screening through posttreatment follow-up—aimed at holding providers responsible for the quality of cancer care delivered. The overarching concept was that public reporting of these measures would lead to informed health-related decision-making by patients, purchasers, and policy makers.

Despite the call to action in these seminal publications, public reporting of measures for cancer care has not reached the planned potential. However, the Affordable Care Act of 2010, together with interest from providers, patients, payers, and organizations such as the National Quality Forum (NQF), has served to intensify this effort.

**Table 2.1** IOM goals and recommendations for cancer care [12]

| |
|---|
| • Provide patients and families with understandable information about prognosis, treatment benefits and harms, palliative care, psychosocial support, and costs |
| • Provide end-of-life care that meets patients' needs, values, and preferences |
| • Ensure coordinated and comprehensive patient-centered care |
| • Ensure that all caregivers have appropriate core competencies |
| • Expand the breadth of data collected in cancer research for older adults and patients with multiple comorbid conditions |
| • Expand the depth of data collected through a common set of data elements that capture patient-reported outcomes, characteristics, and health behaviors |
| • Develop a learning healthcare information technology system that enables real-time analysis of data from patients with cancer in a variety of care settings |
| • Develop a national quality reporting program as part of a learning healthcare system |
| • Implement a national strategy to reduce disparities in access to cancer care for underserved populations by leveraging community interventions |
| • Improve the affordability of cancer care by leveraging existing efforts to reform payment and eliminate |

The NQF is a nonprofit organization that uses a well-defined, consensus-based process to endorse healthcare measures for use in public reporting [13]. In the past decade the NQF conducted several projects to endorse cancer care measures under the guidance of multi-stakeholder committees that represented payer, consumer, quality improvement, provider, and patient perspectives. In 2002 the NQF initiated a project entitled "Cancer Quality of Care Measures" [14]. Phase I created a framework for a core set of cancer care measures and priorities of cancer care: (1) access and cultural competence; (2) communication and care coordination; (3) prevention and screening; (4) diagnosis and treatment of breast, colorectal, and prostate cancers; (5) symptom management; and (6) end-of-life care.

The priorities identified in this phase laid the groundwork for Phase II, which began in 2004. Through this phase, the NQF endorsed 19 voluntary consensus standards addressing breast and colorectal cancers, symptom management, and end-of-life care. Among these were five measures developed through collaboration among the American Society of Clinical Oncology, the National Comprehensive Cancer Network, and the CoC [15].

The NQF directed its attention to an additional project in 2007, in which it endorsed 16 clinician-level measures addressing hematologic and prostate cancers, radiation and medical oncology, and pathology. These measures formed the basis used by CMS to develop the Physician Quality Reporting System (PQRS), which provides incentive payments for eligible physicians who report on quality measures for services furnished to Medicare beneficiaries.

In 2008 the NQF hosted a workshop to build upon previous work and identify a comprehensive set of cancer measures. Workshop participants mapped cancer measures that had been endorsed or approved across an episode of care (the period that includes diagnosis, treatment, and follow-up care) and highlighted key measurement gaps, including patient outcomes, care coordination, shared decision-making, patient and family engagement, and end-of-life care. The subsequent white paper laid the foundation for recent NQF efforts to identify outcome and efficiency measures for cancer [16]. Despite these efforts, considerable gaps persist in cancer-specific measures endorsed for public reporting.

Measures endorsed by the NQF include disease-specific measures for more common cancers such as breast cancer, but few measures for less common cancers, such as ovarian cancer. Many measures address screening and initial cancer treatment, but there are few measures that evaluate posttreatment follow-up and long-term consequences of care. Existing measures focus on physical manifestations of cancer (for example, the amount of time from diagnosis to initiation of therapy), but do not assess the emotional and social consequences of the disease. Overall gaps remain in measures that the ACA identified as meaningful for cancer care, including measures of outcomes, structure, process, costs, efficiency, and patients' perception of care. Outcome measures, frequently regarded as key indicators of healthcare quality, assess the results of health care with regard to recovery, functional restoration, and survival. For patients receiving a cancer diagnosis, survival is the critical outcome and the principal concern. In addition to survival, cancer patients seek to understand the immediate and long-term impacts of their disease and its treatment [17].

Historically, outcome measures focused on short-term results of care, particularly mortality and complications following treatment. That focus has expanded to include immediate and intermediate results relating to quality of life during and after treatment, including functional status and symptom management. Medicare reimbursement is tied to public reporting of certain non-cancer quality measures. The ACA also established a mechanism for a select group of prospective payment system (PPS)-exempt cancer centers and other organizations exempted from quality reporting (such as certain mental health and long-term-care facilities) to begin reporting healthcare quality measures to CMS [18]. Section 3005 of the ACA includes the following stipulations specific to quality reporting by the 11 exempt cancer centers: (1) Beginning in 2014 and thereafter, these cancer centers will be required to submit data to the secretary of health and human services on selected endorsed quality measures. (2) CMS will announce the quality measures for these cancer centers, including measures of outcomes, structure, process, costs, efficiency, and patients' perceptions of care. (3) This information will be reported publicly on the CMS website.

Although this provision specifically addresses the 11 specialized cancer centers, it represents a likely prelude to mandatory public reporting of outcomes, costs, and other measures of cancer care from all cancer centers, leading to greater transparency and scrutiny of the outcomes and costs related to all cancer treatment.

## Organizational Approaches

A variety of organizations use public reporting in their activities. Their efforts are supported by a variety of sources, including grants and contracts from federal and state governments, private foundations, large purchasers of health care, and membership fees. Some of the more prominent of these organizations include the NQF, a nonprofit organization that works with providers, consumer groups, and governments to establish and build consensus for specific healthcare quality and efficiency measures, and the National Committee for Quality Assurance (NCQA), which evaluates and accredits health insurance plans based on quality and value. Other groups involved in public reporting include the Leapfrog Group for Patient Safety (created by employers); the Informed Patient Institute, a group that rates the usefulness of existing online doctor, hospital, and nursing home report cards; and the Commonwealth Fund's www.whynotthebest.org, which allows users to compare hospitals based on specific performance measures using data from a variety of sources, including the Leapfrog Group, the Hospital Quality Alliance, and selected state reporting systems.

In March 2011, AHRQ convened a National Summit on Public Reporting for Consumers [19]. The summit produced a set of recommendations that address how to expand the use of public reports, how to address issues related to content and format of reports, and the methods and data sources needed to implement the system. Hundreds of measures are available to those developing public reports. Many of these have been vetted by the NQF, which has worked since the 1990s to create national consensus standards for measuring and reporting on health system performance. The federal government as well as other major healthcare purchasers uses NQF-endorsed measures to ensure that measures are scientifically sound and to help standardize performance measures.

The choice of measures to be used in any given instance requires consideration of their relevance to the target population, the availability of data (including whether the number of events is sufficient to reliably measure performance), and how the measures will be of use. Although the science of measure development and use has evolved from an exclusive reliance on performance measures to those focused on outcomes, more work is needed to develop measures that will be the most meaningful to consumers at various points in their decision-making process. Physicians and hospitals are particularly concerned that public reports fairly and accurately reflect their performance, and not indicators that are beyond their control, such as the risk profile of the population they treat. For example, a hospital located in a poor urban area may be more likely to treat higher risk patients with more complex medical problems than its suburban counterpart. The outcomes of cancer patients treated will depend on these factors. This problem can be addressed through risk adjustment—statistical methods that adjust scores or values of reported data to account for these factors before results are made public. Since no risk-adjustment technique is perfect, there are concerns that patients may avoid providers whose lower scores may not accurately represent the quality of care they provide, and providers may avoid seeing patients with complex health issues whom they fear might depress their performance scores.

## Data Collection and Use

There is a general consensus that data for performance reports should be obtained automatically as part of ongoing care processes. For example, information can be collected through electronic health records while a patient is visiting the physician's office; it can also be taken from claims that providers send to insurers or other payers requesting payment for care provided. Although use of electronic health records is becoming universal, in part due to federal incentives, it still varies greatly across providers and geographic areas. Many consumers also remain somewhat leery—primarily for privacy reasons—of having their data collected and shared with others especially in view of increased instances of breeches in cyber security. Meanwhile, claims processing systems do not always capture critical elements that are needed for performance measurement. One of the main concerns associated with public reporting is the increasing use by consumers in helping them make informed decisions among healthcare providers. In general, consumers' use of public reporting is low. A 2011 study of 16 community collaboratives in the AHRQ Chartered Value Exchange Program found that some websites comparing hospital performance were used primarily by consumers who were white, college educated, and over 45 years of age [20]. There was little use by vulnerable populations, and only about half of those visiting the sites indicated that they were likely to use the data to choose a hospital. A 2008 poll from the Henry J. Kaiser Family Foundation found that 30% of Americans said that they viewed information comparing the quality of different insurance plans, hospitals, or doctors, but only 14% reported having used such information [21].

Moreover, the information contained in public reports is often not presented in such a way that is understandable and relevant to consumers. A 2007 study of five hospital reporting services found that they used disparate measures and lacked standard definitions for reporting [22]. The obvious conclusion was that consumers were more likely to be confused than informed. In addition, consumers have preexisting ideas about health care that can be difficult to influence through public reporting. An experiment performed by Hibbard and colleagues at the University of Oregon [23] vetted information about providers' costs before 1400 consumers, and found that most assumed that providers' costs were low because they provided low quality. Consumers may be at risk of information overload or are disinclined to make good use of publicly reported information. Much remains to be done to make public reports accessible, understandable, and relevant. Consumer outreach and education are also keys to public reporting success. Consumers not only need to be aware of sources of information and how to access them, but they also need to understand if the information is meaningful.

Participants at AHRQ's 2011 National Summit on Public Reporting discussed strategies to make public reporting more consumer friendly [24]. Among strategies suggested were ongoing campaigns to raise awareness of and demand for quality information among consumers. They also recommended engaging consumers through their providers by involving consumers and their families in practice redesign and improvement. They advocated that development of outcome measures be aimed at consumer needs by understanding their priorities and the information they value at specific decision points, rather than just relying on the data that are available and routinely collected. Finally, they recommended doing research on the best means to present results clearly to consumers and exploring alternative ways to deliver reports using mobile technologies and automated telephone systems.

More work lies ahead if public reporting of cancer outcomes is to meet expectations and fulfill hopes that it can spur broad change in healthcare delivery. A survey of 29 experts and participants at AHRQ's 2011 national summit revealed that, while none doubted the value of public and private investments made in public reporting, most agreed that the information provided so far has had little positive impact on consumers' choices of healthcare providers. The challenge is to make further advances in measurement, data collection, and use of information technology; deliver more consumer-oriented report cards; and accomplish these objectives within the constraints of limited public funding and providers' willingness to be subjected to such scrutiny.

## Examples of Public Reporting of Cancer Outcomes

A current strategy of public reporting of cancer outcomes is provided by the Society of Thoracic Surgeons [25]. Founded in 1964, the Society of Thoracic Surgeons is a not-for-profit organization representing approximately 7200 cardiothoracic surgeons, researchers, and allied healthcare professionals worldwide who are dedicated to ensuring the best possible outcomes for operative procedures involving the heart, lung, and esophagus, as well as other surgical procedures within the chest. The Society's mission is to "enhance the ability of cardiothoracic surgeons to provide the highest quality patient care through education, research, and advocacy." The STS National Database was established in 1989 as an initiative for quality improvement and patient safety among cardiothoracic surgeons. The Database has since grown exponentially and has become an important clinical registry. Participation in the STS National Database is global, currently spanning ten countries on five continents.

The STS National Database has three components, each focusing on a different area of cardiothoracic surgery—Adult Cardiac Surgery, Congenital Heart Surgery, and General Thoracic Surgery. The STS has released the first publicly accessible national report of outcomes after lobectomy for cancer [26]. The surgical outcomes data are from the Society's General Thoracic Surgery Database (GTSD), one of the three components in the STS National Database.

Beginning in 2017, these participant-level outcomes for lobectomy are expected to be publicly reported with comparisons to overall STS and national outcomes. Measures include median postoperative length of stay and a two-domain lobectomy composite measure (including risk-adjusted mortality and major complications) which will be reported for consenting programs. As yet, there is no plan for lung cancer survival data to be publically available. To access the GTSD outcomes directly: http://www.sts.org/thoracic-public-reporting-module-search.

## Adjusting for Disease Severity in Cancer and the Importance of Risk Adjustment

While public reporting of outcomes in cancer care is both appropriate and inevitable, the danger of misinterpreting public disclosure of cancer survival data is heightened when there is absence of effective risk adjustment that hampers the use of data for patient selection and payment strategies. This concept was realized several decades ago when patients in the Veterans Administration system were being compared to the nonveteran cohort. The concern gave rise to the VA National Surgical Quality Improvement Project that highlighted both the need for careful scrutiny of hospital patient data and the reporting of patients using indicators that could level the playing field when disparate groups of patients were compared. This process has been embraced by the American College of Surgeons and has proven to be an important methodology for analyzing surgical data for comparison in all acute care hospitals [27].

The danger inherent in reporting both provider and institutional outcomes for cancer patients is not to mandate the strict use of risk adjustment before such strategies are undertaken. The National Cancer Database (NCDB) [28], which serves as the only national cancer surveillance tool for the United States, has also begun to provide CoC-accredited hospitals with risk-adjusted data in preparation of using NCDB data for effective public reporting. Patient characteristics such as severity of illness and age may greatly influence clinical outcomes, including length of stay and mortality. To ensure equitable comparisons among hospitals, organizations adjust for severity of disease using risk-adjusted methodologies that classify patients according to demographics, diagnoses, severity of illness, mortality risk, and use of resources. However, these models do not account for critical components of cancer outcomes such as cancer type and stage, previous treatment, and coexisting illnesses. Models that ignore these factors result in imprecise outcomes for hospitals with a disproportionate share of high-risk patients who have complex cancers and challenging comorbidities. Therefore, a cancer-specific risk-adjustment model, which accounts for severity of disease and comorbidities, is needed to facilitate public reporting of meaningful measures, to link reimbursement to quality, and to highlight opportunities for improving healthcare delivery for cancer patients.

Once identified, key indicators of cancer outcomes must account for severity of disease using a risk-adjusted methodology. For example, patients with early-stage confined tumors have vastly different expected outcomes than patients who present with a widely metastatic disease that has spread beyond the main tumor site to other organs and tissues. Similarly, those who present with advanced age or multiple serious conditions will not achieve the same outcomes as their younger, healthier counterparts [29, 30]. Current risk-adjustment methodologies are limited in their ability to report accurate cancer outcomes. However, accounting for stage of disease and comorbidities is essential to equitable and meaningful comparisons of cancer outcomes.

## Information Technology and Public Reporting

There is often disconnect between the need to report meaningful outcomes and the data available to support that reporting. Early efforts to report quality measures publicly relied on administrative data because they were widely available. But the interests of providers, patients, and payers were misaligned because the most common measures assessed length of stay, complications of care that could be coded, and mortality. Although these are measures of care, they provide an incomplete view of the quality of healthcare delivery, notably for cancer. Developing systems that capture and analyze extractable data from the electronic health record is fundamental to meaningful quality measurement. Of particular importance are tools that capture patients' perspective of care, such as patient preference and quality of life.

In recent years, providers rushed to implement electronic health records in an effort to capture the data needed to support quality measurement. However, early adopters of these systems observed that the necessary data were embedded in scanned documents or other unsearchable text fields within these systems. For all providers, the common mechanism for collecting data to support quality measurement is to abstract medical records—the process of entering clinical data from a traditional paper or electronic record into an electronic database for clinical or research purposes—which is labor intensive and costly.

Continued adoption and enhancement of electronic systems to support public reporting of meaningful healthcare measures is a vital element of ongoing healthcare reform and quality improvement. For all providers, implementing the technical infrastructure to support this reporting is costly. This is particularly true within the current economic environment, where providers are facing ongoing reimbursement cuts from public and private payers.

## Limitations of Public Reporting of Cancer Outcomes

Although the concept of public reporting has broad support, its implementation has not always been met with approval. There is mixed evidence about the degree to which it has sparked changes within health care or been embraced by consumers. Skeptics of public reporting have a number of concerns, including the accuracy and reliability of the information contained in the reports. For example, only 30% of physicians surveyed believe that quality measures used in public reports were generally accurate [31]. The costs associated with collection, analysis, and dissemination of data can be high, especially for physicians and providers who have not fully implemented electronic health recordkeeping systems. There is also potential for unintended consequences that might result from providers gaming their report card scores, for example, by declining to treat patients with serious conditions that might negatively impact their ratings. Similarly, there is a risk of misinterpretation by consumers if they do not understand the terms used, the intent of an indicator to reveal the quality of care, or whether high or low rates reflect good performance. Despite the degree of investment in developing and implementing public reporting systems, concerns abound as to whether public reporting will improve quality and reduce healthcare costs. Studies have reached different conclusions concerning the degree to which consumers and physicians use public reports, whether providers respond to public reporting of performance measures by changing their behavior, and even whether public reporting improves outcomes [31].

Both supporters and critics recognize the need to address a number of issues in public reporting. These include choice of performance measures, data collection and system capabilities, formatting and content of reports, education and outreach to promote the use of information, and evaluation and continuous refinement to assure that public reporting achieves its objectives rather than becoming an end in itself.

In a 2011 report [32], the IOM stated that although several organizations are attempting to develop quality measures, a proliferation of measures could confuse and fragment the value of meaningful measures. Accordingly, a cohesive set of cancer measures relevant to patients, providers, and payers are essential to improving the quality of cancer care. Short- and long-term outcomes, together with patients' preferences (such as preservation of sexual function following treatment) and patient-reported outcomes, constitute a collection of meaningful measures for patients. For providers, the IOM's six aims for improvement represent six domains of measures useful for evaluating and improving processes [32]. Additionally, in Section 3005, the ACA identifies six categories of measures that are meaningful to payers, particularly as efforts continue to link reimbursement to quality [33].

Frequently, measures based on billing data—for example, length of hospital stay—are limited in their ability to define and influence desired outcomes. Many are measures of convenience, selected because they are reported from existing administrative information systems. In identifying meaningful cancer measures, developers must not allow the logistics of reporting to dictate the selection of the measures. They must instead focus on the following questions: Which health outcomes are providers attempting to deliver? Which outcomes are most important to the patients receiving services? This exercise requires a candid dialogue between providers and patients. Experience suggests that long-term survival and quality-of-life valuations especially regarding cancer are far more important to patients than hospital readmission and infectious complication rates. To date, there has been minimal effort at the national level to support development of measures that are important to patients.

Building a national consensus around measurable cancer outcomes and quality of care will not be a rapid or simple process. Nevertheless, the patient-driven, provider-driven, and payer-driven measurement approaches will define the future path of developing and validating meaningful cancer measures. Viewed as an evolving and iterative effort to link patient, provider, and payer perspectives, it will produce a balanced picture of patient-driven, high-quality cancer care and a model for improving overall healthcare delivery that will ultimately be appropriate for public reporting.

## References


1. Cancer Program Standards. Ensuring patient-centered care. Chicago: American College of Surgeons Commission on Cancer; 2015.
2. Luce JM, Bindman AB, Lee PR. A brief history of health care quality assessment and improvement in the United States. West J Med. 1994;160:263–8.
3. Albright HW, Moreno M, Feeley TW, Walters R, Samuels M, et al. The implications of the 2010 patient protection and affordable care act and the health care and education reconciliation act on cancer care delivery. Cancer. 2011;117(8):1564–74. Epub 2010 Nov 8.
4. McGlynn EA. Identifying, categorizing, and evaluating health care efficiency measures: final report. Rockville, MD: Agency for Healthcare Research and Quality; 2008; (Report No.: 08-0030; Contract No.: 282-00-0005-21).

5. Centers for Medicare and Medicaid Services. Form 7.1: Call for TEP for cancer hospital measures [Internet]. Baltimore, MD: CMS. http://www.cms.gov/MMS/Downloads/MMSCallTEPforPPS.zi.
6. www.hospitalcompare.hhs.gov.
7. www.medicare.gov.
8. Elkin EB, Bach PB. Cancer's next frontier: addressing high and increasing costs. JAMA. 2010;303:1086–7.
9. Siegel RL, Miller KD, Jemal A. Cancer statistics, 2017. CA Cancer J Clin. 2017;67:7–30.
10. Spinks TE, Walters R, Feeley TW, et al. Improving cancer care through public reporting of meaningful quality measures. Health Aff. 2011;30:664–72.
11. United States Institute of Medicine. Committee on quality of health care in America. Crossing the quality chasm: a new health system for the 21st century. Washington, DC: National Academy Press; 2001.
12. Institute of Medicine. Delivering high-quality cancer care: charting a new course for a system in crisis. Washington, DC: National Academies Press; 2013.
13. National Quality Forum. National voluntary consensus standards for quality of cancer care [Internet]. Washington, DC: NQF; 2009. http://www.qualityforum.org/Publications/2009/05/National_Voluntary_Consensus_Standards_ for_Quality_of_Cancer_Care.aspx. [cited 2010 Dec 10]
14. National Quality Forum. Towards a comprehensive cancer measure set: value-based episodes of care [Internet]. Washington, DC: NQF; 2008. http://www.qualityforum.org/Projects/c-d/Cancer_Measure_Set_Value-Based_Episodes_of_Care/Cancer_workshop_summary.aspx.
15. National Quality Forum. Consensus development projects [Internet]. Washington, DC: NQF; 2011. http://qualityforum.org/Projects.aspx. [cited 2011 Mar 21].
16. National Quality Forum. NQF endorsed standards [Internet]. Washington, DC: NQF; 2010. http://www.qualityforum.org/Measures_List.aspx. [cited 2010 Dec 10].
17. Oliver A, Greenberg CC. Measuring outcomes in oncology treatment: the importance of patient-centered outcomes. Surg Clin North Am. 2009;89:17–25.
18. Centers for Medicare and Medicaid Services. Call for quality of care measures for PPS-exempt cancer hospitals [Internet]. Baltimore, MD: CMS; http://www.cms.gov/MMS/Downloads/MMSCallforMeasuresPPS.zip.
19. Bardach NS, Hibbard JH, Dudley RA. Users of public reports of hospital quality: who what why and how? Rockville, MD: Agency for Healthcare Research and Quality; 2011.
20. Ryan AM, Nallamothu BK, Dimick JB. Medicare's public reporting initiative on hospital quality had modest or no impact on mortality from three key conditions. Health Aff (Millwood). 2012;31(3):585–92.
21. Kaiser Family Foundation. 2008 Update on consumers' views of patient safety and quality information. Washington, DC: Kaiser Family Foundation; 2008.
22. Sinaiko AD, Eastman D, Rosenthal MB. How report cards on physicians, physician groups, and hospitals can have greater impact on consumer choices. Health Aff (Millwood). 2012;31(3):602–11.
23. Hibbard JH, Greene J, Sofaer S, Firminger K, Hirsh J. An experiment shows that a well-designed report on costs and quality can help consumers choose high- value health care. Health Aff. 2012;31(3):560–8.
24. Luft HS. Advancing public reporting through a new 'aggregator' to standardize data collection on providers' cost and quality. Health Aff. 2012;31(3):619–26.
25. STS News. Society of Thoracic Surgeons (pub). 2011;16:1–7.
26. Society of Thoracic Surgeons. www.sts.org.
27. American College of Surgeons. National Surgical Quality Improvement Program. Program Overview. https://acsnsqip.org/main/about_overview.asp.
28. Winchester DP, Stewart AK, Phillips JL, Ward EE. The National cancer data base: past, present, and future. Ann Surg Oncol. 2010;17:4–7.

29. Sarfati D, Koczwara B, Jackson C. The impact of comorbidity on cancer and its treatment. CA Cancer J Clin. 2016;66:337–50.
30. Piccirillo JF, Tierney RM, Costas I, et al. Prognostic importance of comorbidity in a hospital-based cancer registry. JAMA. 2004;291:2441–7.
31. James J. Health policy brief. 2012. www.healthaffairs.org/healthpolicybriefs.
32. Institute of Medicine. For the public's health: the role of measurement in action and accountability. Washington, DC: National Academies Press.
33. Burwell SM. Setting value-based payment goals—HHS efforts to improve US health care. N Engl J Med. 2015;372:897–8.

# Chapter 3
# Cancer Statistics: Global and National

**Mary J. Milroy**

> "This is a case of bulging masses I have to contend with … Bulging tumours of the breast mean the existence of swelling on the breast large spreading and hard; touching them is like touching a ball of wrappings or they may be compared to the unripe hemut fruit, which is hard and cool to the touch … Therapy … there is none." Imhotep, Egyptian physician 2625 BC [1].

## Introduction to the Statistics

This ancient manuscript describing "bulging masses" certainly suggests that the fight against cancer dates back throughout human-recorded time. However, when humans struggled for existence and life spans were short, cancer was not a common occurrence. As global public health advances decrease deaths due to communicable diseases and life spans increase, cancer threatens to become a greater global challenge. Deaths from noncommunicable disease (NCD) rose from 65 to 71% between 2005 and 2015 [2]. Increased age is recognized as the greatest risk factor for the development of cancer [3, 4]. "Today, most people, even in the poorest countries, are living longer lives," says Dr. Margaret Chan, Director-General of the World Health Organization [5]. The WHO's news report for the International Day of Older Persons October 1, 2015 predicted that between 2015 and 2050 the proportion of the world's population over 60 years would nearly double from 12 to 22% and reach a total of two billion people. By 2050 this would include 434 million people aged 80 and older and that 80% of older people would be living in low- and middle-income countries. The report also noted that the pace of population aging is much faster than in the past and that all countries will face major challenges to ensure that their health and social systems are ready to make the most

M. J. Milroy
Department of Surgery, Sanford School of Medicine, University of South Dakota, Vermillion, SD, USA



P. Hopewood, M. J. Milroy (eds.), *Quality Cancer Care*,
https://doi.org/10.1007/978-3-319-78649-0_3

of this demographic shift [5]. Knowledge of global and national cancer incidence and mortality will help to guide cancer control efforts.

Cancer is the second leading cause of death throughout the world, second only to cardiovascular disease. In 2015 there were 17.5 million cancer cases and 8.7 million deaths. The Global Burden of Disease Cancer Collaboration analyzed statistics for 32 cancer groups from 195 countries from 2005 to 2015. They observed that cancer cases increased by 33% and nearly 1 in 6 deaths worldwide were due to cancer. They attributed these increases to population aging 16%, population growth 13%, and changes in age-specific rates 4% [2]. While age-standardized incidence rates increased in 174 of the 195 countries analyzed by the Global Burden of Disease Cancer Collaboration, the age-standardized death rates decreased in 140 of the 195 countries analyzed. Countries that did not show a decrease were mostly located on the African continent. This was attributed mainly to late-stage presentation and inaccessible diagnosis and treatment.

The World Health Organization Cancer Fact sheet, updated February 2017, predicts that the number of new cancer cases is expected to rise by about 70% over the next two decades [6]. While mortality figures provide a measurable parameter, the effects of cancer are far broader. Years lived with disability (YLD) is calculated by multiplying prevalence estimates by disability weights. The years of life lost (YLL) are estimated by multiplying age-specific cancer deaths by the reference life expectancy. Disability-adjusted life years (DALY) can then be calculated as the sum of the YLD and the YLL [2]. Globally, for men, prostate cancer had the highest incidence, 1.6 million cases, while tracheal, bronchus, and lung cancers were the leading cause of cancer deaths at 1.2 million deaths and 25.9 million disability-adjusted life years (DALY). For women, breast cancer had the highest incidence at 2.4 million cases, and was also the leading cause of cancer death with 523,000 deaths and 15.1 million DALY. Overall, the most common causes of cancer death were lung, liver, colorectal, stomach, and breast. Worldwide, in 2015, men and women combined had DALYs that totaled 208.3 million [2]. These numbers emphasize the need globally and nationally for an increased focus on cancer control efforts.

The American Cancer Society estimates 1,688,780 new cases of cancer in the United States with 600,920 Americans expected to die of cancer in 2017 [7]. As was seen worldwide, cancer is the second most common cause of death, second only to cardiovascular disease, and accounts for 1 in 4 deaths. Similar to global statistics, in the United States, cancer is strongly associated with aging as 87% of cancer occurs in individuals 50 years of age and older. It is estimated that 41 of 100 men and 38 of 100 women in the United States will develop cancer during their lifetime. Cancer mortality rose in the early twentieth century and peaked in 1991 at 215/100,000 people, but then, due to efforts in prevention, early detection, and treatment, mortality decreased by 2014 to 161/100,000. This represented a 25% decrease and was felt to be due mainly to decreased mortality in lung, colorectal, breast, and prostate cancers. This translated to 2.1 million fewer cancer deaths [7].

## Risk Factors

Unlike aging, many of the risk factors for cancer are controllable. The identification of modifiable risk factors is of prime importance in the effort to decrease both cancer-related mortality and disability. The WHO estimates that one-third of deaths from cancer are due to five leading behavioral and dietary risks: tobacco use, high body mass index, lack of physical activity, low fruit and vegetable intake, and alcohol use [6]. In addition, ultraviolet radiation and chronic viral infection have been identified as modifiable risk factors [8–10].

### *Tobacco Use*

The use of tobacco is the leading risk factor for the development of cancer so the best way to prevent cancer is to not smoke. Worldwide over one billion people smoke and according to the WHO this results in nearly 6 million tobacco-related deaths per year, a tobacco-related death occurs every 6 seconds [6]. In the United States, the CDC estimates that 36.5 million adults currently smoke cigarettes. 480,000 Americans die of a smoking-related disease yearly, and smoking is responsible for 1 in 5 deaths in the United States [11]. More than 16 million Americans live with a smoking-related disease. Current rate of smoking in the United States has declined from nearly 21/100 (20.9%) of adults in 2005 to about 15/100 (15.1%) adults in 2015 [6].

In addition to avoiding exposure to tobacco, the American Cancer Society recognizes the importance of additional, modifiable risk factors and publishes guidelines on nutritional and physical activity for cancer prevention [12]. The ACS states that for nonsmokers, the “most important modifiable determinants of cancer risk are weight control, dietary choices, and level of physical activity” and adds that fully one-third of the cancer death that occurs in the United States each year can be attributed to diet and physical activity habits including overweight and obesity. These same behaviors are particularly important as they impact development of both cardiovascular disease and diabetes. ACS recommendations include (1) achieving and maintaining a healthy weight throughout life, (2) adopting a physically active lifestyle, (3) consuming a healthy diet with an emphasis on plant foods, and (4) limiting consumption if you drink alcoholic beverages. Recommendations for men are to consume no more than two drinks per day and for women no more than one drink per day.

## Body Mass Index

The global Non-Communicable Disease (NCD) Risk Factor Collaborative recognized high body mass index (BMI) as a risk factor for a number of conditions including cardiovascular and kidney disease, diabetes, some cancers, and musculoskeletal disease. A global target goal was set of halting by 2025, the rise in prevalence of obesity at the 2010 level [13]. Unfortunately, their 2016 Lancet publication concluded by saying that "in the past four decades, we have transitioned from a world in which underweight prevalence was more than double that of obesity, to one in which more people are obese than underweight, both globally and in all regions except parts of sub-Saharan Africa and Asia. The rate of increase in BMI since 2000 has been slower than in the preceding decades in high-income countries, where adiposity became an explicit public health concern around this time, and in some middle-income countries. However, because the rate of BMI increase has accelerated in some other regions, the global increase in BMI has not slowed down. If post-2000 trends continue, not only will the world not meet the global target for halting the increase in obesity, but also severe obesity will surpass underweight in women by 2025" [13].

## Low Fruit and Vegetable Intake

The World Health Organization includes low fruit and vegetable intake in the top five preventable causes of cancer. In addition, fruit and vegetable consumption is considered a component of healthy weight control. While mixed results have been obtained from studies looking at the effect fruits and vegetables have on cancer incidence, a number of studies including the European Investigation into Cancer and Nutrition (EPIC) continue to support the role of fruit and vegetable intake and contend that the recommendation to increase intake has a sound basis [14]. Their article concluded by saying, "For the prevention of cancer the primary focus at present should be heightened effort to include smoking and obesity because obesity in the US has become similar in magnitude to smoking as an avoidable cause" [14].

## Ultraviolet Radiation Exposure

Exposure to ultraviolet radiation either from sunlight or from artificial factors such as tanning beds is associated with the development of skin cancers. The Skin Cancer Foundation predicted that 87,110 new cases of invasive melanoma will be diagnosed in the United States in 2017 and 9730 people will die of melanoma [8]. This represents about one person every 54 minutes. The risk of melanoma is doubled with a lifetime history of over five sunburns. Of public health importance is that the regular daily use of SPF sunscreen can decrease the incidence of melanoma by 50% and squamous cell carcinoma by 40% [8]. The Cancer Council Australia's Sid the Seagull launched a public health campaign in 1981 of *Slip* on a shirt, *Slop* on sunscreen, and *Slap* on a hat. In 2007 it was modified to add *Seek* shade and *Slide* on wraparound sunglasses [9]. Australia has the highest rate of skin cancer in the world with 50% of Australians expected to develop skin cancer during their lifetime. Melanoma was the third leading cause of cancer death and was responsible for the highest cost to the healthcare system. After launching the campaign, public opinion about tanning changed. Follow-up studies reported that the number of Australians liking to tan went from 61% in 1988 to 35% in 1998 and there was reported to be a 50% decrease in sunburns. Results are still emerging but rates of skin cancer are beginning to plateau after decades of sharp increase [15].

## Chronic Viral Infection

Chronic viral infection by either DNA or RNA viruses is associated with development of cancer. The most common viruses responsible are *Helicobacter pylori*, hepatitis viruses B and C, human papilloma virus (HPV), and Epstein–Barr virus [10]. The WHO estimates that chronic virus infection is responsible for up to 25% of cancer cases in low- and middle-income countries and a significant cause of cancer in more developed countries [6]. *Helicobacter pylori* is related to gastric cancer, and hepatitis viruses B and C are risk factors for the development of cirrhosis of the liver and the development of hepatocellular carcinoma (HCC). Globally these infections are responsible for more than 1.3 million deaths per year. "Liver cancer is the second leading cause of cancer-related death worldwide, with HCC representing approximately 90% of all primary liver cancer cases" [16]. Treatment of chronic hepatitis virus infection is effective and can prevent the development of both cirrhosis and HCC. Enhanced detection and treatment programs for chronic hepatitis viral infection would markedly decrease the incidence of HCC. The Annual Report to the Nation in 2013 focused on HPV-related cancers [17]. Although over 150 types of HPV have been identified high-risk HPV 16 and 18 are strongly associated with the development of cancer. High-risk HPV is responsible for nearly all cases of cervical cancer and also responsible for 90% of oropharyngeal cancers [18] and 40% of cancers of the anus, vagina, vulva, and penis [17]. Epstein–Barr virus is associated with Burkitt's lymphoma [10]. While there are no vaccines against *H. pylori* and Epstein–Barr viruses, vaccines do exist for hepatitis B and C and for HPV [19]. A recent meta-analysis of 20 high-income countries with at least a 50% vaccination rate in girls aged 13–19 showed a 68% reduction in HPV prevalence from pre- to postvaccination data and a 61% decrease in anogenital warts [20]. This suggests strong population effect of vaccination and promises a future impact on HPV-related cancer incidence. Unfortunately, vaccination rates in the United States have remained below Healthy People 2020 targets and lag behind vaccination rates for other childhood vaccines suggesting missed vaccination opportunities [21]. Increasing vaccinationc rates for both boys and girls represent an important opportunity for cancer prevention in the United States.

## Summary

Although cancer remains a major cause of death both nationally and globally with factors such as age being unmodifiable, there are opportunities for cancer prevention activities to have a major impact on cancer incidence and mortality. The Cancer Prevention Study II Nutrition Cohort enrolled 111,966 nonsmoking men and women from 1992 to 1993. After 14 years this cohort was reevaluated to see if adhering to the American Cancer Society's cancer prevention guidelines on body mass index, physical activity, diet, and alcohol consumption would impact cancer mortality. Their study concluded that yes, a statistically significant decrease in cancer, cardiovascular disease, and all-cause mortality was observed in nonsmokers following the American Cancer Society's guidelines [22]. This is encouraging news for cancer control efforts.

## Following Cancer Prevention Guidelines Can Decrease Incidence of Cancer

Facing the challenge of increasing cancer incidence is a major component of cancer control efforts. Cancer represents the second leading cause of death nationally and globally. In the face of an increasingly aging population at increased risk for cancer, this represents a major challenge for healthcare systems. Fortunately modifiable risk factors do exist and have been shown to decrease mortality. Avoidance of smoking, adherence to a healthy lifestyle with normal body mass index, adequate physical activity, healthy diet, moderate alcohol consumption, sun safety, and obtaining recommended vaccinations can go far to decrease the incidence and mortality from cancer.

## References

1. Mukherjee S. The emperor of all maladies, a biography of cancer. Scr Theol. 2011:40–1.
2. Global Burden of Disease Cancer Collaboration, Fitzmaurice C, Allen C, Barber RM, Barregard L, Bhutta ZA, Brenner H, et al. Global, regional, and national cancer incidence, mortality, years of life lost, years lived with disability, and disability-adjusted life-years for

32 cancer groups, 1990 to 2015: a systematic analysis for the global burden of disease study. JAMA Oncol. 2017;3(4):524–48.
3. Li D, de Glas NA, Hurria A. Cancer and aging: General principles, biology, and geriatric assessment. Clin Geriatr Med. 2016;32(1):1–15.
4. Serrano M. Unraveling the links between cancer and aging. Carcinogenesis. 2016;37(2):107.
5. WHO: Number of people over 60 years set to double by 2050; major societal changes required. www.who.int/mediacentre/news/releases/2015/older-persons-day-en/.
6. WHO Cancer Fact sheet updated February 2017. 2017. http://www.who.int/mediacantre/factsheets/fs297/en/.
7. Siegel R, Miller K, Jemal A. Cancer statistics, 2017. CA Cancer J Clin. 2017;67:7–30.
8. Skin Cancer Foundation. http://www.skincancer.org/skin-cancer-information/skin-cancer-facts#melanoma.
9. Cancer Council Australia. http://www.cancer.org.au/preventing-cancer/sun-protection/campaigns-and-events/slip-slop-slap-seek-slide.html.
10. Plummer M, de Martel C, Vignat J, Ferlay J, Bray F, Franceschi S. Global burden of cancers attributable to infections in 2012: a synthetic analysis. Lancet Oncol. 2012;4(9):e609–16.
11. CDC-Fact Sheet. Current cigarette smoking among adults in the U.S. www.cdc.gov/tobacco/data_cig_smoking/index.html.
12. Kushi L, Doyle C, McCullough M, Rock C, Demark-Wahnefried W, Bandera E, et al. ACS Guidelines on nutrition and physical activity for cancer prevention. CA Cancer J Clin. 2012;62(1):30–67.
13. NCD Risk Factor Collaboration. Trends in adult body mass index in 200 countries from 1975 to 2014: a pooled analysis of 1678 population-based measurement studies with 19.2 million participants. Lancet. 2016;387(10026):1377–96.
14. Boffetta P, Couto E, Wichmann J, Ferrari P, Trichopoulos D, Bueno-de-Mesquita HB, et al. Fruit and vegetable intake and overall cancer risk in the European prospective investigation into cancer and nutrition (EPIC). J Natl Cancer Inst. 2010;102(8):529–37.
15. Montague M, Borland R, Sinclair C. Sun smart-twenty years on 1980 to 2000: skin cancer control and 20 years of population based campaigning. Health Educ Behav. 2001;28(3):290–305.
16. Ringehan M, McKeating JA, Protzer U. Viral hepatitis and liver cancer. Philos Trans R Soc Lond Ser B Biol Sci. 2017;372(1732):20160274.
17. Jemal A, Simard EP, Dorell C, et al. Annual report to the nation on the status of cancer, 1975–2009, featuring the burden and trends in human papillomavirus (HPV)-associated cancers and HPV vaccination coverage levels. J Natl Cancer Inst. 2013;105(3):175–201.
18. Chaturvedi AK, Engels EA, Pfeiffer RM, et al. Human papillomavirus and rising oropharyngeal cancer incidence in the United States. J Clin Oncol. 2011;29(32):4294–301.
19. Gillison ML, Chaturvedi AK, Lowy DR. HPV prophylactic vaccines and the potential prevention of noncervical cancers in both men and women. Cancer. 2008;113(10 Suppl):3036–46.
20. Drolet M, Benard E, Boily MC, Ali H, Baandrup L, Bauer H, et al. Population-level impact and herd effects following human papillomavirus vaccination programmes: a systematic review and meta-analysis. Lancet Infect Dis. 2015;15(5):565–80. Epub 2015 Mar 3
21. Reagan-Steiner S, Yankey D, Jeyarajah J, et al. National, regional, state and selected area vaccination coverage among adolescents aged 13-17 years-United States 2015. MMWR Morb Mortal Wkly Rep. 2016;65:850–8.
22. McCullough ML, Patel AV, Kushi LH, Patel R, Willett W, Doyle C, et al. Following cancer prevention guidelines reduces risk of cancer, cardiovascular disease, and all-cause mortality. Cancer Epidemiol Biomark Prev. 2011;20(6):1089–97.

# Chapter 4
# Understanding the Social Determinants of Cancer: Challenges, Opportunities, and Pathways to Success

**Neil Maniar, Tracy Wiedt, and Richard Wender**

"In any discussion of social equity and justice, illness and health must figure as a major concern …. Health inequity cannot be concerned only with health, seen in isolation. Rather it must come to grips with the larger issue of justice in social arrangements, including economic allocations, paying appropriate attention to the role of health in human life and freedom."—Amartya Sen, Nobel Laureate.

## Introduction

The causes and correlates of cancer cross a broad spectrum of biological, social, environmental, and economic determinants. Many of our most significant advances in the battle against cancer have been the product of research at the molecular level; however, to sustainably reduce the burden of cancer and achieve ambitious goals in cancer survival rates we must also address the social, environmental, and economic determinants of cancer. The conditions in which individuals live, learn, work, play, and pray [1] can exert a particularly strong influence across the cancer continuum. Importantly, early life experiences and exposures can have significant effects on risk of poor health outcomes later in life [1]. These social determinants of health include but are not limited to housing status and conditions, environmental exposures, educational attainment, employment opportunities, access to healthy and affordable nutrition, and access to quality health care.

N. Maniar (✉)
Bouvé College of Health Sciences, Northeastern University, Boston, MA, USA
e-mail: s.maniar@northeastern.edu

T. Wiedt · R. Wender
American Cancer Society, Atlanta, GA, USA
e-mail: tracy.wiedt@cancer.org; richard.wender@cancer.org

 
P. Hopewood, M. J. Milroy (eds.), *Quality Cancer Care*,
https://doi.org/10.1007/978-3-319-78649-0_4

In the context of cancer prevention, social determinants may impact the extent to which individuals can access and utilize effective cancer screening tools. Furthermore, the ability of an individual to reduce their risk for cancer can also be a function of access to nutrition, the types of employment opportunities available to them, the degree to which they live in areas that are conducive to physical activity, and their level of health literacy. In this chapter, we explore in greater depth how specific social and economic determinants play a pivotal role in efforts to reduce cancer incidence and increase cancer screening rates.

Social determinants also influence what happens once an individual hears the three words that many of us fear the most: "you have cancer." Access to health care, health literacy, economic and employment factors, and barriers such as transportation can have a profound impact on the treatment options following a cancer diagnosis, adherence to the treatment regiment, access to clinical trials, and outcomes following the completion of treatment. There are an increasing number of options available to help patients and caregivers mitigate the impact of these determinants and enhance outcomes following cancer diagnoses. In this chapter, we explore the impact of patient navigation, transportation programs, and other efforts to help empower, educate, and engage patients and caregivers as they progress through their cancer journey. In addition, we also examine the role of financial toxicity both during and after cancer treatment and the lasting impact of this determinant for many cancer survivors and their caregivers.

Social determinants also lie at the root of many of the persistent disparities that exist across the cancer continuum. Disparities in vital opportunities for cancer prevention including adoption of health-promoting behaviors, access to cancer screening, and early detection and timely initiation of treatment are often observed in parallel with disparities in employment rates, food security, educational attainment, and environmental factors. This association is not a coincidence. As we see across many health outcomes, disparities in key social determinants are not only concentrated in certain communities, but they also underlie disparities across a broad range of health outcomes. This observation is central to the concept that one's zip code may be more important than one's genetic code [2]. Lifelong exposure to environmental toxins, exposure to hazards in the home, and limited access to healthy and affordable food all play important roles in elevating the risk for many different types of cancer. Educational attainment is a key predictor of employment opportunities, and it can also impact levels of health literacy. In the absence of adequate educational attainment, individuals may be restricted to working in fields that expose them to workplace toxins and other environmental hazards and they may make lower wages, impacting their ability to live healthy lifestyles and complying with cancer treatment regimens. In addition, employment is an important correlate of access to health care, particularly with respect to health insurance and paid sick leave.

There is clear and compelling evidence demonstrating the importance of not only understanding the influence of social determinants across every facet of the cancer continuum, but also developing effective and sustainable strategies to mitigate the impact of negative determinants and enhance the influence of positive ones in order to improve cancer prevention, detection, and treatment outcomes. Over the course of this chapter, we highlight the mechanisms through which social determinants influence cancer outcomes and identify strategies that can be replicated across a diverse array of settings.

## Defining Social Determinants of Health

Both conceptually and practically, the concept of social determinants of health is complex and multidimensional. In order to fully comprehend this construct, it is important to first define several related terms.

- *Health disparities* are "differences in health outcomes and their determinants between segments of the population, as defined by social, demographic, environmental, and geographic attributes" [3]. Health disparities data are used to measure progress towards achieving health equity. For example, black females have 14% higher cancer death rates than non-Hispanic white females despite 6% lower cancer incidence rates [4].
- *Health equity* is "attainment of the highest level of health for all people. Achieving health equity requires valuing everyone equally with focused and ongoing societal efforts to address avoidable inequalities, historical and contemporary injustices, and the elimination of health and healthcare disparities" [5]. Health equity "means that everyone has a fair and just opportunity to be as healthy as possible. This requires removing obstacles to health such as poverty, discrimination, and their consequences, including powerlessness and lack of access to good jobs with fair pay, quality education and housing, safe environments, and health care" [6].
- *Health inequities* are "health differences that are avoidable, unnecessary, and unjust" [7]. Embedded within this definition is the concept of social justice and the impact of inequities across a spectrum of social constructs on health outcomes. For example, differential access to cancer screening may lead to a higher proportion of individuals within a particular group who are diagnosed with cancer at a later stage relative to another group.
- *Social determinants of health* are "conditions in the environment in which people are born, live, learn, work, play, worship, and age and affect a wide range of health, functioning, and quality of life outcomes and risks" [8]. The World Health Organization has focused on social determinants of health for two decades and suggests "these circumstances are shaped by the distribution of money, power, and resources at global, national, and local levels. The social determinants of health are mostly responsible for health inequities" [9].

On April 26, 2016, Dr. Leandris Liburd—Associate Director for Minority Health and Health Equity for the Centers for Disease Control and Prevention's Office of Minority Health and Health Equity—used the below illustration during her health

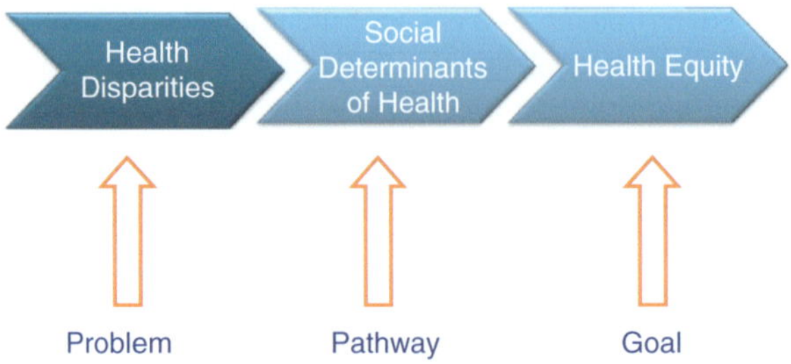


**Fig. 4.1** Dr. Liburd's model of health disparities, social determinants of health, and health equity [10]. Reprinted with permission by Dr. Leandris Liburd, 2017, Centers for Disease Control and Prevention, Atlanta, Georgia

equity presentation at the American Cancer Society (see Fig. 4.1) [10]. Dr. Liburd noted that if health disparities are the problem, and health equity is the goal, then addressing the social determinants of health is the pathway to the goal of ensuring that the highest level of health is attained for all.

## *Social Determinants of Health Frameworks*

It is widely documented that social, economic, and environmental factors are more significant predictors of health than access to care [11–13]. These factors shape opportunities for health at both an individual and community level, and they may either encourage healthy choices or impose barriers to these choices that result in unhealthy lifestyles. Where you live, meaning what opportunities you have and what resources are available, impacts your health and life expectancy [14], and there is increasing evidence that, in predicting the health of a population, where individuals live may be more important in predicting health than genetic factors [2].

The following models further illustrate determinants of health. The University of Wisconsin Population Health Institute's County Health Rankings & Roadmaps' Model of Population Health uses more than 30 health outcomes and health factors to rank the health of every county in the United States (see Fig. 4.2) [12]. Each year, new measures are included to study their impact on health. In 2015, County Health Rankings & Roadmaps added income inequality to examine the gap between the poor and the affluent. Income inequality can increase risk of mortality and contribute to poor health [15]. The University of Wisconsin Population Health Institute found that higher income households have 5.4 times higher, or in some cases almost 10 times, the income of lower income households in a county [16]. The unhealthiest counties had higher income inequality ratios. Counties found in large metropolitan areas and those located in the Southeast, Southwest, Appalachia, and the Plains had the highest income inequity ratios.

The US Department of Health and Human Services' Healthy People 2020 Social Determinants of Health Framework focuses on five key determinants to promote good health for all Americans [8]. They are (see Fig. 4.3):

- Economic stability (e.g., poverty, employment, food security, housing stability)
- Education (e.g., high school graduation, enrollment in higher education, language, and literacy)
- Health and health care (e.g., access to health care, access to primary care, health literacy)
- Neighborhood and built environment (e.g., access to healthy foods, crime and violence, and environmental conditions)
- Social and community context (e.g., social cohesion, civic participation, discrimination)

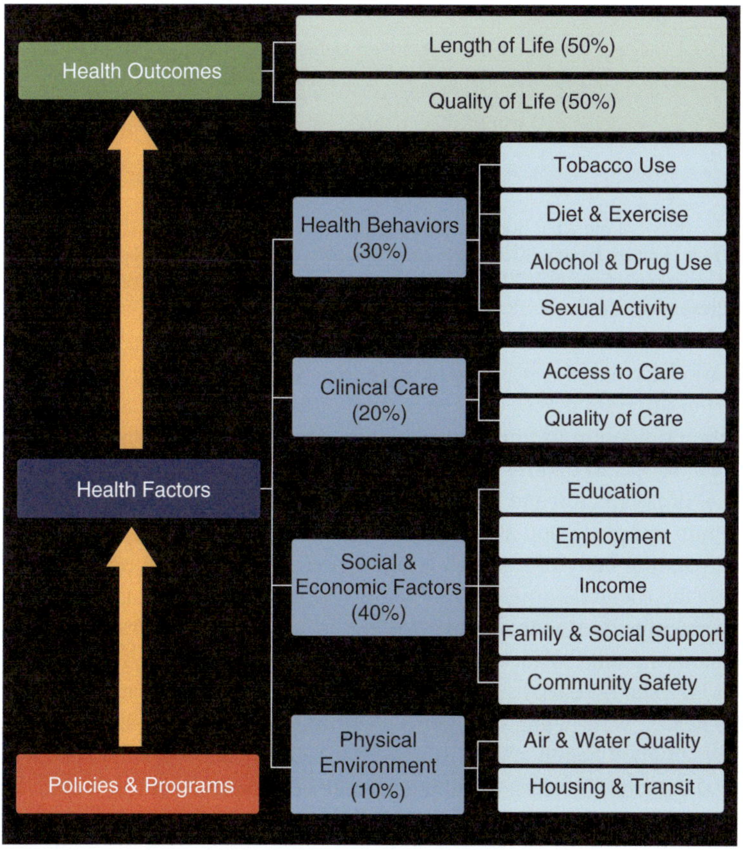


**Fig. 4.2** County Health Rankings & Roadmaps Determinants of Health Model [12]. Reprinted with permission from University of Wisconsin Population Health Institute. *County Health Rankings & Roadmaps* 2017. www.countyhealthrankings.org

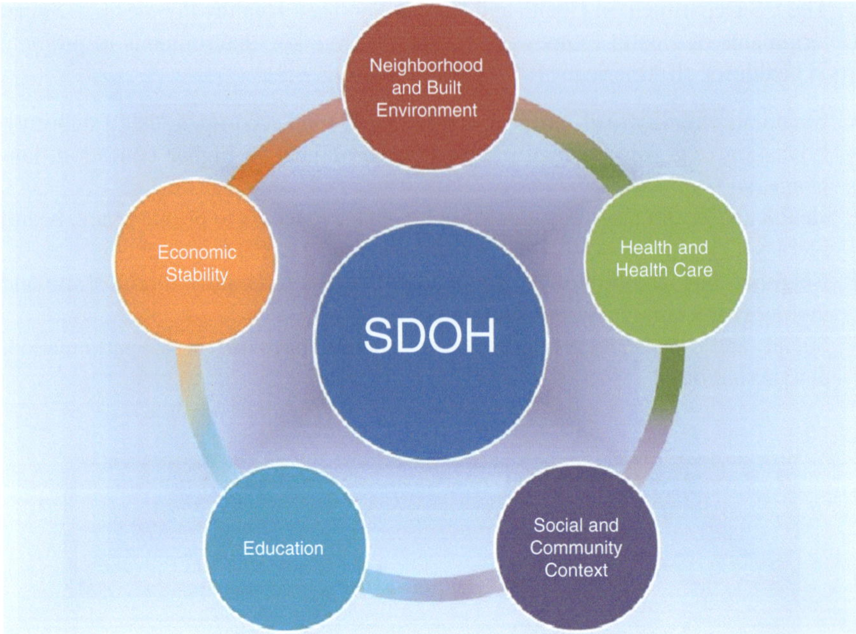


**Fig. 4.3** Healthy People 2020 Social Determinants of Health Framework [8]. Reprinted with permission from Healthy People 2020 [https://www.healthypeople.gov/2020/topics-objectives/topic/social-determinants-of-health], 2017, by US Department of Health and Human Services, Office of Disease Prevention and Health Promotion, Washington, D.C.

This model emphasizes understanding how conditions (e.g., social, economic, physical) in different places (e.g., neighborhood, school, workplace) impact health of specific population groups. For example, better understanding of how housing conditions, access to quality education, or availability of healthy foods impacts an individual or population and addressing social and physical barriers impeding good health could improve population health outcomes (Fig. 4.3).

An expanding body of research and practice is documenting effective strategies to address the social determinants of health and health equity. For example, County Health Rankings & Roadmaps provide policy and program strategies to address determinants in the "What Works" section on their website. The Robert Wood Johnson Foundation uses its Culture of Health framework as a national agenda to improve health, well-being, and equity. A Culture of Health is "broadly defined as one in which good health and well-being flourish across geographic, demographic, and social sectors; fostering healthy equitable communities guides public and private decision making; and everyone has the opportunity to make choices that lead to healthy lifestyles" [17]. Earlier this year, *Communities in Action: Pathways to Health Equity*, a report from the National Academy of Sciences, Engineering, and Medicine and commissioned by the Robert Wood Johnson Foundation was released, which outlines solutions to address health equity. Their conceptual model for community-based solutions to promote health equity is provided here (see Fig. 4.4) [18]. Among the conclusions of this report is the finding that "community-driven solutions should address at least one of the nine social determinants—education, employment, health systems and services, housing, income and wealth, physical environment, public safety, social environment, and transportation—and be: community-driven, multi-sectoral and evidence informed" [18].

## *Cancer Prevention and Early Detection*

In 2015, cancer death rates were about 26% lower in the United States than they were in 1990. The United States achieved about one-half of the American Cancer Society's challenge goal to reduce cancer mortality by 50%, over a 25-year period [19]. This decline in cancer mortality is attributable to many factors including:

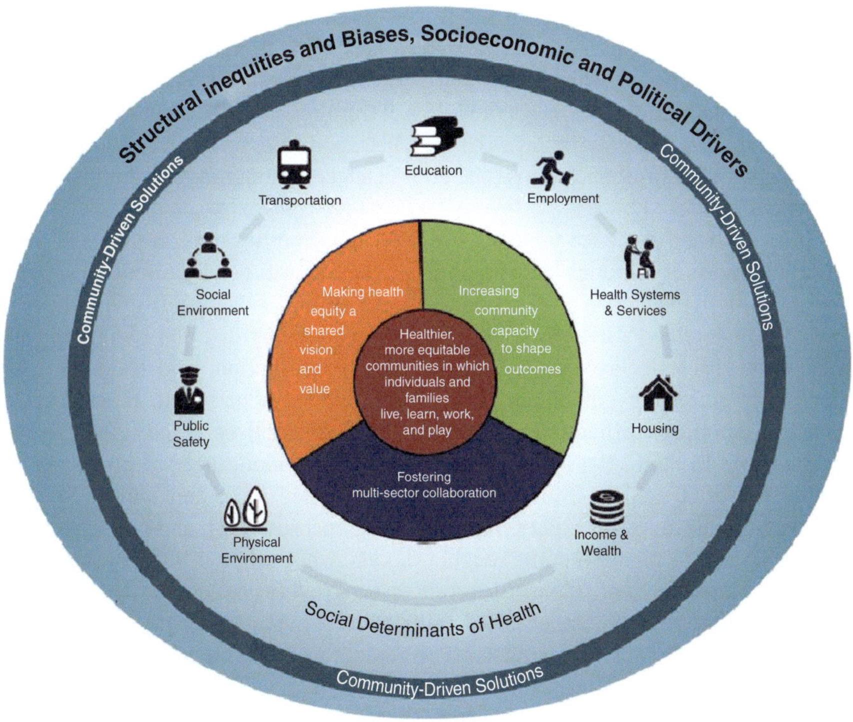


**Fig. 4.4** NASEM's conceptual model for community-based solutions to promote health equity [18]. Reprinted with permission from Fig. S-1, Communities in Action: Pathways to Health Equity, 2017, by the National Academy of Sciences, Courtesy of the National Academies Press, Washington, D.C.

1. Adoption of policies and interventions that reduce tobacco use and exposure
2. The introduction and adoption of new approaches to cancer screening, including mammography, PSA screening for prostate cancer, and colon cancer screening tests
3. Broader provision of health insurance coverage
4. Advances in cancer treatment [19, 20]

However, the authors evaluating progress towards ACS's challenge goals noted that in order to achieve the 50% reduction in cancer mortality, all sectors of civil society—including those focused on determinants of health such as income, availability of care, and many other social and environmental factors affecting cancer-reducing programs and policies—need to be involved [19]. Furthermore, we must also focus on the root causes of health disparities including inequities in employment opportunities, wealth, education, housing, and overall standard of living, as well as social barriers to high-quality cancer prevention, early detection, and treatment services [4].

Individuals living in poor neighborhoods often face many challenges when seeking quality health care and taking advantage of opportunities for prevention. Residents of these neighborhoods often live on a fixed income and may not have access to transportation and other resources necessary to make healthier lifestyle and healthcare choices. This assessment underscores the need for a concerted and multidisciplinary effort to address the full spectrum of social determinants of health including income, neighborhood environments, food insecurity, and availability of health care and their impact across the entire cancer continuum from prevention to survivorship.

There is strong evidence underscoring key opportunities to reduce cancer incidence and mortality through the adoption of a healthier lifestyle. About 50% of all cancer deaths in the United States could be avoided if individuals did not use tobacco products, maintained a healthy weight by eating a healthy diet and living a physically active lifestyle, avoided/reduced alcohol consumption, and followed age-appropriate screening guidelines [21]. Unfortunately, adhering to these healthy behaviors can prove difficult depending upon where one lives or the resources one has available to them. If you live in a poor neighborhood, tobacco products and alcohol are often widely available [22] and marketed [23], and unhealthy food options are plentiful [24], highly marketed [25], cost less [26], and are convenient [27], compared to higher income neighborhoods. Choosing a healthy option when unhealthy options are both plentiful and cheap can be very challenging, thus increasing the risk for cancer and other poor health outcomes. Making healthy foods available is also insufficient; changing food preferences requires a comprehensive and sustained approach to culture change.

In the United States, an estimated 20% of cancers are due to the collective effects of excess alcohol consumption, poor nutrition, physical inactivity, and excess weight [28]. Barriers that contribute to increase obesity include limited access to healthy affordable foods; marketing and advertising of foods and beverages high in calories, fat, and added sugar, particularly to kids; schools and worksites that are not conducive to good health; community design that hinders physical activity and promotes sedentary behavior; and economic and time restraints [4].

The American Cancer Society's Guidelines on Nutrition and Physical Activity for Cancer Prevention provide recommended solutions [29]. The recommendations for community action suggest public, private, and community organizations work collaboratively at national, state, and local levels to implement policy and environmental changes that:

- Increase access to affordable, healthy foods in communities, worksites, and schools, and decrease access to and marketing of foods and beverages of low nutritional value, particularly to youth.
- Provide safe, enjoyable, and accessible environments for physical activity in schools and worksites, and for transportation and recreation in communities.

Income level impacts the opportunities and decisions that can lead to either good or poor health. Income influences access to safe and affordable housing and the stress associated with a disproportionate amount of household income being consumed by housing costs versus other expenses. Income can also influence access to housing that is free of lead or mold, whether the neighborhood is safe and conducive for being physically active, availability of transportation to access for a healthy lifestyle, proximity of job opportunities, and access to other basic needs and resources that can impact health.

Access to health care is an important determinant of health. Evidence-based cancer screening reduces mortality by both finding and treating cancer precursors and by finding cancer in an earlier and more treatable stage, increasing the likelihood of effective cancer management and treatment and raising the odds of survival. However, certain types of cancer screening such as colonoscopy or mammography may require individuals to take time off from work beyond time required for office visits. Furthermore, the fear of a positive finding and the burden of cancer treatment, including extended sick leave, sometimes prevent individuals from getting screened. The disparities in access to sick leave and their impact on cancer screening and treatment can be significant. An estimated 38% of employed adults do not have paid sick leave [30]. Paid sick leave, a social determinant that is a function of employment, appears to be associated with increased use of preventive services, including mammography, Pap test, and endoscopy, compared to people who do not have paid sick leave [30]. Workers who were less likely to report having sick leave included those in service or production occupations, those in the private sector, and those in smaller firms with fewer years on the job. Participation in cancer screening is highly sensitive to out-of-pocket cost [31, 32]. The perception that screening will be expensive and the actual costs associated with screening are major deterrents to participation.

*In New York, most public employees are provided 4 h of separate paid leave for breast and prostate cancer screenings. This leave is separate from other leave benefits such as sick, vacation, or personal leave. In addition to the time covered under New York State law for breast and prostate cancer screenings, Schenectady, New York added four additional hours of paid leave for cancer screenings (e.g., colon cancer) for its county employees.* The New York State Department of Health Bureau of Cancer Prevention and Control is working with organizations and municipalities throughout the state on 28 projects to permit paid time off for cancer screening [33]. Eight municipalities and five organizations have adopted or expanded their paid leave policies for cancer screenings since the fall of 2016.

Patient navigation strategies are also effective in removing barriers to healthcare access for breast, cervical, and colorectal cancer screenings. Interventions to increase community demand (e.g., client/patient reminders, one-on-one education), increase community access (e.g., reducing structural barrier or client out-of-pocket costs), and increase provider delivery of screening services (e.g., provider feedback, provider reminders) are examples of effective strategies to increase cancer screening uptake [34].

When financial resources are scarce, adults are likely to forego a doctor's visit when needed; one out of every four Latino adults and one out of every five African-American adults did not visit a doctor in the last year when needed due to cost [35]. This could mean that preventive measures such as the cancer vaccine for adolescents to prevent several cancers associated with the human papillomavirus or screening exams for breast or colorectal cancers are either never pursued or are delayed. The Patient Protection and Affordable Care Act is helping mitigate the cost barrier preventing patients from pursuing preventive screening exams. Under the law, private insurance plans are required to cover recommended preventive services without patients sharing the cost, including cancer screening exams [36].

The Patient Protection and Affordable Care Act of 2010 also requires not-for-profit hospitals to conduct a community health needs assessment every 3 years and for these hospitals to act on strategies aimed at addressing the needs identified in their assessments. Some hospitals are assessing the social determinants of health needs in their communities and exploring how to address these factors. For example, Dana-Farber Cancer Institute is using a social determinant of health framework for their community health needs assessment and implementation activities. They are also examining this work through a health equity lens. Their community health needs assessment found poverty, physical/built environment, and affordable housing as determinants that were of concern and in need of attention [37].

Opportunities exist for national and cross-sector collaborative actions that support civic engagement and community-driven approaches to address the social determinants of health and advance health equity. Organizations—no matter how large or small—at all levels of society are needed to embrace the concept of social determinants of health. Education of the constructs is needed for those sectors that don't impact health directly. Engagement and inclusion of organizations that do not primarily impact health are critical. Organizations like the American Cancer Society can play an important role by continuing to raise awareness on this critical subject; embracing and taking action to address social determinants related to cancer, including advocating for policy and system-level approaches and building community capacity; and serving as a convener of diverse sectors to help foster cross-sector collaborations and mobilize action. We must remain vigilant and be bold if we are to prevent cancer, save lives, and diminish suffering from cancer, including better integrating strategies to address social, economic, and environmental factors into our work.

## Access to Care in the Context of Cancer Treatment

The availability of high-quality health care isn't often enough to ensure a good outcome following a cancer diagnosis. In fact, some of the nation's leading cancer centers are located in cities that have long-standing disparities in cancer outcomes. In these cities, residents living in communities that are often within the shadow of cancer centers face a multitude of barriers that undermine their ability to receive timely and state-of-the-art cancer treatment. Why does this paradox exist? The answer lies, at least in part, within the realm of social determinants of health and their influence on access to health care.

The Institute of Medicine defines access to health care as having "the timely use of personal health services to achieve the best health outcomes" [38]. According to the Agency for Healthcare Research and Quality, access to high-quality health care is the product of three steps:

1. Gaining entry into the healthcare system
2. Accessing sites where needed services are available
3. Finding providers who can not only meet the needs of patients, but also develop stable and trusting relationships [39]

Social determinants influence each of these steps in a number of independent and also interrelated ways. Having healthcare coverage that enables patients to receive care at cancer centers that are best equipped to treat a particular diagnosis can facilitate gaining entry into the healthcare system. In the wake of a cancer diagnosis, timely access to a healthcare provider can impact both quality of life and survival rates across a range of cancer outcomes. However, timely access to care may be impeded by financial barriers, lack of sufficient sick leave, lack of transportation, and difficulty navigating the healthcare system [40]. Similarly, access to sites that provide needed care can also be a function of the same social determinants of health that influence the ability of a patient to gain entry into the healthcare system. The specialized care that is required to treat certain cancers, for example bone marrow transplant, is often concentrated within a handful of healthcare institutions in a region. Therefore, patients must have the ability to not only physically access these sites, but also advocate for specialized treatment when appropriate. For some of these sites, cancer care also requires lodging over a long period of time and for cancer patients and their caregivers the burden of cancer treatment can be exacerbated by a lack of social support. Finding providers with whom patients can develop a relationship grounded in trust and proper communication may also require a base of culturally concordant providers in an area [41].

Social determinants of health including education, transportation, income, employment, and social support influence the quality and type of treatment that cancer patients receive through several distinct mechanisms. Education levels can mediate the level of satisfaction that patients have with cancer treatments by influencing their ability to synthesize information related to cancer diagnosis and treatment options and by influencing patient-provider communication [42]. Patients who are more informed may also be more likely to advocate for the most advanced cancer treatment available and for both patients and caregivers access to information and the ability to process information can improve quality of life both during and after cancer treatment. In some cases, income and other financial resources can also be critical facilitators or barriers when patients are trying to access certain treatment options. Some cancer centers will only accept specific forms of insurance and in many cases the cost of treatment even with Medicare or Medicaid can impose a significant financial burden on patients and caregivers.

## *The Role of Health Literacy*

Health literacy has become a fundamental factor in our conceptualization of how specific social determinants of health influence a broad range of health behaviors and health outcomes. According to the CDC, the Patient Protection and Affordable Care Act of 2010 defines health literacy as "the degree to which an individual has the capacity to obtain, communicate, process, and understand basic health information and services to make appropriate health decisions" [43]. Embedded within this definition is the idea that in order for health literacy to exist, individuals must first have the potential to meaningfully absorb health-related information and that the information itself must exist in format that is accessible by a diverse array of populations with varying baseline literacy levels. In the 2010 Department of Health and Human Services' report, a National Action Plan to Improve Health Literacy, Assistant Secretary for Health Dr. Howard Koh notes that "too often, there exists a chasm of knowledge between what professionals know and what consumers and patients understand. Basic health literacy is fundamental to the success of each interaction between healthcare professionals and patients – every prescription, every treatment, and every recovery" [44].

As patients begin to chart their course for cancer treatment, several critical decisions are often required on the part of patients and their caregivers: What is the best initial treatment course? What side effects are the patient willing to tolerate? Can the patient travel for treatment? What are the patient and caregiver goals over the course of treatment? What aspects of their care do patients value most? How much will the treatment cost? For each of these decisions, there are often multiple sources of information to help guide the decision-making process. In the midst of the stress and emotional turbulence that surrounds a cancer diagnosis, synthesizing this information can be challenging for even the most health-literate individuals. Furthermore, in order to advocate effectively for themselves and their loved ones, patients and caregivers must also know about different treatment protocols and potential advances in treatment so that they can fully engage in the shared decision-making process [45].

Health literacy itself can be shaped by multiple social determinants including education, social support, and environmental factors. Low levels of health literacy can significantly influence engagement in adverse health behaviors early in life, thus increasing cancer risk, reducing the likelihood of engaging in prevention and early detection opportunities, and increasing risk for other comorbid health outcomes (diabetes, obesity, heart disease) that further exacerbate the health literacy gap [46].

## *Financial Toxicity and the Cost of Treatment*

A key theme of our discussion of how social determinants of health exert influence across the cancer continuum focuses on the role of income and employment as facilitators and barriers for cancer prevention, early detection, treatment, and survivorship. The escalating cost of cancer treatment coupled with a shifting landscape of healthcare access and coverage imposes further burdens on patients and caregivers who are already dealing with an exceptionally stressful life circumstance. The cost of cancer treatment includes both the direct costs of treatment and indirect costs associated with reduced employment or lack of employment, increased debt burden, and transportation and lodging costs associated with certain types of cancer treatment. In recent years, a new term has been developed to describe the adverse effects of the direct and indirect cost of cancer treatment: financial toxicity. Zafar and Abernethy note that "an expanding body of evidence suggests that cancer patients with insurance are dealing with cost implications as a part of their cancer experience [and] out-of-pocket expenses related to treatment are akin to physical toxicity, in that costs can diminish quality of life and impede delivery of the highest quality care [47]." The prevalence of financial distress among cancer patients, particularly elderly cancer patients, is significant. Studies suggest that 50% of elderly cancer patients pay over 10% of their income towards cancer expenses [48] and patients with cancer have greater out-of-pocket expenses compared to patients with other chronic illnesses [48]. A study in Washington state demonstrated that individuals with cancer are 2.7 times more likely to declare bankruptcy than individuals without cancer [49]. Another study found that 79% of patients with cancer report moderate to catastrophic financial burden resulting from cancer care [50].

The impact of financial toxicity may be amplified in the presence of low levels of health literacy. Poor understanding of coverage options, including appropriate deductibles, and treatment options lead patients and caregivers to not only underestimate the cost of cancer treatment, but also pursue treatment options that may be financially devastating. Zafar and colleagues note that a nationally representative survey of 3500 participants revealed that only 16% could calculate out-of-pocket costs for out-of-network lab tests and out of the 52% who expressed an interest in discussing costs with their provider only 19% did so [48]. To tackle the intersection of health literacy and financial toxicity, Zafar and colleagues proposed a modified version of the *socio-ecological framework to identify barriers associated with health cost literacy*. Figure 4.5 addresses opportunities to improve health cost literacy at the individual level through increased education, at the interpersonal level by focusing on the patient-provider relationship, and at the health system level by providing timely financial assistance [48].

The cluster of factors referred to as social determinants are powerful and consistent predictors of health across virtually all measures of health status, including all major risk factors for premature mortality and all disease types. Social determinants account for a substantial fraction of health disparities. While health disparities are often reported based on continent of origin, national roots, and skin color, social determinants are far more important predictors of health status. African-Americans, Hispanic/Latinos, Native Americans, and Asian-Americans, as well as immigrants and refugees, are more likely to confront lower incomes, lower levels of educational achievement, and difficulty in accessing health care. When these social determinants are not present, health disparities as measured by usual categories are greatly diminished.

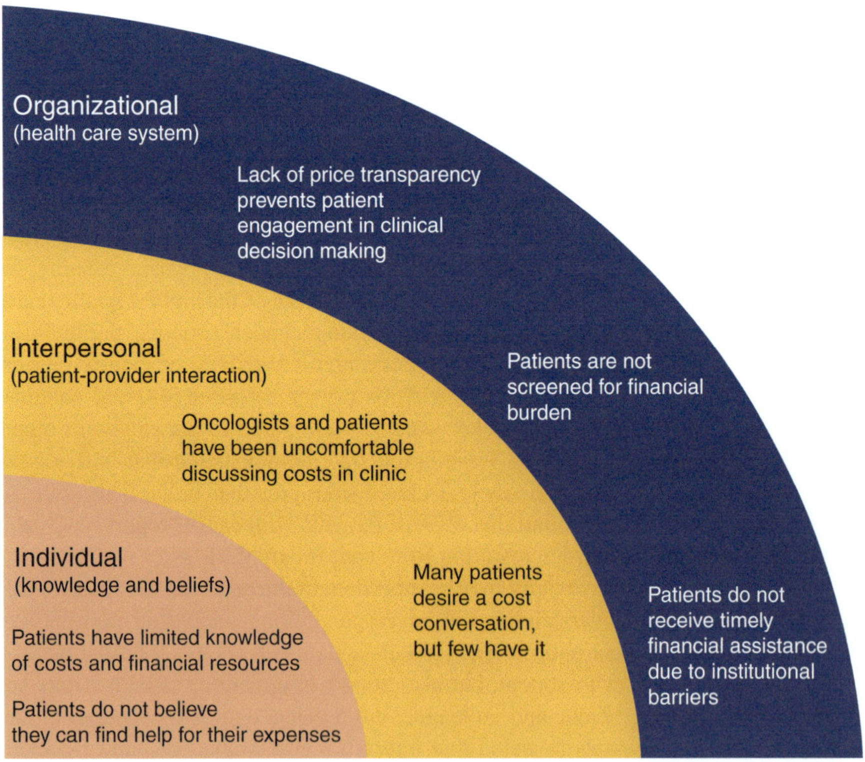


**Fig. 4.5** Modified socio-ecological framework to identify barriers associated with health cost literacy [48]. Reprinted with permission. © (2015) American Society of Clinical Oncology. All rights reserved. Zafar SY, Ubel PA, Tulsky JA, et al. Journal of Oncology Practice, Vol. 11, Issue 3, 2015:171–173

Recognition that social factors are critical determinants of health is a necessary but not sufficient step to stimulate and guide efforts to address these issues. In fact, confronting the complexity of these factors can have a paralyzing effect; feeling overwhelmed and being unaware of proven interventions or even a starting point to stimulate change are persistent deterrents to meaningful engagement and action. This task is rendered more difficult by two facts: our inability to clearly prioritize the importance of each social determinant, and a paucity of proven interventions to bring about lasting change. Attempts to prioritize the impact of each factor consistently reveal that social determinants are tightly associated with each other. Each of them is independently associated with poorer health, but each of them is also associated with other determinants of health and they often act synergistically to produce a compound effect. While low educational achievement is a particularly strong predictor of poor health outcomes, lower educational achievement is also strongly associated with poverty, higher social isolation, and risky health behaviors. Attempts to independently address level of educational achievement or any other single factor have proven to be difficult; changing one determinant without addressing the cluster of social issues that contribute to health may be unrealistic and unproductive. While recognizing the interdependence of these factors, a reasonable argument can be made that low income is likely to be the most important and persistent determinant of poor health. Income disparity has grown in the United States. From 1979 through 2008, wealth actually declined in the poorest quintile. Most growth in wealth occurred in the wealthiest 20% of individuals, and particularly in the wealthiest 5% [51].

## Creating a Framework for Action

While acknowledging that few proven interventions to produce sustained improvement in social determinants have been identified, we propose seven elements that should be considered in designing a framework to guide action to address social determinants of health. First, differentiating interventions intended to bridge health disparities from interventions intended to lessen the impact of adverse social determinants is necessary. Numerous studies and models as well as clinical experience have guided efforts to prospectively identify individuals who are likely to experience less desirable health outcomes, based on factors like education, income, and social support. Interventions such as social service consultation, programs to address financial barriers to care, and navigation are proven to improve outcomes for individuals, but they do not actually alter the social circumstances in which patients and their caregivers live. Our proposed framework is specifically intended to address social determinants of health at the population or community level. The framework reflects an aspirational thought and hypothesis, a guide to direct action and collection of evidence. These interventions are complex and difficult, but simple solutions will not effectively address the deeply ingrained aspects of society that must be addressed to catalyze lasting change.

## *Place: A Unifying Principle for Social Determinants*

The work of numerous experts and organizations is increasingly highlighting the importance of community-level factors and where individuals live as proximal determinants of health. Life expectancy is vastly different based on where an individual is born and lives; life expectancy in the United States is 20 years longer in the longest-lived counties than in the counties with the lowest life expectancy [52]. Factors related to socioeconomic and race/ethnicity factors (e.g., income, unemployment), behavioral and metabolic risk (e.g., obesity prevalence, smoking prevalence), and health care (e.g., access to health care and healthcare quality) explained 60%, 74%, and 27% of county-level variation in life expectancy, respectively [52]. There are also large variations in cancer mortality rates among US counties [53]. These data point us towards interventions designed to improve the health-promoting facets of communities while attempting to lessen or diminish the factors that impede achievement of health. All of the modifiable factors that contribute to or impede health are potential targets for intervention. We propose seven steps (elements) that must be considered when constructing a framework to guide action. Making meaningful change in any one of these facets may be important and effective, but working on the first three, ideally in the order they appear, may lead to a higher likelihood of real change (Box 4.1).

**Box 4.1 Seven Steps (Elements) That Must Be Considered**
*When constructing a framework to guide action*

1. Solutions must be designed and implemented at the community level, one community at a time.
2. Efforts to address social determinants of health are facilitated by engagement of, and preferably, leadership provided by residents of the community.
3. Leaders and champions, embedded within or deeply engaged with a community, often determine the level of success of interventions.
4. Engagement of all sectors, including private, public, government, and non-governmental organizations, is typically required to create lasting change.
5. Change requires relentless, long-lasting engagement, often spanning more than a decade.
6. Strategies to address specific structural elements of communities and to implement policies that reduce barriers to health should be identified and pursued.
7. The ability to measure and periodically assess progress is an important predictor of success.

### Solutions Must Be Designed and Implemented at the Community Level, One Community at a Time

Although local, state, and national policies can both facilitate or impede efforts to reduce the social determinants of cancer (and their importance should not be underestimated), the most sustainable change is rooted in community-level efforts that are fueled by genuine community engagement and leadership. Examples include structural changes such as changes in the built environment, availability of transportation, technology, healthy foods, places to exercise, housing, and health care, as well as changes in services and opportunities, such as access to good jobs, jobs with good benefits that support, and health care. A shared vision, created, owned, and implemented *with* the community is essential.

### Efforts to Address Social Determinants of Health Are Facilitated by Engagement of, and Preferably, Leadership Provided by Residents of the Community

Many well-meaning individuals, groups, and institutions have designed and attempted to implement programs in our poorest communities without conducting full needs assessments or engaging community residents. While these programs are occasionally beneficial, they often fail as a result of inadequate engagement of residents and at times loss of community trust is an unfortunate result. The growing focus on community health needs assessment (CHNA), community health assessments by local health departments, health equity assessments, and networks of community coalitions and other existing community-organizing efforts can be powerful facilitators of successful efforts to address social determinants of health. These approaches are designed to be community-driven efforts and strategies to address identified health needs and often intersect with many different social determinants of health. To successfully address the barriers communities and neighborhoods face in seeking health and improving cancer outcomes, community members should be authentically engaged in discussions and decisions. This could include being involved in data collection to better understand barriers and strategy development and implementation and engaging nontraditional partners in efforts to improve outcomes.

In a recently published study, Cole and colleagues describe the effectiveness of leveraging the patient navigation model and a community partner to increase colonoscopy screening rates among black men in New York City. The authors of the study spent a significant amount of time building relationships with barbershop employees to determine their relevance in efforts to tackle cancer-related disparities. The authors then implemented a randomized trial design with three arms, with two of the arms receiving patient navigation and a control arm that only received advice about blood pressure control. The results of the study revealed significant improvements in colorectal cancer screening rates once navigation entered the picture. The percentage of men within the two intervention arms who got screened for colorectal cancer screening (CRC) within 6 months was more than double the percentage in the control arm [54]. A central factor in the success of this intervention was the role of the barbershop employees as trusted members of the community.

### Leaders and Champions, Embedded Within or Deeply Engaged with a Community, Often Determine the Level of Success of Interventions

Numerous examples highlight the vital role played by individuals committed to improving the health of community residents. While direction from leaders is usually necessary to ensure sustained engagement of an organization, individual champions, the people who fight to improve community life as a routine part of their work and of their purpose in life, often become the key drivers of sustained change. These individual champions provide a valuable perspective in every stage of program development and they also bring both the experience and trust needed to successfully implement sustainable interventions to address social determinants of health.

### Engagement of All Sectors, Including Private, Public, Government, and Nongovernmental Organizations, Is Typically Required to Create Lasting Change

Due to the complexity of and interrelationships of social determinants of health, most successful change results from engaging numerous and diverse individuals and organizations that share a commitment to improving the health of a community. While roles may differ, from philanthropy to provision of specific services and to community organization, meaningful engagement by numerous individuals and organizations is more likely to result in sustained and committed effort. Building nontraditional partnerships that bridge sectors can help overcome some of the persistent barriers that have hindered previous efforts. The multidisciplinary nature of social determinants requires active and sustained partnerships across a diverse array of sectors and constituents including, but not limited to, health care, education, economic development, business, housing, law enforcement, community development, and philanthropy.

### Change Requires Relentless, Long-Lasting Engagement, Often Spanning More than a Decade

Specific interventions designed to address a single determinant of health and spanning only a few years rarely produce lasting change. The road to improving the health of communities is never predictable, uninterrupted, or linear. Community improvement requires a sustained effort usually spanning generations. This commitment applies to both the partnerships that will drive change and the organizational priorities that will ensure the availability of funding to support and achieve lasting change. Exogenous factors including changes in the healthcare landscape, a shift in the prevailing political ideology, or economic crises can derail or set back efforts to tackle social determinants. Because some efforts will not yield the intended result for years, if not decades, it is also sometimes difficult to navigate an environment that is oriented towards short-term results.

### Strategies to Address Specific Structural Elements of Communities and to Implement Policies That Reduce Barriers to Health Should Be Identified and Pursued

While short-lived, single-focus interventions usually don't result in meaningful reduction in barriers to health, successful efforts do require careful assessment of community needs and priorities, and specific, often complex, interventions designed to assess a series of specific problems or issues, such as technology, transportation, food insecurity, housing, and health care. Addressing the built environment and other structural characteristics of communities can be a daunting task, particularly in resource-constrained environments. However, leveraging other efforts in the community, including the community health needs assessments that are conducted by all nonprofit hospitals and many FQHCs and health departments, can provide insight into common structural elements that can be the focus of a collaborative effort.

### The Ability to Measure and Periodically Assess Progress Is an Important Predictor of Success

Like any other aspect of quality improvement, change requires measurement of the impact of interventions. Choosing appropriate measures of progress can be challenging, but is, nevertheless, critically important. Several national surveys and instruments measure various aspects of social determinants of health, such as high school graduation rates, employment rates, having health insurance, and measures of healthy food access. However, gathering these data at the local level and in a timely way poses a challenge. One solution to this barrier is to leverage measures that are already in use at the local level. Through the partnerships described in element 4 above, it may be possible to access data that will provide timely local data across a broad range of performance measures.

Milwaukee, Wisconsin, is an example that brings to life some of these elements. The 2017 County Health Rankings ranked Milwaukee county 71 out of 72 counties, meaning it had the second worst health outcomes in the state [55]. Milwaukee also ranked 71 out of 72 counties for socioeconomic status, physical environment, and health behaviors. The city of Milwaukee has higher than state average rates of breast, cervical, lung, and prostate cancer [56].

The metropolitan Milwaukee, Wisconsin area, has the largest gap in unemployment between blacks and whites in the country—17.3% of blacks were unemployed compared to 4.3% of whites [57]. Milwaukee has the second largest income gap in the country—the median household income for blacks was $25,600 compared to $62,600 for whites. Employment is important because there is a greater chance someone will have access to health insurance, increasing their ability to access cancer screening and care. Furthermore, being diagnosed with cancer can negatively impact one's ability to remain employed. In one study, nearly 33% of women in Detroit and Los Angeles diagnosed with early-stage breast cancer who were working when they began treatment were unemployed 4 years later [58].

Recently, the Milwaukee Health Department embarked on a community-wide survey and community and stakeholder meetings with more than 3000 residents and 200 partners to better understand health issues. The issues that mattered most to the respondents were (1) crime and neighborhood safety (42.8%), (2) access to affordable and healthy food (39.9%), (3) jobs and income/wages (33.8%), (4) education (29.8%), and (5) access to basic human needs (27.8%) [56]. The community ranking for access to health care was tenth.

After an extensive community health assessment, asset mapping, surveys, focus groups, a photo-voice campaign, and stakeholder interviews, the city of Milwaukee completed a prioritization process. Since then, the city has embarked on a journey to elevate Milwaukee as the healthiest city in the nation. This bold effort, aptly named, *Milwaukee Elevate*, has advanced an overarching goal of building safe and healthy neighborhoods in the city through a community-driven approach. This goal will be achieved by ensuring economic security, fostering an inclusive and fair society, and supporting positive mental health. For more than a year, the American Cancer Society has been working with community volunteers in Milwaukee to focus on the determinants of health and is well positioned to play an important role. Through ACS's diverse community partnerships, the capacity of and leadership in government, business, health systems, universities, and others can be leveraged to add value to *Milwaukee Elevate.* Efforts like this can help address the underlying issues that impact cancer outcomes in communities.

## Getting Started: The Critical First Steps

Although efforts to improve the health of communities can be initiated through a variety of pathways, most successful and sustained projects are catalyzed when like-minded individuals come together and agree to pursue an important community-based and -driven goal. Efforts to engage people who live in the community as leaders and co-facilitators are always critical, even when it is difficult. The first steps to success often begin with small, achievable plans that harness the collective commitment and effort and ensure that they are sustained. Securing funding through grants and philanthropy is also necessary as is the willingness and commitment to pursue new dollars, year after year, throughout the life course of the intervention. Finally, local, state, and national advocacy to support programs that address social determinants of health is usually instrumental to support whatever community initiatives are pursued.

## Healthcare Institutions: Key Partners for Success

Hospitals and other healthcare institutions have the potential to catalyze, lead, and/or be a partner in improving health for communities they serve. Despite a growing focus on meaningful programs to address social determinants of health, many hospitals have not elevated community health improvement to the top of their agenda. The focus on improving the health of the community can sometimes take a back seat to fiscal priorities or other patient management efforts, even though social determinants have a powerful impact on a hospital's bottom line. We contend that all hospitals have a responsibility to:

1. Identify the communities they serve that experience poor health outcomes due to social determinants of health
2. Establish improving community health as a top organizational priority and dedicate human and financial resources to address this priority
3. Identify leaders, champions, and partners
4. Implement specific programs to address needs
5. Measure and report progress
6. Keep working to address community needs year after year

While recognizing that this call to action is a tall task, some hospitals consistently address the needs of underserved communities they serve and, ultimately, almost every hospital has the capacity to consider social determinants of health in planning their work and goals. If every hospital demonstrated commitment to address social determinants of health as a core institutional priority, substantial improvements in health are likely to occur.

## Conclusion

The numerous factors that comprise the social determinants of health are powerful predictors of the health of individuals. Poverty, lack of educational achievement, social isolation, inadequate access to healthy foods and safe places to exercise, inadequate access to lodging, transportation, and technology, along with other social factors, form a set of seemingly intractable barriers to the achievement of optimal health. Identifying obstacles to changing the social determinants of health is not difficult, but perhaps no obstacle is more limiting than complacency. All healthcare providers and institutions have the opportunity and, we would argue, the obligation to elevate the elimination of health disparities that result from social determinants to being a top agenda and goal. Knowing how to get started can seem difficult, but a good place to start is to form real attachments to people living in communities and understanding the barriers preventing them from making healthier choices. Leaders and champions should be encouraged and nurtured. Efforts should be sustained. With shared effort and conviction, fueled by reason and passion, meaningful change and improved health can be realized.

## References


1. Braveman P, Egerter S. Overcoming obstacles to health: report from the Robert Wood Johnson Foundation to the commission to build a healthier America. Princeton, NJ: Robert Wood Johnson Foundation; 2008.
2. Roeder A. Zip code better predictor of health than genetic code. Harvard Gazette; 2014. https://wwwhsphharvardedu/news/features/zip-code-better-predictor-of-health-than-genetic-code/. Accessed 26 July 2017.
3. Truman B, Smith CK, Roy K, Chen Z, Moonesinghe R, Zhu J, et al. Rationale for regular reporting on health disparities and inequalities—United States. MMWR Morb Mortal Suppl. 2011;60(01):3–10.
4. American Cancer Society. Cancer Facts & Figures. Atlanta: American Cancer Society; 2017. https://www.cancer.org/research/cancer-facts-statistics/all-cancer-facts-figures/cancer-facts-figures-2017.html. Accessed 2 May 2017.
5. National Partnership for Action to End Health Disparities. National Stakeholder Strategy for Achieving Health Equity. Rockville, MD: U.S. Department of Health & Human Services, Office of Minority Health; 2011. https://minorityhealth.hhs.gov/npa/templates/content.aspx?lvl=1&lvlid=33&ID=286. Accessed 27 April 2017.
6. Braveman P, Arkin E, Orleans T, Proctor D, Plough A. What is health equity? And what difference does a definition make? Princeton, NJ: Robert Wood Johnson Foundation; 2017.
7. Whitehead M. The concepts and principles of equity and health. Int J Health Serv. 1992;22:429–45.
8. Healthy People 2020. Washington, DC: U.S. Department of Health and Human Services, Office of Disease Prevention and Health Promotion. http://www.healthypeople.gov/2020/topics-objectives/topic/social-determinants-health?topicid=39. Accessed 27 Apr 2017.
9. World Health Organization website. 2017. http://www.who.int/social_determinants/sdh_definition/en/. Accessed 28 Apr 2017.
10. Liburd L. Model of health disparities, social determinants of health, and health equity. Presentation 2016. Atlanta, GA: Accessed Centers for Disease Control and Prevention; 2017.
11. Heiman HJ, Artiga S. Beyond Health Care: the role of social determinants in promoting health and health equity. Issue Brief by the Henry J Kaiser Family Foundation. 2015. http://kff.org/disparities-policy/issue-brief/beyond-health-care-the-role-of-social-determinants-in-promoting-health-and-health-equity/. Accessed 2 May 2017.
12. University of Wisconsin Population Health Institute. County Health Rankings & Roadmaps. 2017. www.countyhealthrankings.org. Accessed 28 Apr 2017.
13. McGinnis M, Williams-Russo P, Knickman JR. The case for more active policy attention to health promotion. Health Aff (Millwood). 2002;21(2):98–3.
14. Chetty R, Stepner M, Abraham S, Lin S, Scuderi B, Turner N, et al. The association between income and life expectancy in the United States, 2001–2014. JAMA. 2016;315(16):1750–66.
15. Pickett KE, Wilkinson RG. Income inequality and health: a causal review. Soc Sci Med. 2015;128:316–26.
16. University of Wisconsin Population Health Institute. 2015 County Health Rankings – Key Findings Report 2015. http://www.countyhealthrankings.org/sites/default/files/resources/CHR%26R%202015%20Key%20Findings.pdf. Accessed 28 Apr 2017.

17. Robert Wood Johnson Foundation website. http://www.evidenceforaction.org/what-culture-health. Accessed 29 Apr 2017.
18. National Academies of Sciences, Engineering, and Medicine. Communities in action: pathways to health equity. Washington, DC: The National Academies Press; 2017. https://doi.org/10.17226/24624.
19. Byers T, Wender RC, Jemal A, Baskins AM, Ward EE, Brawley OW. The American Cancer Society challenge goal to reduce US cancer mortality by 50% between 1990 and 2015: results and reflections. CA Cancer J Clin. 2016;66(5):359–69.
20. Marks JS, Orleans CT, Gerlach KK. On the threshold of a dream. Cancer. 2016;107(2):217–20.
21. Siegel R. Strategic Director, Surveillance Information Services at the American Cancer Society, Personal Communication on Monday, 30 January 2017.
22. Rodriguez D, Carlos H, Adachi-Mejia AM, et al. Predictors of tobacco outlet density nationwide: a geographic analysis. Tob Control. 2013;22(5):349–55.
23. Seidenberg A, Caughey R, Rees V, et al. Storefront cigarette advertising differs by community demographic profile. Am J Health Promot. 2010;24(6):e26–31.
24. Powell LM, Slater S, Mirtcheva D, Bao Y, Chaloupka FJ. Food store availability and neighborhood characteristics in the United States. Prev Med. 2007;44(3):189–95.
25. Powell LM, Wada R, Kumanyika S. Racial/ethnic and income disparities in child and adolescent exposure to food and beverage television ads across U.S. media markets. Health Place. 2014;29:124–31.
26. Krukowski RA, West DS, Harvey-Berino J, Prewitt TE. Neighborhood impact on healthy food availability and pricing in food stores. J Community Health. 2010;35(3):315–20.
27. Ver Ploeg M, Mancino L, Todd JE, et al. Where do Americans usually shop for food and how do they travel to get there? Initial findings from the National Household Food Acquisition and Purchase Survey. Washington, DC: U.S. Department of Agriculture, Economic Research Service; 2015. https://www.ers.usda.gov/webdocs/publications/eib138/eib138_errata.pdf?v=42636. Accessed 27 Apr 2017
28. World Cancer Research Fund and American Institute for Cancer Research. Continuous Update Project. 2017. http://www.wcrf.org/int/research-we-fund/continuous-update-project-cup. Accessed 1 May 2017.
29. Kushi LH, Doyle C, McCullough M, Rock CL, Demark-Wahnefried W, Bandera EV, et al. American Cancer Society guidelines on nutrition and physical activity for cancer prevention: reducing the risk of cancer with healthy food choices and physical activity. CA Cancer J Clin. 2012;62(1):30–67.
30. Peipins LA, Soman A, Berkowitz Z, White MC. The lack of paid sick leave as a barrier to cancer screening and medical care-seeking: results from the National Health Interview Survey. BMC Public Health. 2012;12(1):520.
31. Pignone M, Bucholtz D, Harris R. Patient preferences for colon cancer screening. J Gen Intern Med. 1999;14(7):432–7.
32. National Colorectal Cancer Roundtable. 80% by 2018 Communications Guidebook: Recommended messaging to reach the unscreened 2017. http://nccrt.org/tools/80-percent-by-2018/80-by-2018-communications-guidebook/. Accessed 31 May 2017.
33. New York State Department of Health. Developing a paid leave policy for cancer screenings. Albany (NY). 2016. www.health.ny.gov/diseases/cancer/educational_materials/docs/developing_paid:leave_policy.pdf. Accessed 29 April 2017.
34. Community preventive services task force, task force finding and rationale statement. 2016. https://www.thecommunityguide.org/sites/default/files/assets/Cancer-Screening-Multicomponent-Interventions.pdf. Accessed 2 May 2017.
35. Wiedrich K, Sims Jr L, Weisman H, et al. The steep climb to economic opportunities for vulnerable families. Corporation for Enterprise Development. 2016. http://assetsandopportunity.org/assets/pdf/2016_Scorecard_Report.pdf. Accessed 27 Apr 2017.
36. Library of Congress. Patient Protection and Affordable Care Act: Public Law 111-148, 2010. www.congress.gov/bill/111th-congress/house-bill/3590/text/pl?overview=closed. Accessed 2 May 2017.

37. Dana-Farber Cancer Institute. Preliminary Report – 2016 Community Health Needs Assessment. 2016. www.dana-farber.org/uploadedFiles/Library/about-us/community-outreach/chna-preliminary-report-2016.pdf. Accessed 2 May 2017.
38. Millman M, editor. Institute of Medicine (US) Committee on Monitoring Access to Personal Health Care Services. Washington, DC: National Academies Press (US); 1993.
39. 2011 National Healthcare Quality Report. Content last reviewed October 2014. Rockville, MD: Agency for Healthcare Research and Quality. http://www.ahrq.gov/research/findings/nhqrdr/nhqr11/index.html
40. Mandleblatt J, Yabroff K, Kerner J. Equitable access to cancer services: a review of barriers to quality care. Cancer. 1999;86(11):2378–90.
41. Cooper LA, Powe NR. Disparities in patient experiences, health care processes, and outcomes: the role of patient-provider racial, ethnic, and language concordance. Discussion Paper. The Commonwealth Fund; 2004.
42. Martinez L, Schwartz J, Freres D, Fraze T, Hornik R. Patient-clinician information engagement increases treatment decision satisfaction among cancer patients through a feeling of being informed. Patient Educ Couns. 2009;77(3):384–90.
43. Centers for Disease Control and Prevention's Health Literacy Website – https://www.cdc.gov/healthliteracy/learn/index.html. Accessed 26 July 2017.
44. U.S. Department of Health and Human Services. Office of Disease Prevention and Health Promotion. Washington, DC: National Action Plan to Improve Health Literacy; 2010.
45. Kehl K, Landrum M, Arora N, Ganz P, van Ryn P, Mack J, Keating N. Shared decision making in cancer care: the association of actual and preferred decision roles with patient-reported quality. JAMA Oncol. 2015;1(1):50–8.
46. Rowlands G, Shaw A, Jaswal S, Smith S, Harpham T. Health literacy and the social determinants of health: a qualitative model from adult learners. Health Promot Int. 2017;31(1):130–8.
47. Zafar S, Abernethy A. Financial toxicity, Part I: A new name for a growing problem. Oncology. 2013;27(2):80–149.
48. Zafar S, Ubel P, Tulsky J, Pollack K. Cost-related health literacy: a key component of high-quality cancer care. J Oncol Pract. 2015;11(3):171–3.
49. Ramsey SD, Blough DK, Kirchhoff AC, et al. Washington state cancer patients found to be at greater risk for bankruptcy than people without a cancer diagnosis. Health Aff. 2013;32(6):1143–52.
50. Ramsey SD, Bansal A, Fedorenko CR, et al. Financial insolvency as a risk factor for early mortality among patients with cancer. J Clin Oncol. 2016;34(9):980–6.
51. United for a Fair Economy. Comparing the Growth of Family Incomes Illustration. http://www.faireconomy.org/comparing_family_incomes. Accessed 28 July 2017.
52. Dwyer-Lindgren L, Bertozzi-Villa A, Stubbs RW, Morozoff C, Mackenbach JP, van Lenthe FJ, et al. Inequalities in life expectancy among US counties, 1980 to 2014: temporal trends and key drivers. JAMA Intern Med. 2017;177(7):1003–11.
53. Mokdad AH, Dwyer-Lindgren L, Fitzmaurice C, Stubbs RW, Bertozzi-Villa A, Morozoff C, et al. Trends and patterns of disparities in cancer mortality among US Counties, 1980–2014. JAMA. 2017;317(4):388–406.
54. Cole H, Thompson H, White M, Brown R, Trinh-Shevrin C, Braithwaite S, et al. Community-based, preclinical patient navigation for colorectal cancer screening among older black men recruited from barbershops: the MISTER B trial. Am J Public Health. 2017;107(9):1433–40.
55. University of Wisconsin Population Health Institute. County Health Rankings. 2017. http://www.countyhealthrankings.org/app/wisconsin/2017/rankings/milwaukee/county/outcomes/overall/snapshot. Accessed 17 Oct 2017.
56. City of Milwaukee. 2016. http://city.milwaukee.gov/ImageLibrary/Groups/healthAuthors/Accredit/MKEelevate/PriorityIssueSurveyResults12-4-16.pdf. Accessed 17 Oct 2017.
57. National Urban League. 2016 State of black America locked out: education, jobs & justice. http://soba.iamempowered.com/soba-books. Accessed 17 Oct 2017.
58. Jagsi R, Hawley ST, Abrahamse P, Li Y, Janz NK, Griggs JJ, et al. Impact of adjuvant chemotherapy on long-term employment of survivors of early-stage breast cancer. Cancer. 2014;120:1854–62.

# Chapter 5
# How Prevention and Screening Programs Can Be Identified Through a Community Health Needs Assessment

**Peter Hopewood**

## Introduction

Hippocrates and Osler have said that we need to focus on the type of patient with a disease rather than the disease the patient has. Looking at the Centers for Disease Control (CDC) mortality data for cancer state by state there is a wide range or variability (Fig. 5.1) [1]. I am sure that all the hospitals in red are providing evidence-based cancer care. If so, why are the cancer mortality rates in California and Washington DC so different? As Hippocrates and Osler noted 2400 and 100 years ago, focus on the type of patient with a disease, the population served.

Place the patient in the center of their own diagnosis. This is patient-centered care redux. Their lifestyle may have caused or contributed to their disease as innocent victims or knowing accomplices.

For example, before 1850 the average life expectancy was 36 years old. The leading causes of death until 1850 were infectious and communicable diseases. Living conditions and nutrition were poor. Many people lived in close quarters. Diphtheria and tuberculosis were rampant. Water supplies were contaminated with pathogens. Gastrointestinal infectious diseases like cholera killed many. As living conditions and nutrition improved, there has been a significant shift in the causes of death to chronic diseases especially cancer and heart disease. Between 1850 and 2010, life expectancy has more than doubled in developed countries. Now the leading cause of death is chronic disease. Many of these chronic diseases are preventable.

Since the 1900s there has been a tripling in cancer-related deaths. The causes of this are multifactorial. People are living longer but have less active lifestyles. They tend to have more sedentary work and less leisure or playtime. Obesity is reaching epidemic levels in developed countries (Fig. 5.2) and tobacco use has skyrocketed

P. Hopewood
American College of Surgeons Commission on Cancer, Falmouth, MA, USA
e-mail: peterhopewood@comcast.net



P. Hopewood, M. J. Milroy (eds.), *Quality Cancer Care*,
https://doi.org/10.1007/978-3-319-78649-0_5

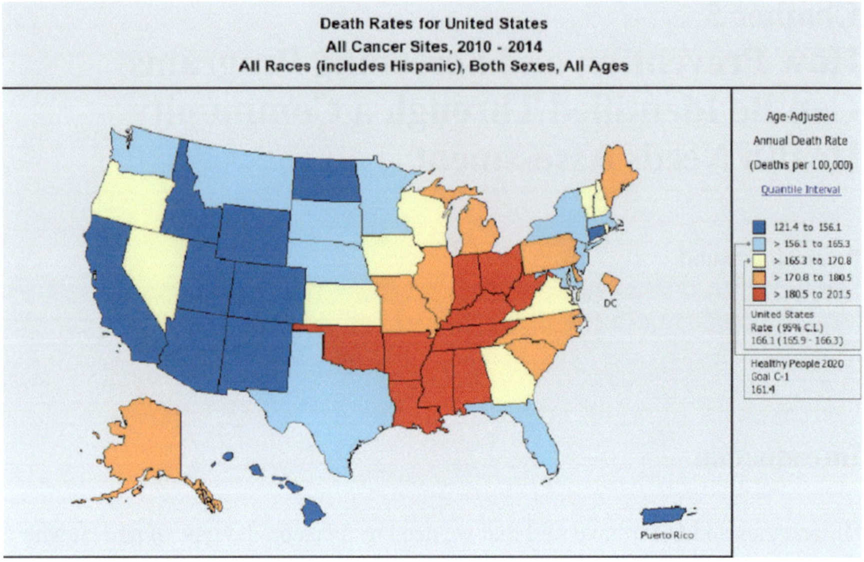


**Fig. 5.1** Mortality data by state [1]. Reprinted from National Cancer Institute, CDC, State cancer profiles at https://statecancerprofiles.cancer.gov/map/map.withimage.php?00&001&001&00&0&02&0&1&5&0#results

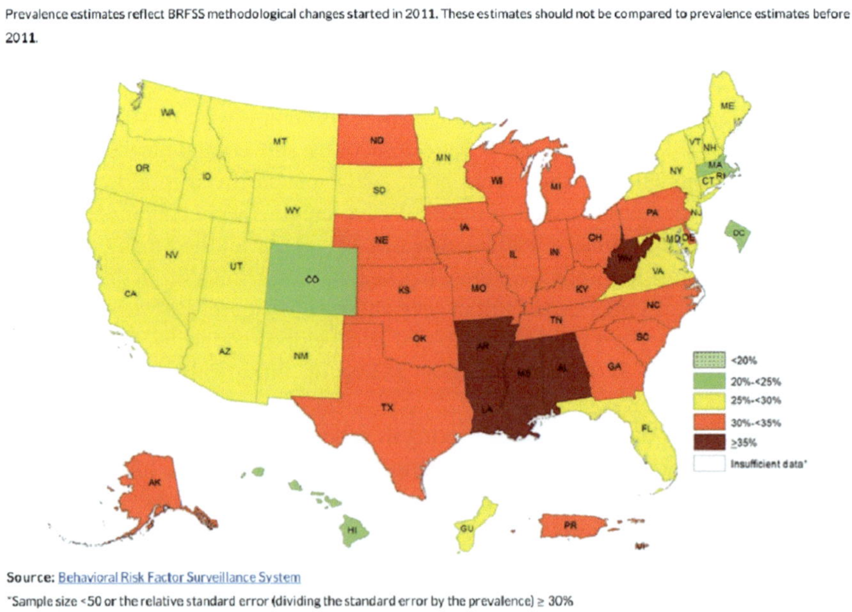


**Fig. 5.2** Self-reported obesity by state and territory [2]. Reprinted from CDC at https://www.cdc.gov/obesity/data/prevalence-maps.html

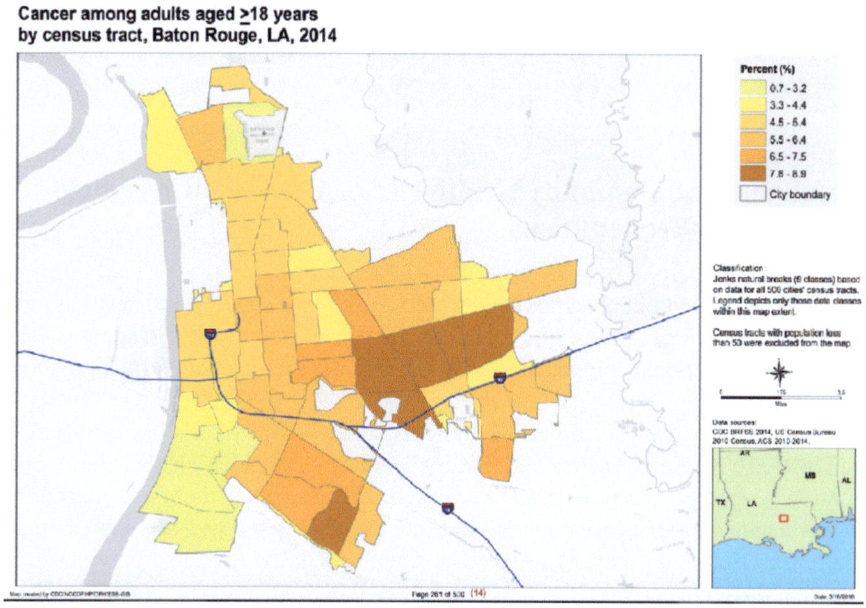


**Fig. 5.3** Cancer among adults by census tract Baton Rouge [3]. Reprinted from CDC 500 Cities Project. https://nccd.cdc.gov/500_Cities/rdPage.aspx?rdReport=DPH_500_Cities.InteractiveMap&islCategories=HLTHOUT&islMeasures=ARTHRITIS&islStates=22&rdRnd=4071

over the past 200 years. Lifestyle, nutrition, obesity, and tobacco contribute to more than 50% of all deaths in the United States. These are all behavioral factors which become ingrained during childhood. The root causes of cancer need to be better publicized. Only then can we stop them by prevention programs and identify them earlier through screening programs.

What is a patient's ancestry? Where did they grow up? What did they eat? What water did they drink? What neighborhood did they live in (Fig. 5.3)? Basic demographic data coupled with social environment have a lot to do with the cancers people develop, and their ability to complete treatment and follow a survivorship care plan.

The community health needs assessment (CHNA) is a review of a community's patient population and its health. As part of the Affordable Care Act, a CHNA and implementation strategy is required of tax-exempt hospitals every 3 years. These review general health needs and barriers to care. This should give hospitals the information they need to provide programs that meet the needs of their communities. Usually this is accomplished as a survey of a random group of patients throughout multiple locations in a service area.

Since cancer is the leading cause of death in the United States among people under 85, you would think that cancer prevention and screening questions would dominate CHNAs. They don't!

Many CHNAs do not ask questions about the root causes of cancer, e.g., low HPV vaccination or low colonoscopy rates. Fortunately, many identify contributing factors such as access to care, tobacco use, and obesity but fall short in providing transportation, tobacco cessation, nutrition/exercise, or other needed programs (Fig. 5.3).

## Developing a Community Health Needs Assessment Weighted with Cancer-Related Items

As noted, not-for-profit hospitals need to perform a community health needs assessment (CHNA) every 3 years. Some of these are stock off the shelf and administered by contracted national companies. These vendors have no inside information about a healthcare systems' service area or population. Other CHNAs are developed and analyzed by the involved healthcare systems. Both groups look at many different variables. To have an effective community health needs assessment as regards cancer trends, specific questions need to be asked. The answers to these questions need to be mapped onto census tracks. Zip codes of respondents accomplish this. Outreach efforts can then be directed to those locations. As noted previously in Fig. 5.3, there are certain areas in Baton Rouge with higher cancer incidences than others. When this CHNA was performed, the patient responder locations were noted by ZIP codes. Data like this shows specific areas within Baton Rouge that have the highest cancer rates. When more deeply analyzed, these tracts or neighborhoods have multiple social determinants of health predicting high cancer rates.

Asking the right questions can allow you to better understand the cancer demographics of your service area. This will lead to specific prevention and screening programs for your healthcare system. Several examples include transportation issues, distance to grocery stores and fresh produce, elderly people living alone, tobacco use, active lifestyles, health insurance status, employment/unemployment, poverty, etc. A robust CHNA will identify the locations of patients with barriers to access, e.g., inability to get transportation to receive health care. A healthcare system could then target that location for an outreach such as mobile mammography or house call care.

To fine-tune your CHNA, there are several public access databases which can be used to create more detailed questions. The remainder of this chapter discusses each of these databases.

## US Census

The US census is updated every 10 years. It will be updated again in 2020. It includes interim data from 2015. The US census is a treasure chest of information. It shows county, state, and national data [4]. It can also show city data. All of these can be compared. As an example, Bibb County, Georgia, can be compared to Jones and Monroe Counties, Georgia, and the United States (Fig. 5.4).

A population changes up or down over a decade. The census subdivides population changes by age, e.g., is a county population gaining elderly or losing young people. It also shows ethnicity population changes for Caucasian-Americans, African-Americans, Hispanic-Americans, Asian-Americans, Native Americans, Native Hawaiian, and Pacific Islanders (Fig. 5.5). We are told that the American population is aging and becoming more diversified. That may be true for the nation as a whole but not in all cities, counties, or states as illustrated in Figs. 5.4 and 5.5.

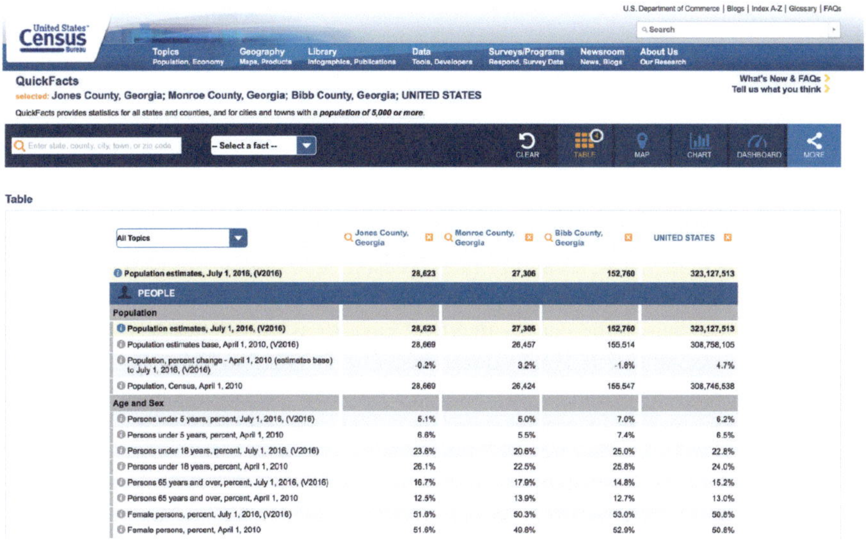


| All Topics | Jones County, Georgia | Monroe County, Georgia | Bibb County, Georgia | UNITED STATES |
|---|---|---|---|---|
| Population estimates, July 1, 2016, (V2016) | 28,623 | 27,306 | 152,760 | 323,127,513 |
| PEOPLE | | | | |
| Population | | | | |
| Population estimates, July 1, 2016, (V2016) | 28,623 | 27,306 | 152,760 | 323,127,513 |
| Population estimates base, April 1, 2010, (V2016) | 28,669 | 26,457 | 155,514 | 308,758,105 |
| Population, percent change - April 1, 2010 (estimates base) to July 1, 2016, (V2016) | -0.2% | 3.2% | -1.8% | 4.7% |
| Population, Census, April 1, 2010 | 28,669 | 26,424 | 155,547 | 308,745,538 |
| Age and Sex | | | | |
| Persons under 5 years, percent, July 1, 2016, (V2016) | 5.1% | 5.0% | 7.0% | 6.2% |
| Persons under 5 years, percent, April 1, 2010 | 6.6% | 5.5% | 7.4% | 6.5% |
| Persons under 18 years, percent, July 1, 2016, (V2016) | 23.6% | 20.6% | 25.0% | 22.8% |
| Persons under 18 years, percent, April 1, 2010 | 26.1% | 22.5% | 25.8% | 24.0% |
| Persons 65 years and over, percent, July 1, 2016, (V2016) | 16.7% | 17.9% | 14.8% | 15.2% |
| Persons 65 years and over, percent, April 1, 2010 | 12.5% | 13.9% | 12.7% | 13.0% |
| Female persons, percent, July 1, 2016, (V2016) | 51.6% | 50.3% | 53.0% | 50.8% |
| Female persons, percent, April 1, 2010 | 51.6% | 49.8% | 52.9% | 50.8% |

**Fig. 5.4** Three county population comparisons, central Georgia [5]. Reprinted from US Census Bureau. .https://www.census.gov/quickfacts/fact/table/jonescountygeorgia,monroecountygeorgia,bibbcountygeorgia,US/PST045216

| All Topics | Jones County, Georgia | Monroe County, Georgia | Bibb County, Georgia | UNITED STATES |
|---|---|---|---|---|
| Population estimates, July 1, 2016, (V2016) | 28,623 | 27,306 | 152,760 | 323,127,513 |
| Race and Hispanic Origin | | | | |
| White alone, percent, July 1, 2016, (V2016) (a) | 72.7% | 74.3% | 41.1% | 76.9% |
| Black or African American alone, percent, July 1, 2016, (V2016) (a) | 25.0% | 23.0% | 55.0% | 13.3% |
| American Indian and Alaska Native alone, percent, July 1, 2016, (V2016) (a) | 0.3% | 0.3% | 0.3% | 1.3% |
| Asian alone, percent, July 1, 2016, (V2016) (a) | 0.6% | 1.0% | 2.0% | 5.7% |
| Native Hawaiian and Other Pacific Islander alone, percent, July 1, 2016, (V2016) (a) | Z | Z | 0.1% | 0.2% |
| Two or More Races, percent, July 1, 2016, (V2016) | 1.2% | 1.3% | 1.5% | 2.6% |
| Hispanic or Latino, percent, July 1, 2016, (V2016) (b) | 1.5% | 2.3% | 3.2% | 17.8% |
| White alone, not Hispanic or Latino, percent, July 1, 2016, (V2016) | 71.6% | 72.4% | 38.8% | 61.3% |

**Fig. 5.5** Three county ethnicity comparisons, central Georgia [5]. Reprinted from US Census Bureau. https://www.census.gov/quickfacts/fact/table/jonescountygeorgia,monroecountygeorgia,bibbcountygeorgia,US/PST045216

| All Topics | Jones County, Georgia | Monroe County, Georgia | Bibb County, Georgia | UNITED STATES |
|---|---|---|---|---|
| Population estimates, July 1, 2016, (V2016) | 28,623 | 27,306 | 152,760 | 323,127,513 |
| **Race and Hispanic Origin** | | | | |
| White alone, percent, July 1, 2016, (V2016) (a) | 72.7% | 74.3% | 41.1% | 76.9% |
| Black or African American alone, percent, July 1, 2016, (V2016) (a) | 25.0% | 23.0% | 55.0% | 13.3% |
| American Indian and Alaska Native alone, percent, July 1, 2016, (V2016) (a) | 0.3% | 0.3% | 0.3% | 1.3% |
| Asian alone, percent, July 1, 2016, (V2016) (a) | 0.6% | 1.0% | 2.0% | 5.7% |
| Native Hawaiian and Other Pacific Islander alone, percent, July 1, 2016, (V2016) (a) | Z | Z | 0.1% | 0.2% |
| Two or More Races, percent, July 1, 2016, (V2016) | 1.2% | 1.3% | 1.5% | 2.6% |
| Hispanic or Latino, percent, July 1, 2016, (V2016) (b) | 1.5% | 2.3% | 3.2% | 17.8% |
| White alone, not Hispanic or Latino, percent, July 1, 2016, (V2016) | 71.6% | 72.4% | 38.8% | 61.3% |

**Fig. 5.6** Three county education level, health insurance, and poverty comparisons, central Georgia [6]. Reprinted from US Census Bureau three county population comparisons central Georgia. Reprinted from US Census Bureau. https://www.census.gov/quickfacts/fact/table/peachcountygeorgia,jonescountygeorgia,monroecountygeorgia,US/PST045216

Additional information in the census includes education level, employment status, unemployment status, disability rates, persons without health insurance, travel time to work, median income, and poverty rates (Fig. 5.6).

The detailed data in the census makes it easy to ask more pointed community health needs assessment (CHNA) questions. The answers to these questions will focus prevention, screening, and outreach programs towards disparate groups related to ethnicity, age, insurance status, income levels, and education.

## County Health Rankings & Roadmaps

County Health Rankings & Roadmaps is another public access source with information concerning county data as regards health [7].

It looks at health outcomes and health factors and ranks counties in a state. This data is updated annually. Some of its major topics include length of life, quality of life, health behaviors, clinical care, social and economic factors, and physical environment. Figures 5.7, 5.8, and 5.9 use Rockingham County, NH, as an example.

There is some overlap between County Health Rankings & Roadmaps and US census data, but there's also additional information and corroborating information to identify barriers and community health needs. As shown in Fig. 5.7, note the increased days of poor physical and mental health for Rockingham County, NH. In Fig. 5.8 we see that smoking, obesity, and excessive alcohol intake are increased in this county compared to the rest of the state and top US performers. Physical and environmental issues noted in Fig. 5.9 include drinking water violations, air pollution, housing, driving alone to work, and long commutes to work. All of these factors identify ideas for prevention programs, e.g., smoking cessation, weight, and alcohol control.

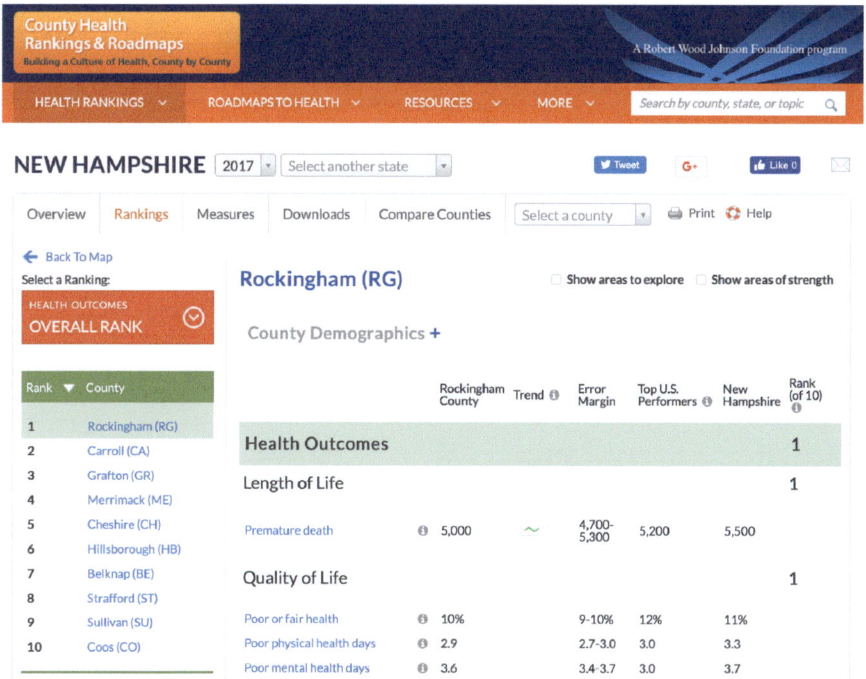


**Fig. 5.7** Introductory page for Rockingham County, NH [8]. Reprinted from University of Wisconsin Population Health Institute. County Health Rankings & Roadmaps 2017. http://www.countyhealthrankings.org/app/new-hampshire/2017/rankings/rockingham/county/outcomes/overall/snapshot

## State Cancer Profiles

The CDC in Atlanta sponsors State Cancer Profiles which can be viewed by trend, graph, or map [9]. If you have not had a chance to access the site, I would highly recommend it. It is an interactive look at our nation, state, and counties as regards cancer and many of its underlying causes. If you are a visual learner, these pictures and graphics are worth a thousand words. The CDC provides quick-pick topics about demographics, screening and risk factors, cancer knowledge, incidence, and mortality. You can view the entire United States by state and county. The CDC has recently added their "500 cities project" which looks at data from 500 cities throughout the United States in more detail [10]. This site is discussed later in the chapter.

The demographic section of the CDC State Cancer Profiles can search for crowding, education, income levels, mobility, insurance, non-English language spoken, population, poverty, and workforce. Many of these are true determinants of health previously known as socioeconomic status then social determinants of health. These are reviewed in more detail in Chap. 4.

| | Rockingham County | Trend | Error Margin | Top U.S. Performers | New Hampshire | Rank (of 10) |
|---|---|---|---|---|---|---|
| **Health Behaviors** | | | | | | 2 |
| Adult smoking | 14% | | 13-14% | 14% | 16% | |
| Adult obesity | 26% | | 24-28% | 26% | 28% | |
| Food environment index | 8.6 | | | 8.4 | 8.4 | |
| Physical inactivity | 19% | | 18-21% | 19% | 20% | |
| Access to exercise opportunities | 86% | | | 91% | 84% | |
| Excessive drinking | 19% | | 18-19% | 12% | 18% | |
| Alcohol-impaired driving deaths | 37% | | 32-41% | 13% | 31% | |
| Sexually transmitted infections | 209.9 | | | 145.5 | 271.0 | |
| Teen births | 9 | | 9-10 | 17 | 15 | |
| Additional Health Behaviors (not included in overall ranking) + | | | | | | |
| **Clinical Care** | | | | | | 3 |
| Uninsured | 9% | | 8-10% | 8% | 11% | |
| Primary care physicians | 1,210:1 | | | 1,040:1 | 1,060:1 | |
| Dentists | 1,420:1 | | | 1,320:1 | 1,410:1 | |
| Mental health providers | 510:1 | | | 360:1 | 390:1 | |
| Preventable hospital stays | 47 | | 45-49 | 36 | 45 | |
| Diabetes monitoring | 91% | | 88-94% | 91% | 90% | |
| Mammography screening | 72% | | 69-75% | 71% | 71% | |

**Fig. 5.8** Health behaviors and clinical care for Rockingham County, NH [8]. Reprinted from University of Wisconsin Population Health Institute. County health rankings & roadmaps. http://www.countyhealthrankings.org/app/new-hampshire/2017/rankings/rockingham/county/outcomes/overall/snapshot

Let's take a look at one of these parameters—immigration. It is listed as mobility for people moving into a state from outside the United States (Fig. 5.10). As shown, several states have higher rates of immigration than others.

Using the online version, you can click on any state to get the rates by county. I have illustrated this for the counties of Washington in Fig. 5.11. It shows four counties in Washington that have a population at risk for a disparity in care due to immigrant status.

Note that this CDC data as well as the other data sources reviewed in this chapter are frequently updated. Therefore, some of the data presented may have changed from the time this manuscript was submitted for publication.

| | Rockingham County | Trend | Error Margin | Top U.S. Performers | New Hampshire | Rank (of 10) |
|---|---|---|---|---|---|---|
| **Social & Economic Factors** | | | | | | 1 |
| High school graduation | 91% | | | 95% | 88% | |
| Some college | 75% | | 72-77% | 72% | 69% | |
| Unemployment | 3.6% | | | 3.3% | 3.4% | |
| Children in poverty | 7% | | 5-8% | 12% | 11% | |
| Income inequality | 3.8 | | 3.6-3.9 | 3.7 | 4.3 | |
| Children in single-parent households | 23% | | 20-25% | 21% | 28% | |
| Social associations | 9.2 | | | 22.1 | 10.5 | |
| Violent crime | 126 | | | 62 | 200 | |
| Injury deaths | 62 | | 58-66 | 53 | 68 | |
| Additional Social & Economic Factors (not included in overall ranking) + | | | | | | |
| **Physical Environment** | | | | | | 10 |
| Air pollution - particulate matter | 8.7 | | | 6.7 | 7.8 | |
| Drinking water violations | Yes | | | | | |
| Severe housing problems | 16% | | 15-16% | 9% | 16% | |
| Driving alone to work | 84% | | 83-85% | 72% | 81% | |
| Long commute - driving alone | 44% | | 43-46% | 15% | 38% | |

Note: Blank values reflect unreliable or missing data

**Fig. 5.9** Social and economic factors and physical environment for Rockingham County, NH [8]. Reprinted from University of Wisconsin Population Health Institute. County health rankings & roadmaps. http://www.countyhealthrankings.org/app/new-hampshire/2017/rankings/rockingham/county/outcomes/overall/snapshot

Here is an example of language isolation or non-English-speaking populations in the United States by state (Fig. 5.12).

If we focus on Maine and look at its counties (Fig. 5.13), note that Knox County has the highest rate of non-English spoken at home in the state. This is on the Canadian-American border and they speak French.

When a language barrier is identified within a healthcare system service area, there is a need for translation services and diversity among healthcare providers to care for and communicate with these patients. As you can guess, these non-English-speaking people may have different cultural and religious attitudes regarding their personal and family healthcare needs.

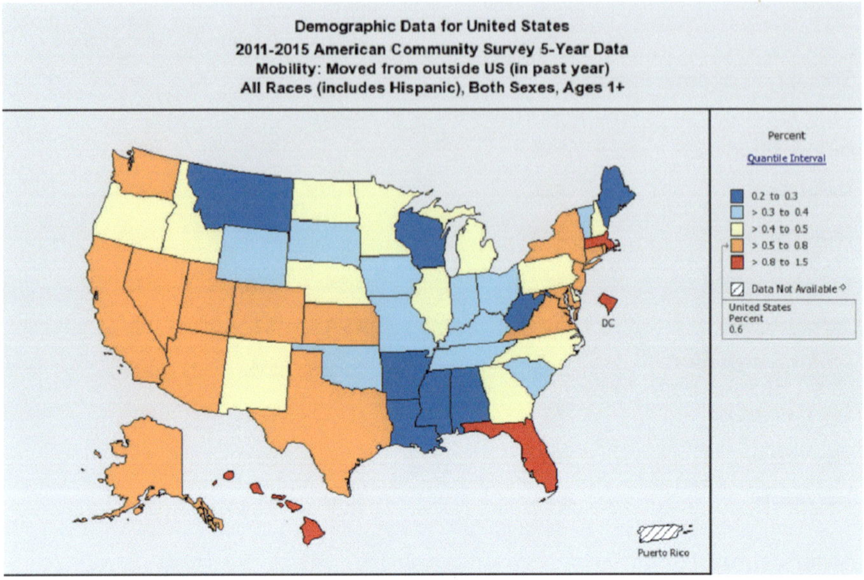


**Fig. 5.10** In-migration data from outside the US data by state [11]. Reprinted from National Cancer Institute, CDC, State Cancer Profiles. https://statecancerprofiles.cancer.gov/map/map.withimage.php?00&901&00021&00&0&3&0&1&5&0#results

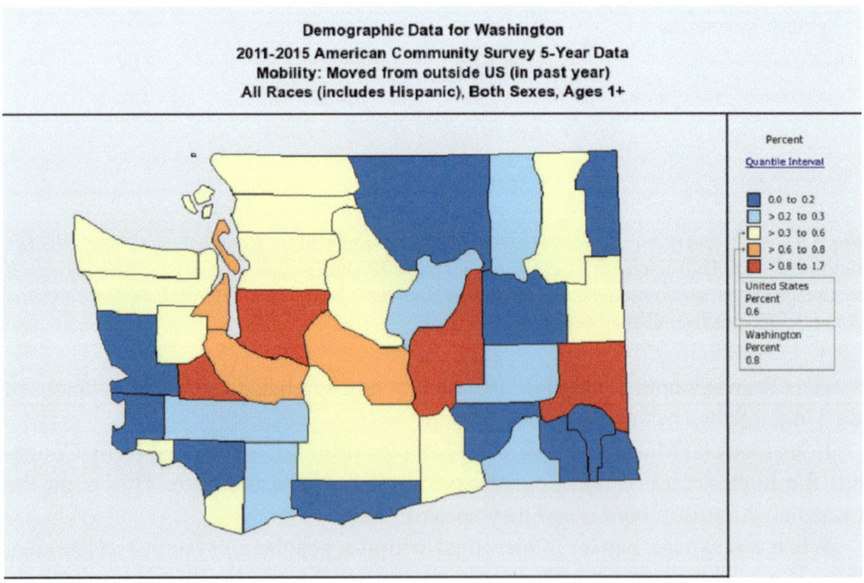


**Fig. 5.11** In-migration rates by Washington counties [12]. Reprinted from National Cancer Institute, CDC, State Cancer Profiles. https://statecancerprofiles.cancer.gov/map/map.withimage.php?53&901&00021&00&0&3&0&1&5&0#results

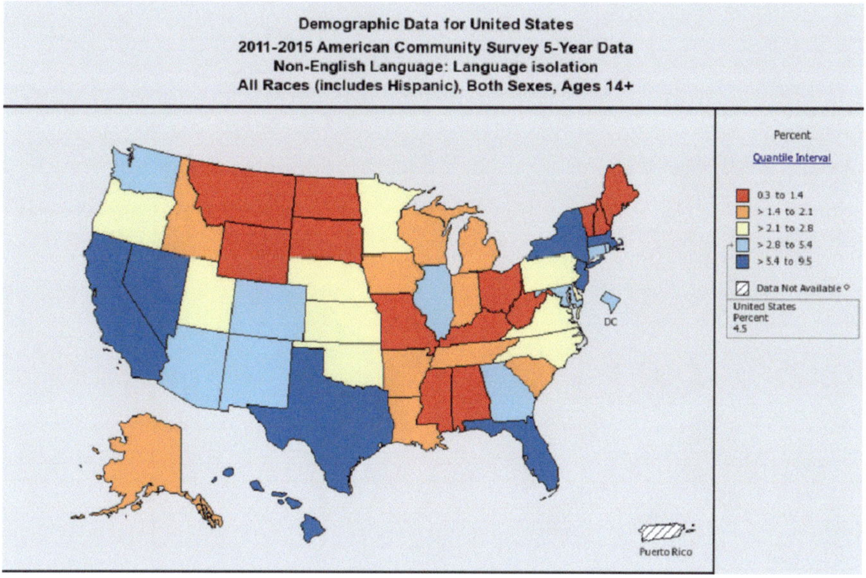


**Fig. 5.12** Language isolation or non-English language spoken at home [13]. Reprinted from National Cancer Institute, CDC, State Cancer Profiles. https://statecancerprofiles.cancer.gov/map/map.withimage.php?00&914&00015&00&0&3&0&1&5&0#results

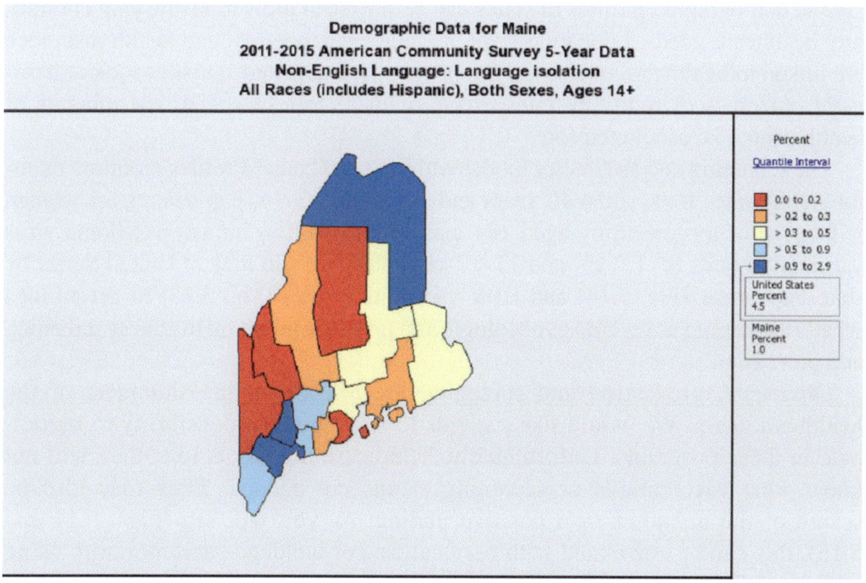


**Fig. 5.13** Non-English language spoken at home for Maine by counties [14]. Reprinted from National Cancer Institute, CDC, State Cancer Profiles. https://statecancerprofiles.cancer.gov/map/map.withimage.php?23&914&00015&00&0&3&0&1&5&0#results

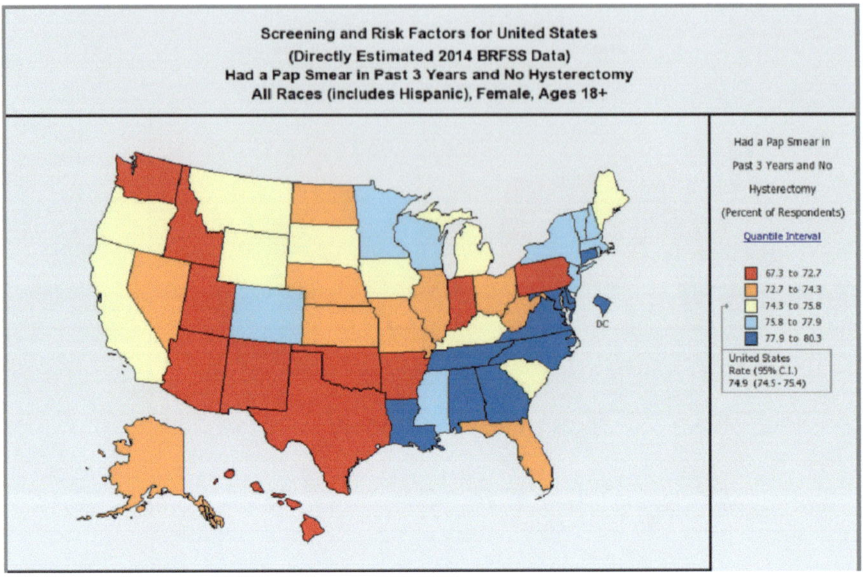


**Fig. 5.14** Pap smear during past 3 years for women 18 years or older not having prior hysterectomy by state [15]. Reprinted from National Cancer Institute, CDC, State Cancer Profiles. https://statecancerprofiles.cancer.gov/map/map.withimage.php?00&918&999&00&2&11&0&1&5&0#results

The demographic profiles of states can be powerful tools in identifying community healthcare needs. Education level, income level, poverty, and health insurance are linked to healthcare outcomes. Even when risk-adjusted statistics look at treatment outcomes or mortality rates, many of these true or social determinants of health cannot be accounted for.

The screening and risk factor model within State Cancer Profiles monitors mammography rates for women 40 years and older and 50–74, Pap smears for women without prior hysterectomy aged 18+ and 21+, as well as human papilloma virus vaccination rates for 13–15- and 13–17-year-olds. We can look at United States by state Pap smear (Fig. 5.14) and HPV vaccination rates (Fig. 5.15) to get an idea what's happening as regards gynecologic and pediatric attention to cancer screening and prevention.

Obviously, prevention and screening are not all on the shoulders of the healthcare team. We would like patients to take some responsibility to participate in these programs. Unfortunately, healthcare literacy is low; they will not know what vaccinations or screening exams are needed. They may also be scared of the unknown or a positive finding. As you will see (Figs. 5.14 and 5.15), this can be correlated with cervical cancer incidence and mortality using additional CDC data.

The CDC provides cancer knowledge maps which look at knowledge and attitudes towards cancer. These are public opinion poll taken by the CDC concerning

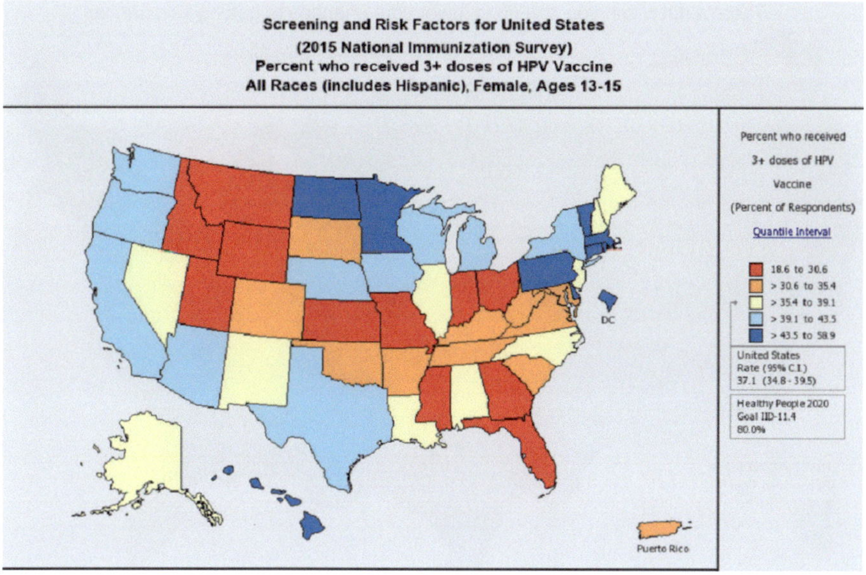


**Fig. 5.15** Percent of women receiving 3+ doses of HPV vaccine aged 13–15 [16]. Reprinted from National Cancer Institute, CDC, State Cancer Profiles. https://statecancerprofiles.cancer.gov/map/map.withimage.php?00&315&999&00&2&70&0&1&5&0#results

cervical, colorectal, lung, prostate, and skin cancers. They ask simple questions such as these: “Have you ever heard about HPV?” “Is there anything you can do to prevent cervical cancer?” Here are two national maps with the results of asking “is there’s anything you can do to prevent skin cancer?” (Fig. 5.16) and “is sun exposure linked to skin cancer?” (Fig. 5.17).

Unbelievably, certain parts of the country don’t recognize the association between sun exposure and skin cancer. I think the message about tanning booths causing skin cancer is getting more attention than sun exposure. Melanoma rates in northern latitude states for example Washington (check out the CDC incidence maps for melanoma) are elevated and promoted by these attitudes and low healthcare literacy. To counter this, in southern Maine, there’s a best practice of educating middle school children about sun exposure and its importance. In Texas, MD, Anderson has produced a sunwise educational program for pre-K, kindergarten, and first graders called “The Sunbeatables.”

There is a very interesting pattern developing as regards melanoma incidence, age, and gender. What is becoming apparent is that melanoma incidence is higher in young women, which progressively decreases, whereas in men it progressively increases with age. This is felt to be due to sun exposure and tanning booths in young women and occupational, recreational, and cumulative sun exposure in men. I will review this information at the end of this chapter using the password-protected National Cancer Database.

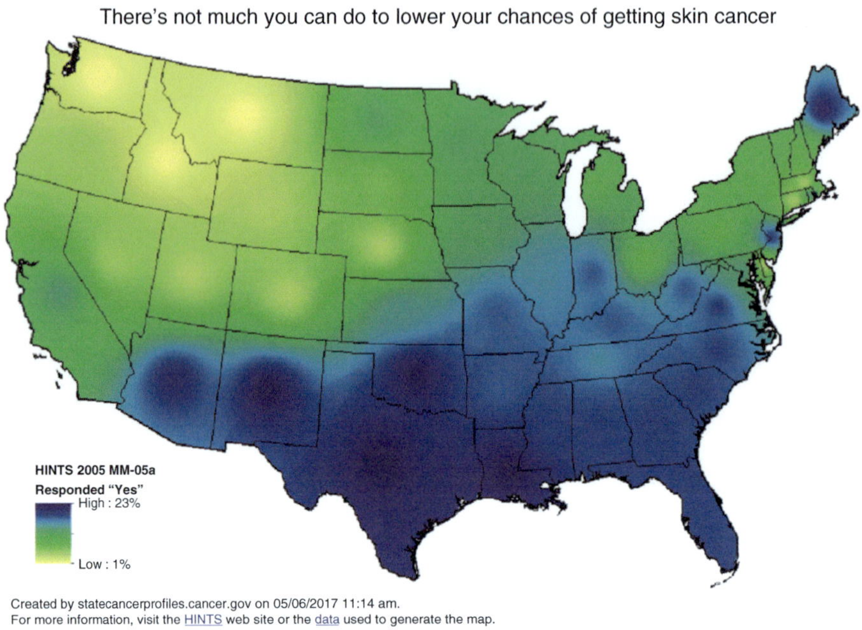


**Fig. 5.16** US knowledge survey map about decreasing risk of getting skin cancer [17]. Reprinted from National Cancer Institute, CDC, State Cancer Profiles. https://statecancerprofiles.cancer.gov/cancerknowledge/index.php?topic=skin&question=q16&age=001&type=hints#results

The CDC also has cancer incidence and mortality rates for 22 specific cancer sites. This can be searched by state, county, ethnicity, gender, and age. Most healthcare systems involve a county and surrounding areas. The CDC county maps can be used to identify opportunities for new program development by using a combination of graphs and maps to understand cancer trends. Here is a good example. Liver and bile duct cancers are increasing in frequency (Fig. 5.18) and mortality (Fig. 5.19) throughout our country. Note that a hash mark "#" represents a statistically significant change.

Now, let us look at Hawaii. Honolulu County has increasing rates for both (Figs. 5.20 and 5.21).

In my naïveté, I assumed this was due to the increased risk of liver cancer in Asian and Pacific Americans living in Hawaii. When you focus more deeply into the CDC data, you find that it was among the white non-Hispanics! This presents an opportunity for healthcare systems in Honolulu to develop hepatology programs, assure high hepatitis B vaccination rates, expand infectious disease programs for hepatitis B and C, and strengthen programs to decrease alcohol consumption. You may have seen national advertising from the CDC recommending a hepatitis C serology for all baby boomers. Baby boomers are those born between 1945 and 1965 and one in fifty will have a positive hepatitis C serology. The vast majority of these are among citizens without known risk factors for hepatitis C, e.g., transfusions and IV drug abuse. It is suspected that the increase in hepatitis C among baby boomers is related to inadequate sterilization of medical instruments, dental drills,

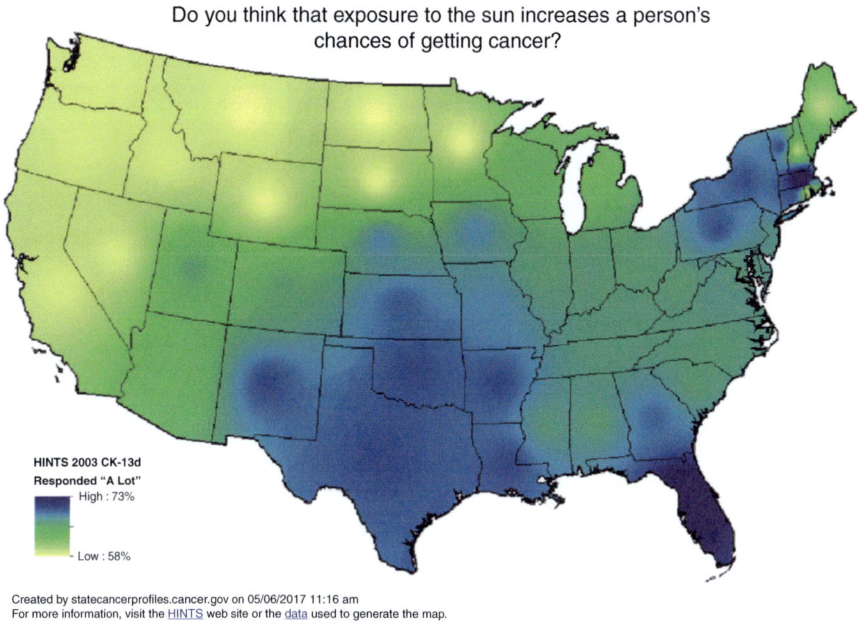


**Fig. 5.17** US survey knowledge map asking if sun exposure increases risk of getting cancer [18]. Reprinted from National Cancer Institute, CDC, State Cancer Profiles. https://statecancerprofiles.cancer.gov/cancerknowledge/index.php?topic=skin&question=q11&age=001&type=hints#results

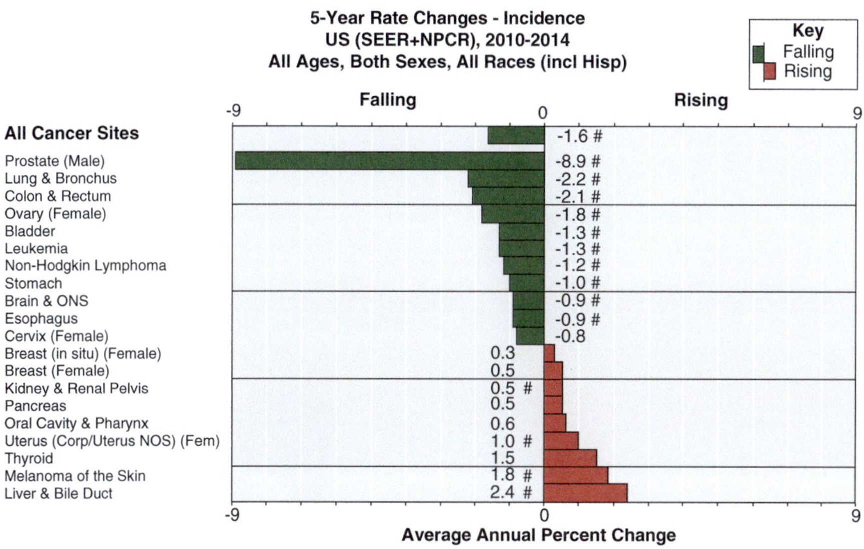


**Fig. 5.18** Cancer incidence 5-year rate changes for the United States [19]. Reprinted from National Cancer Institute, CDC, State Cancer Profiles. https://statecancerprofiles.cancer.gov/recenttrend/index.php?0&00&0&9599&001&999&00&0&0&0&1#results

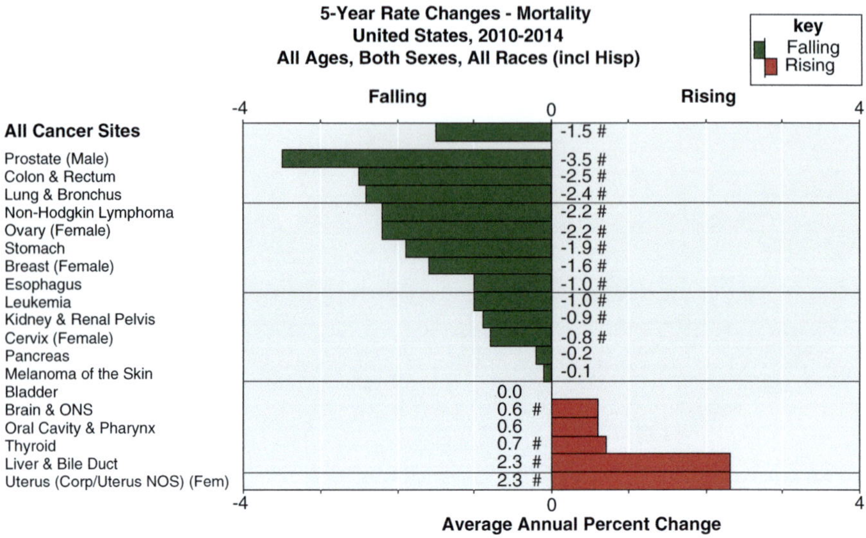


**Fig. 5.19** Cancer mortality 5-year rate changes for the United States [20]. Reprinted from National Cancer Institute, CDC, State Cancer Profiles. https://statecancerprofiles.cancer.gov/recenttrend/index.php?0&00&0&9599&001&999&00&0&0&0&2#results

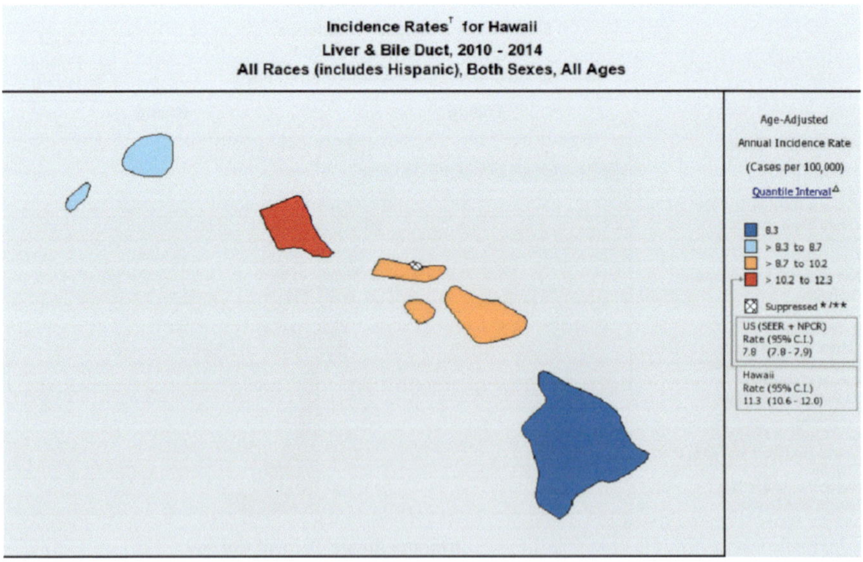


**Fig. 5.20** Incidence of liver cancer Hawaii by county from 2010 to 2014 [21]. Reprinted from National Cancer Institute, CDC, State Cancer Profiles. https://statecancerprofiles.cancer.gov/map/map.withimage.php?15&001&035&00&0&01&0&1&5&0#results

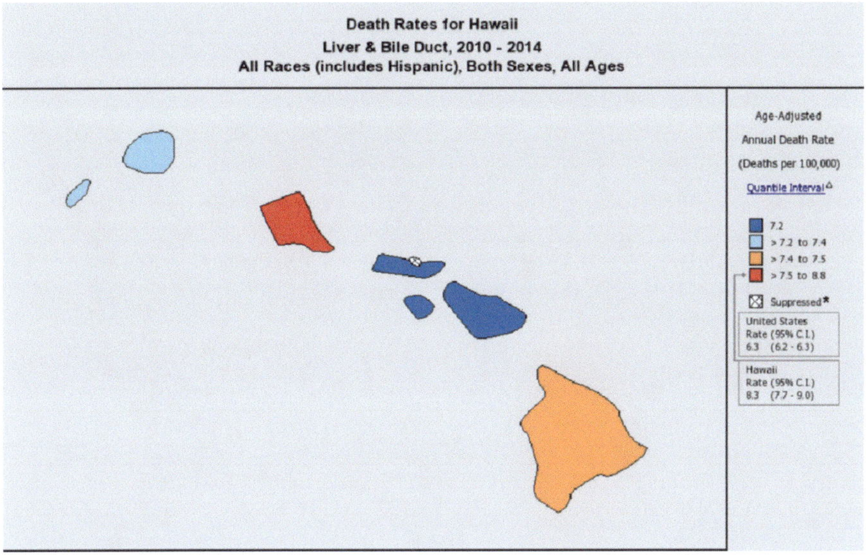


**Fig. 5.21** Mortality rate liver cancer Hawaii by county from 2010 to 2014 [22]. Reprinted from National Cancer Institute, CDC, State Cancer Profiles. https://statecancerprofiles.cancer.gov/map/map.withimage.php?15&001&035&00&0&02&0&1&5&0#results

and vaccinations during their childhood. Since there is an effective treatment for hepatitis C, identifying patients with asymptomatic hepatitis C has become a public health imperative and can prevent liver cancer.

## 500 Cities Project: Local Data for Better Health

During 2017, the CDC released a new module called 500 Cities Project: Local Data for Better Health [10]. This is a collaboration between the CDC, Robert Wood Johnson Foundation, and the CDC Foundation. It chose 500 cities (Fig. 5.22) and provides detailed information concerning health outcome prevention and unhealthy behaviors.

This database looks at smaller areas and census tracts within cities. It identifies areas within a city with risk factors for poor health and identifies the risks as well. Regarding cancer information, it includes physical health, insurance status, rates of annual checkups, mammography, Pap and colorectal cancer screening rates, binge drinking, current smoking, physical activity levels, and obesity. I showed you one of these at the beginning of this chapter (Fig. 5.3). Here's how it works. If you selected Boston as the city, you can see detailed maps with small areas individually outlined showing cancer (Fig. 5.23), health insurance (Fig. 5.24), and smoking rates (Fig. 5.25). These details allow cancer programs to target outreach activities to specific areas within their service area for prevention and screening programs.

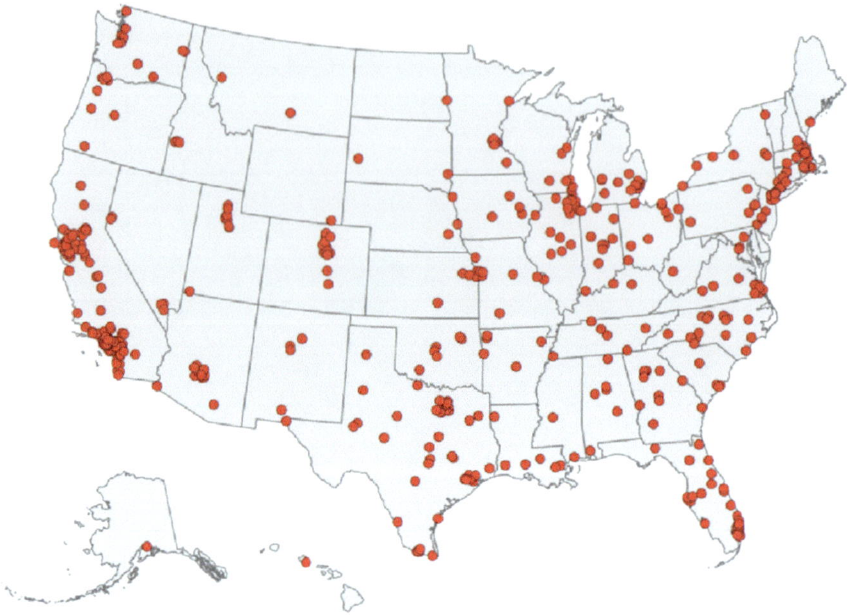

**Fig. 5.22** 500 Cities project from the CDC looks at local data for better health. These are the 500 cities chosen [23]. Reprinted from CDC 500 cities project https://www.cdc.gov/500Cities/

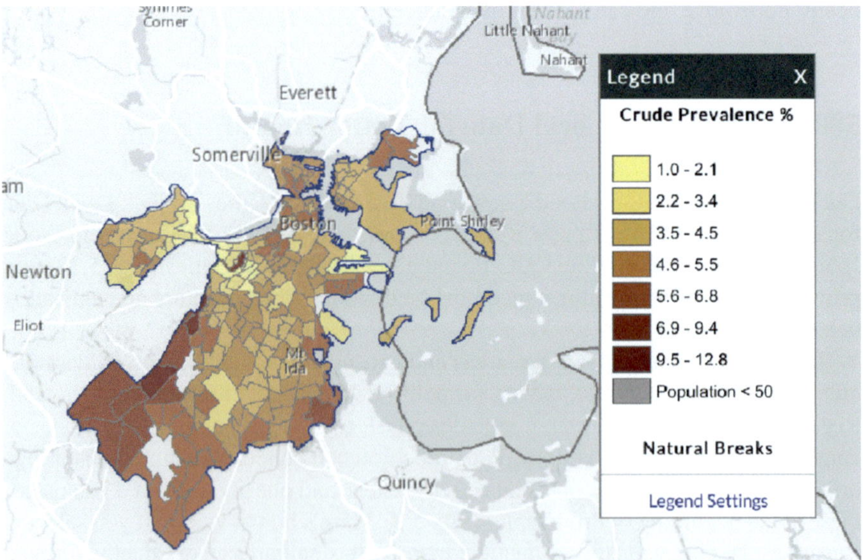


**Fig. 5.23** 500 City cancer incidence circa Boston by local census tracts [10]. Reprinted from CDC 500 Cities project. https://nccd.cdc.gov/500_Cities/rdPage.aspx?rdReport=DPH_500_Cities.InteractiveMap&islCategories=HLTHOUT&islMeasures=ARTHRITIS&islStates=22&rdRnd=40715

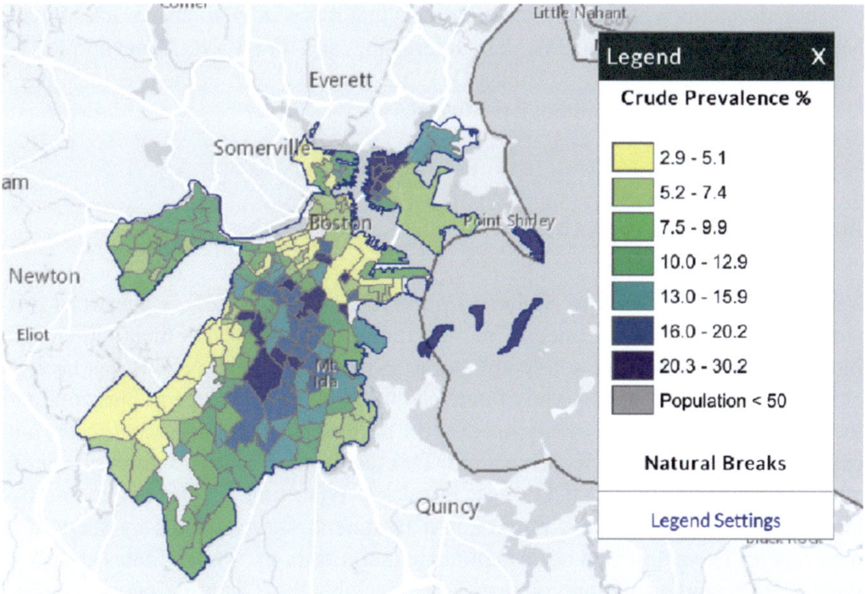


**Fig. 5.24** 500 City health insurance rates Boston by local census tracts [23]. Reprinted from CDC 500 Cities project. https://nccd.cdc.gov/500_Cities/rdPage.aspx?rdReport=DPH_500_Cities.InteractiveMap&islCategories=HLTHOUT&islMeasures=ARTHRITIS&islStates=22&rdRnd=40715

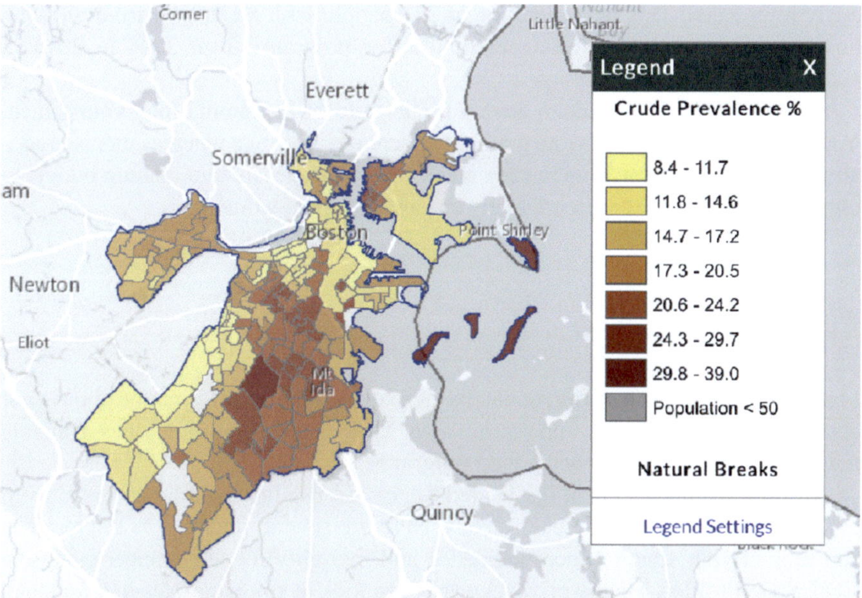


**Fig. 5.25** 500 City unhealthy behavior smoking from the CDC: 500 Cities project: local data for better health [24]. Reprinted from CDC 500 Cities project. https://nccd.cdc.gov/500_Cities/rdPage.aspx?rdReport=DPH_500_Cities.InteractiveMap&islStates=59&islCategories=UNHBEH&islMeasures=CSMOKING

There is so much online public access data that it is so hard to keep track of it all. Many other sites have complementary, interesting, and timely data, for example The American Cancer Society and Breast Q. What you have seen in the previous pages is available to everyone without a password.

## National Cancer Database

Very detailed data from the National Cancer Database (NCDB) is password protected. Commissioner on Cancer (CoC)-accredited programs enter their patient data into this database and are solely able to access this data. The NCDB has been in existence since 1989 and is jointly funded by the American College of Surgeons and the American Cancer Society. It has over 34 million patients within its servers and captures 250 data points for each patient. This database includes 75 different cancer sites, demographic data, AJCC stage, histologic type, time to first treatment, distance traveled for treatment, type of first treatment, survival rates by stage, and many more. There are 5564 acute healthcare facilities in the United States and more than 1500 hospitals nationwide are accredited by the Commission on Cancer. Seventy percent of all cancer patients are treated within CoC-accredited programs. This is a powerful database which allows a deeper dive into cancer trends which can be correlated with other databases, e.g., CDC and SEER.

Here is the example using NCDB melanoma incidence by gender and age previously referenced. This data includes 54,231 people with melanoma from all 1466 hospitals who were Commissioner on Cancer programs from 2004 to 2014 in Fig. 5.26.

As depicted, young women have a higher rate of melanoma than young men. Young women's melanoma rate gradually decreases with age whereas men's gradually increases. Men catch up as they reach 50. Sun exposure and tanning booths to obtain beautiful tanned skin are likely causes for young women.

## Conclusions

I have shown you many different databases to obtain cancer information about your country, state, county, city, and service area. More detailed information is available to Commission on Cancer-accredited programs.

All healthcare systems in the United States can use these public access sites to assess their cancer-related health needs. Here are several practical examples. You can look at your state's cancer incidence and mortality for lung cancer using the CDC State Profiles. Then work backwards and look at smoking rates in your state, county using Healthcare Rankings, and if covered 500 Cities Project data. Additional data may be available from your department of public health (Comprehensive Cancer Control Prevention Plan) about tobacco smoking rates by age, pregnant

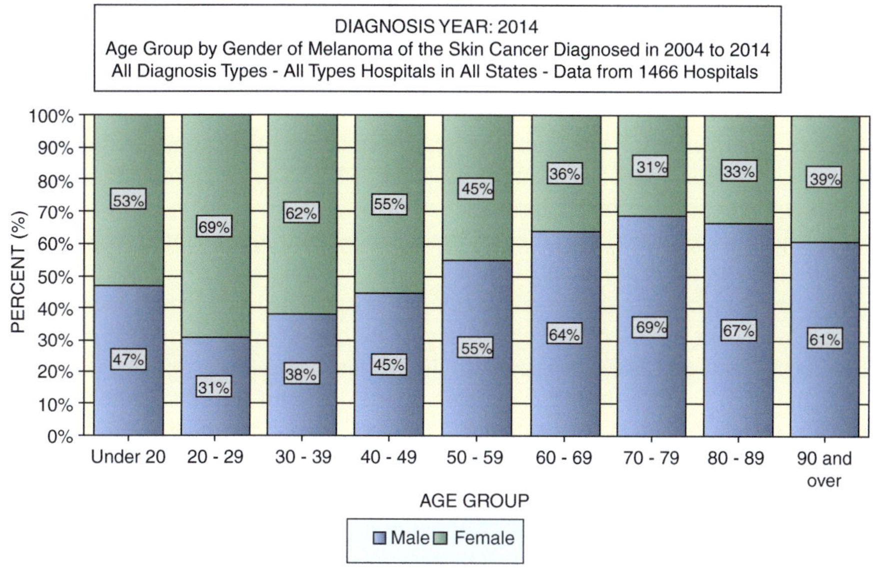


**Fig. 5.26** NCDB melanoma incidence by age and gender [25]. Information was derived from the American College of Surgeons' National Cancer Database. https://www.facs.org

women smoking, and smokeless tobacco. For areas with increased mortality, targeted programs for smoking cessation can be implemented. A best practice I have seen monitored smoking cessation program success by using a carbon monoxide meter (breath-analyzer meter). You can measure the level of carbon monoxide in smokers at baseline. Everyone knows that carbon monoxide is a poison and people die of carbon monoxide poisoning in their homes from inadequate ventilation with heating units. What people fail to recognize is that carbon monoxide is also in their blood with smoking. The more or less you smoke the more or less carbon monoxide is in your blood, respectively. This level can be followed serially as smoking cessation program participants decrease their rate of smoking. This is a great way to document success or failure of a smoking cessation program.

Remember we need to keep it simple. Healthcare literacy doesn't allow too many chances to get a point across. Here is a way to say it in plain language. Carbon monoxide kills people; the more you smoke the more carbon monoxide is in your blood and the more likely you will die. Simple and to the point.

Smoking kills 443,000 people each year, of which 128,900 die of lung cancer and another 92,900 from emphysema. It would be easy to screen smokers at a county fair with a carbon monoxide meter. Checking carbon monoxide levels and telling them that this is in their blood may be the impetus they need to quit smoking. Another simple measurement of smoking-related lung damage is respiratory spirometry. We can show a smoker that their lung capacity is falling and at a certain level you can't breathe. Spirometry testing with a disposable mouthpiece, e.g., at a county fair, could give smokers another tangible reason to stop smoking.

Triennial community health needs assessments (CHNA) have been mandated for tax-exempt hospitals by the government through the Affordable Care Act. This gives healthcare systems the opportunity to evaluate their community demographics and determinants of health. Some of these assessments are developed in-house whereas others are contracted out. I've seen both but most are contracted out. The quality of the report depends upon the questions asked. The programmatic response to the report depends upon the healthcare system.

If a healthcare system uses the databases presented in this chapter, they will be able to make up the cancer-related questions that need to be answered. As an example, a western Massachusetts rural community hospital needed to know more about access issues for its elderly patients. They asked questions concerning transportation, cost, distance traveled for care, ability to leave an elderly spouse, and their own ability to travel to health care. This is a very useful information to identify barriers to care among elderly patients. In another part of the country, food deserts (an area more than a mile from where you live to the grocery store) limited access to food and fresh produce was identified as an issue. Both of these are common problems for rural areas and people without transportation but can also be an issue in non-rural areas. County Health Rankings has a surrogate for this called food insecurity. This is an inclusive parameter which includes food deserts and income as regards the affordability of food. The Rankings also measures limited access to healthy foods.

Once you have reviewed and used the databases outlined above, you should be able to:

- Use this data to identify multiple barriers and determinants of health which contribute to cancer incidence and mortality in your service area.
- Write your own cancer-weighted CHNA.
- Identify cancers in your service area with increased incidence and mortality.
- Propose new or enhanced prevention and screening programs.
- Target specific neighborhoods and populations to maximize the effectiveness of these programs.

## References

1. Mortality Data by State. National Cancer Institute, CDC, State Cancer Profiles at https://statecancerprofiles.cancer.gov/map/map.withimage.php?00&001&001&00&0&02&0&1&5&0#results.
2. Self-reported obesity by state and territory. CDC at https://www.cdc.gov/obesity/data/prevalence-maps.html.
3. Cancer among adults by census tract Baron Rouge. CDC 500 Cities Project. https://nccd.cdc.gov/500_Cities/rdPage.aspx?rdReport=DPH_500_Cities.InteractiveMap&islCategories=HLTHOUT&islMeasures=ARTHRITIS&islStates=22&rdRnd=4071.
4. Census quick facts. https://www.census.gov/quickfacts/table/PST045216/00.
5. Three County Population Comparisons Central Georgia. US Census Bureau. https://www.census.gov/quickfacts/fact/table/jonescountygeorgia,monroecountygeorgia,bibbcountygeorgia,US/PST045216.

6. Three county education level, health insurance and poverty comparisons central Georgia. US Census Bureau. https://www.census.gov/quickfacts/fact/table/peachcountygeorgia,jonescountygeorgia,monroecountygeorgia,US/PST045216.
7. http://www.countyhealthrankings.org/rankings/data.
8. Introductory page for Rockingham County NH. University of Wisconsin Population Health Institute. County Health Rankings & Roadmaps. 2017. http://www.countyhealthrankings.org/app/new-hampshire/2017/rankings/rockingham/county/outcomes/overall/snapshot.
9. State cancer profiles. https://statecancerprofiles.cancer.gov/index.html.
10. CDC 500 cities project. https://www.cdc.gov/500Cities/.
11. In-Migration data from outside the US Data by State. National Cancer Institute, CDC, State cancer profiles. https://statecancerprofiles.cancer.gov/map/map.withimage.php?00&901&00021&00&0&3&0&1&5&0#results.
12. In-migration rates by Washington Counties. National Cancer Institute, CDC, State cancer profiles. https://statecancerprofiles.cancer.gov/map/map.withimage.php?53&901&00021&00&0&3&0&1&5&0#results.
13. Language isolation or non-English language spoken at home. National Cancer Institute, CDC, State cancer profiles. https://statecancerprofiles.cancer.gov/map/map.withimage.php?00&914&00015&00&0&3&0&1&5&0#results.
14. Non-English language spoken at home for Maine by Counties. National Cancer Institute, CDC, State cancer profiles. https://statecancerprofiles.cancer.gov/map/map.withimage.php?23&914&00015&00&0&3&0&1&5&0#results.
15. Pap Smear during past 3 years for women 18 years or older not having prior hysterectomy by State. National Cancer Institute, CDC, State cancer profiles. https://statecancerprofiles.cancer.gov/map/map.withimage.php?00&918&999&00&2&11&0&1&5&0#results.
16. Percent of women receiving 3+ doses of HPV vaccine ages 13–15. National Cancer Institute, CDC, State cancer profiles. https://statecancerprofiles.cancer.gov/map/map.withimage.php?00&315&999&00&2&70&0&1&5&0#results.
17. US Knowledge survey map about decreasing risk of getting skin cancer. National Cancer Institute, CDC, State cancer profiles. https://statecancerprofiles.cancer.gov/cancerknowledge/index.php?topic=skin&question=q16&age=001&type=hints#results.
18. US survey knowledge map asking if sun exposure increases risk of getting cancer. National Cancer Institute, CDC, State cancer profiles. https://statecancerprofiles.cancer.gov/cancerknowledge/index.php?topic=skin&question=q11&age=001&type=hints#results.
19. Cancer incidence 5 year rate changes for the US. National Cancer Institute, CDC, State cancer profiles. https://statecancerprofiles.cancer.gov/recenttrend/index.php?0&00&0&9599&001&999&00&0&0&0&1#results.
20. Cancer mortality 5 year rate changes for the US. National Cancer Institute, CDC, State cancer profiles. https://statecancerprofiles.cancer.gov/recenttrend/index.php?0&00&0&9599&001&999&00&0&0&0&2#results.
21. Incidence of liver cancer Hawaii by County from 2010–2014. National Cancer Institute, CDC, State cancer profiles. https://statecancerprofiles.cancer.gov/map/map.withimage.php?15&001&035&00&0&01&0&1&5&0#results.
22. Mortality rate liver cancer Hawaii by County from 2010–2014. National Cancer Institute, CDC, State cancer profiles. https://statecancerprofiles.cancer.gov/map/map.withimage.php?15&001&035&00&0&02&0&1&5&0#results.
23. 500 Cities project CDC local data for better health: Boston cancer incidence and health insurance rates. CDC 500 cities project. https://nccd.cdc.gov/500_Cities/rdPage.aspx?rdReport=DPH_500_Cities.InteractiveMap&islCategories=HLTHOUT&islMeasures=ARTHRITIS&islStates=22&rdRnd=40715.
24. 500 Cities project CDC local data for better health: unhealthy smoking behavior. CDC 500 cities project. https://nccd.cdc.gov/500_Cities/rdPage.aspx?rdReport=DPH_500_Cities.InteractiveMap&islStates=59&islCategories=UNHBEH&islMeasures=CSMOKING.
25. NCDB melanoma incidence by age and gender (information was derived from the American College of Surgeons' National Cancer Database). https://www.facs.org.

# Chapter 6
# The Role of Quality Metrics in Improving Oncologic Survival

**Matthew A. Facktor**

Clinical quality metrics have become ubiquitous in modern health care. The primary goal is to improve patient care delivery and overall outcomes, but they have also been tied to reimbursement and general quality improvement efforts. Numerous organizations have developed and/or promoted the use of quality metrics, including many for oncology. Ultimately, the hope is that increased use of well-conceived quality metrics will lead to improved survival. This chapter outlines the approach taken by the American College of Surgeons Commission on Cancer (CoC), and highlights recent data on the relationship between quality measures and improvements in survival.

## Overview of the Commission on Cancer and the National Cancer Database

The Commission on Cancer (CoC) is a consortium of multidisciplinary professional organizations dedicated to improving survival and quality of life for cancer patients through standard setting, prevention, research, education, and monitoring of comprehensive quality care [1]. One of the best known efforts of the CoC on its mission to improve the quality of cancer care has been the development of multiple quality measures using its large internal database.

The National Cancer Database (NCDB) was created jointly in 1989 by the American College of Surgeons Commission on Cancer (CoC) and the American Cancer Society. As of the end of 2017, the NCDB contains information on more than 37 million patients, with approximately 250 clinical data points for each patient, covering 74 types of cancer. Using various Web-based data applications,

M. A. Facktor
Department of Thoracic Surgery, Geisinger Health System, Danville, PA, USA
e-mail: mafacktor@geisinger.edu



P. Hopewood, M. J. Milroy (eds.), *Quality Cancer Care*,
https://doi.org/10.1007/978-3-319-78649-0_6

CoC-accredited institutions have access to a wealth of information. The data tools allow users to obtain survival reports, hospital comparisons (local, regional, national, etc.), quality measure performance, and many other types of reports. More than 1500 CoC-accredited hospitals across the United States contribute clinical oncologic data to the NCDB, which represents approximately 70% of newly diagnosed cancers. Realizing the size and maturity of the NCDB, the CoC began leveraging the power of this database in 2003 to improve cancer care by developing a variety of quality measures.

All current CoC quality measures are process measures, which means they address how and/or when a particular part of clinical care is delivered (e.g., did the patient get the recommended treatment for their stage of disease). The measures are evidence based, using peer-reviewed literature sources, including some studies utilizing NCDB data. The "best" studies are well-designed randomized controlled trials supporting a specific area of oncology care. The first measures developed involved breast and colon cancers, with several other disease sites added thereafter. With additional measures being released soon, the CoC currently monitors and reports on 23 separate quality measures covering ten different disease sites [2].

## Quality Measure Development at the CoC

The Quality Integration Committee (QIC) of the Commission on Cancer partners with internal and external clinical experts to develop quality measures. The development and approval of quality measures rely on the specialized expertise of members of the QIC and CoC member organizations. To that end, the CoC has worked in conjunction with the Society of Surgical Oncology (SSO), the Society of Gynecologic Oncology (SGO), the Society of Urologic Oncology (SUO), and the American Urologic Association (AUA).

## Types of Quality

There are three types of measures approved by the CoC: accountability, quality improvement, and surveillance [2]. Evidence-based measures (accountability) promote improvements in care delivery and are the highest standard for measurement. These measures demonstrate provider accountability, influence payment for services, and promote transparency. Quality improvement measures monitor the need for quality improvement or remediation and are based upon slightly less rigorous scientific data. Generally, these measures are for individual program use rather than national comparisons. Surveillance measures are used to identify the status quo, generate information for decision-making, and/or monitor patterns and trends of care. These measures are based upon less stringent data in conjunction with expert consensus. Table 6.1 summarizes these three types of CoC quality measures.

**Table 6.1** Three types of Commission on Cancer quality measures

| Measure type | Measure definition and use |
|---|---|
| Accountability | High level of evidence supports the measure, including multiple randomized control trials. These measures can be used for such purposes as public reporting, payment incentive programs, and selection of providers by consumers, health plans, or purchasers. |
| Quality improvement | Evidence from experimental studies, not randomized control trials, supports the measure. These are intended for internal monitoring of performance within an organization. |
| Surveillance | Limited evidence exists that supports the measure or the measure is used for informative purposes to accredited programs. These measures can be used to identify the status quo as well as monitor patterns and trends of care in order to guide decision-making and resource allocation. |

## Current CoC Reporting Tools/Activities

The CoC reports quality measure data back to its accredited cancer centers using tools readily available to members on a secure online portal. Data reporting applications include NCDB Hospital Comparison Benchmark Reports (demographic, cancer identification, treatment, and administrative data), NCDB Survival Reports (AJCC stage-stratified, 5-year observed survival rates for all cancer sites filtered by primary site of the cancer and diagnosis period), and Cancer Program Practice Profile Reports ($CP^3R$; adherence to and consideration of standard of care therapies for major cancers). Individual institutions can view their own data at the hospital level, and are able to compare their data with peer institutions in their region or with those across the entire country. Comparison data are currently updated once annually, but available anytime online for analysis. A more rapid data feedback tool known as the Rapid Quality Reporting System (RQRS) was developed to assist CoC-accredited cancer programs in promoting evidence-based cancer care at the local level. The RQRS is a Web-based, systematic data collection and reporting system that advances evidence-based treatment through a prospective alert system, allowing programs to close any open quality measure care gaps in somewhat real time. If a breast cancer patient undergoes breast-conserving surgery, for example, and is due to receive radiation therapy within 1 year (a CoC quality measure), then the rapid reporting tool automatically reminds the caregivers of the "open loop" until initiation of radiation therapy is documented in the cancer registry. This process promotes higher reliability in maintaining the standard of care as promulgated by the quality measures.

Expected estimated performance rates (EPR) for all of the accountability and quality improvement measures are established annually. The CoC standards require programs to meet or exceed these performance levels annually in order to maintain CoC accreditation. The EPRs are set high (generally between 80 and 90%), but not typically at 100% given that there are many reasonable clinical justifications for not satisfying a quality measure every single time (a patient decides after extensive discussions, for example, not to have the recommended breast radiation). In this manner, all 1500+ accredited programs in the CoC work constantly to strive for, maintain, and improve upon a high level of evidence-based oncology care delivery.

## Examples of Specific Quality Measures

Details, descriptions, and supporting literature for all active CoC quality measures are openly available online [2]. One of the earliest developed accountability measures is the following: radiation therapy is administered within 1 year of diagnosis for women under age 70 receiving breast-conserving surgery for breast cancer. This measure is based upon randomized controlled trials demonstrating a reduced risk of local recurrence in women receiving adjuvant radiation [3–5]. Two additional measures for stage I-B to III breast cancer recommend either combination chemotherapy for hormone receptor-negative disease or hormone (endocrine) therapy for hormone receptor-positive disease. These two measures are based upon multiple randomized controlled trials demonstrating both recurrence and survival advantages [4, 6–8], and they have both received ongoing endorsement by the National Quality Forum (NQF), a testament to the strength of data upon which they are based [9, 10]. Two CoC colon cancer quality measures are also NQF endorsed [11, 12]. The first of these measures (accountability) recommends adjuvant chemotherapy for patients with stage III (lymph node positive) disease [2]. The second of these measures (quality improvement) recommends the harvest and pathologic evaluation of at least 12 regional lymph nodes at the time of colon resection [2].

One final example relates to surgical management of stage I and II non-small cell lung cancer. This measure (surveillance) recommends the removal and pathologic examination of at least ten lymph nodes at the time of pulmonary resection, and is based upon somewhat weaker data [2, 13–15]. There is controversy in the thoracic surgery community surrounding the merits of this particular measure because lymph node counts may be misleading. During lung cancer surgery, lymph nodes can easily fragment when handled and/or processed, which if not meticulously documented leads to potentially erroneous numbers (one true node could be accidentally counted as two or three or even more nodes on the final pathology report). Many surgeons argue that it would be better for us to count the number of different lymph node stations harvested rather than the exact number of lymph nodes themselves [16]. Regardless of how thoracic lymph nodes are counted, the thoracic oncology community uniformly agrees upon the importance of an adequate lymph node harvest. This recommendation is graded as a "surveillance" measure for these reasons (CoC-accredited institutions are not held accountable), and at the very least is providing an ever-clarifying picture of the status of lymph node dissection for lung cancer in the United States.

The aforementioned examples are all process measures, which tend to be easier to measure in real-world clinical practice and with current readily available national databases such as the NCDB. Compliance with these and other quality measures tends to increase over time, with the presumption that overall survival improvements follow thereafter. Whether or not this is actually true, however, has been somewhat difficult to firmly establish.

## Improving Quality and Survival in the NCDB (Lymph Nodes in Lung Cancer)

There is a growing body of literature supporting the relationship between higher numbers of lymph nodes harvested and improved quality of care (nodal upstaging and survival) in early-stage non-small cell lung cancer. The following discussion summarizes two recent example articles from both inside and outside of the NCDB.

Dr. Krantz and his colleagues at NorthShore University Health System just outside of Chicago published a large NCDB analysis in 2017 looking at the relevance of clinical trials and guidelines on improving lymph node harvest at the time of curative intent pulmonary resection [17]. The study included more than 51,000 patients in the NCDB between the years 2004 and 2013 who underwent curative intent pulmonary resection for clinical stage I non-small cell lung cancer. The first important finding was that the mean number of lymph nodes assessed increased significantly from 8.1 to 10 ($p < 0.001$) over that time period. The second important finding was that academic centers were statistically less likely to harvest only 0–5 nodes when compared to community centers (27.2 vs. 43.6%; $p < 0.001$).

While it is interesting to note that more lymph nodes were harvested over time and at academic centers, it is even more important to note the beneficial effect this has on clinical outcomes. Dr. Krantz and his colleagues demonstrated a higher likelihood of nodal upstaging in patients with more than 14 nodes harvested compared to those with 1–14 lymph nodes harvested (17.9% vs. 10.9%, respectively; $p < 0.001$). Overall survival advantages were also discovered in a couple of different scenarios. In the first comparison, patients with zero lymph nodes harvested had worse overall survival versus those with at least one node assessed. Among those who were upstaged, patients with more than 14 nodes assessed showed a survival advantage over patients with fewer than 14 nodes assessed (3.87 vs. 4.32 years, respectively; $p = 0.0058$). This led them to conclude, parenthetically, that at least 14 nodes should be assessed to maximize the probability that node-positive patients are correctly identified. The current CoC quality measure, as mentioned previously in this chapter, recommends that at least ten lymph nodes are removed and pathologically reviewed. Multivariate analysis enabled the authors to support their conclusion that the number of nodes harvested impacts survival.

A second important and somewhat similar study was published in 2017 by Dr. Smeltzer and his colleagues at the University of Memphis in Tennessee [18]. This research was conducted using the Mid-South Quality of Surgical Resection cohort, which is a database of curative intent pulmonary resections performed in northern Mississippi, eastern Arkansas, and western Tennessee. This particular study included patients from 2009 to 2016 and aimed to examine whether survival was affected by sequentially more stringent definitions of pathologic nodal staging quality (i.e., numbers and locations of lymph nodes harvested at surgery).

Dr. Smeltzer and his colleagues divided the population into eight different groups depending upon the stringency of lymph node dissection, starting with those who had zero lymph nodes harvested (representing lowest quality) and ending with those who had at least one hilar node, at least ten total nodes, and at least three mediastinal nodal stations harvested (highest quality). The current CoC quality measure (ten or more nodes harvested and pathologically assessed) was Group #4 in this particular study, meaning it was considered "middle of the pack" in regard to the overall level of lymph node harvest quality. The groups considered higher in quality than those that meet the current CoC quality measure were defined much more specifically than what is possible using the NCDB. In other words, this research group had the ability within their dataset to examine not just the raw number of lymph nodes harvested, but also the number of different nodal stations, the number of hilar stations/nodes, and the number of mediastinal stations/nodes. Although the CoC cannot currently be this granular (which is the primary criticism of the quality measure), many of the patients in the NCDB meeting the ten-lymph node requirement will indeed have multiple hilar and mediastinal nodal stations included, which represents the highest quality lymph node dissection.

The primary finding from Dr. Smeltzer and his colleagues was that survival improved with increasing quality of lymph node dissection. Specifically, there was better survival curve separation between pN0, pN1, and pN2 tumors (all were M0) as the degree of mediastinal nodal examination was defined more stringently. The authors concluded that mandating examination of at least ten lymph nodes (the CoC quality measure) was associated with the biggest increase in pN0 survival, which in effect is a reflection of retrieving a larger quantity of N1 (hilar) nodes. They also concluded that requiring dissection of a minimum of at least three different mediastinal nodal stations resulted in the biggest increase in pN1 survival. Similar to Dr. Krantz's group, these authors were able to support their conclusions with statistically significant data specific to the effect of nodal dissection. Ultimately, they recommend examining at least ten lymph nodes with sampling from at least three different mediastinal nodal stations [18].

When clinical stage I lung cancer patients are upstaged to either pathologic stage II (pN1) or III (pN2) postoperatively, they tend to receive adjuvant chemotherapy (and sometimes adjuvant mediastinal radiation) with the goal of improving their chances of survival. These are the current recommendations of the National Comprehensive Cancer Network [19]. The two studies mentioned in the paragraphs immediately above help support the notion that higher quality lymph node dissection (e.g., higher numbers of nodes/stations harvested) specifically and reliably increases the chances that a patient is more accurately staged. More accurate staging leads to more accurate and/or aggressive therapy (e.g., adjuvant chemotherapy for node-positive disease), which leads to increased overall survival. As more effective adjuvant systemic therapies are developed, this survival benefit will increase even further, which makes adequate lymph node dissection even more important. More and more studies, such as those two mentioned above, are demonstrating the importance and benefits of adhering to evidence-based quality measures.

## Comparing Survival as a Quality Metric in the NCDB (Breast and Lung Cancer)

Using survival as a measure of the quality of cancer care seems logical. One of the main criticisms of this hypothesis, however, is that unadjusted survival measurements may inherently flaw comparisons between institutions. A recent large study using the NCDB helps provide clarity to the question of whether or not survival is the ultimate measure of cancer care. Dr. Shulman and his colleagues at the CoC published an article in 2017 using the NCDB as the reference dataset to evaluate whether unadjusted and risk-adjusted survival could be used as quality indicators for individual hospitals [20]. Their primary aims were to (1) evaluate survival differences across CoC hospitals with risk adjustment and (2) compare survival after risk adjustment across different types of institutions. Risk adjusted in this study means the data was adjusted for diagnosis, year, stage, age, gender, ethnic background, insurance status, and comorbidities.

There are four different program types within the CoC: community cancer programs, comprehensive community cancer programs, academic comprehensive cancer programs, and NCI-designated comprehensive cancer centers. The NCI designation speaks for itself, while the other three program types are defined by the number of cancer cases seen each year and the presence or absence of postgraduate education programs. All program types are expected to participate in cancer-related clinical research. The community cancer programs are the smallest, defined by seeing 100–500 newly diagnosed cancer cases per year. Comprehensive community cancer programs see more than 500 newly diagnosed cancer cases per year, which is the same requirement for academic comprehensive cancer programs. Academic programs also provide postgraduate medical education [21].

Dr. Shulman's study targeted two different survival scenarios involving breast and lung cancers. In general, as the authors summarized, breast cancer has a high 5-year survival rate and treatments are relatively standard/stable, so they asked whether or not there are differences in survival at different program types. On the other hand, and in general terms, non-small cell lung cancer (NSCLC) has poor survival, but newer molecular diagnostics and targeted therapies may be beginning to improve survival. The research group examined these two groups of patients using the NCDB and focused on differences in survival between cancer program types, as defined by the CoC. Using the NCDB, the authors felt that the outcomes would reflect "real-world" data rather than the more typically "ideal" datasets obtained in strictly defined randomized controlled trials [20].

Looking specifically at stage III breast cancer survival, Dr. Shulman and his group noted that in fact most programs are "average," with a few programs statistically better, and a few programs statistically worse than average. Comparing unadjusted survival by hospital type, NCI-designated comprehensive cancer centers have the highest survival probability. Comparing risk-adjusted survival further limited the numbers of survival outliers (best and worst performers) as compared to unadjusted survival. The NCI programs maintained better risk-adjusted survival when compared to both community and comprehensive community programs [20].

For NSCLC, the researchers looked at advanced disease (stages III-B and IV). The results were similar to those found with stage III breast cancer. Most programs are average when looking at unadjusted survival, with a relatively small number of statistically significant best and worst outliers. Unadjusted survival comparisons by hospital type again reveal that the best survival probability is at NCI-designated comprehensive cancer centers. Risk adjustment further limits the numbers of best and worst outliers (most programs remain average). NCI programs have statistically better risk-adjusted survival when compared to both community and comprehensive community programs.

The authors draw several conclusions from their analysis. First, they maintain that NCDB survival data are useful for looking at national trends, across different hospital types, by diagnosis, stage, and year of diagnosis. Similarly, NCDB survival data gives “real-life” data on patient survival to be compared with Phase III randomized trials. Secondly, recognizing that unadjusted survival comparisons are not justified, risk-adjusted survival remains an approximation because it is not possible to include all potential variables given the limits of any particular dataset. Third, very few hospitals have risk-adjusted survivals that are statistically significantly better or worse than average. Fourth, there are differences in risk-adjusted survival by hospital type in the aggregate (NCI programs perform best, followed by academic programs, and then followed by both comprehensive community and community program types). Finally, they suggest that it may be important to correlate survival outcomes with adherence to quality metrics to determine if they truly will reflect important factors in care. The ultimate recommendation from the study is that we must be careful in using survival as a definitive discriminator of hospital quality, given that this NCDB data suggest that most programs perform equally well [20].

## Future Direction

As the data from the use of quality measures matures, it will likely allow more robust survival and other outcome analyses. The CoC is uniquely positioned in this regard, given its ongoing maintenance and development of quality measures based upon the NCDB. Although survival seems appealing as an “ultimate” quality measure, we must use caution as noted by Dr. Shulman and his colleagues [20] when comparing survival across institutions without appropriate forms of risk adjustment. Even with risk adjustment, it appears in the “real world” of NCDB survival data that most institutions perform similarly to each other. Over time, however, and with increasing compliance on quality measures, overall survival should continue to improve even if most institutions perform equally well. Further research will be needed to continue to fine-tune the relationship between quality measure compliance and oncologic survival.

## References


1. American College of Surgeons: Commission on Cancer. https://www.facs.org/quality-programs/cancer/coc. Accessed 6 Feb 2018.
2. American College of Surgeons: Commission on Cancer, National Cancer Database, CoC Quality of Care Measures. https://www.facs.org/quality-programs/cancer/ncdb/qualitymeasures. Accessed 6 Feb 2018.
3. Early Breast Cancer Trialists' Collaborative Group (EBCTCG), Darby S, McGale P, Correa C, et al. Effect of radiotherapy after breast-conserving surgery on 10-year recurrence and 15-year breast cancer death: meta-analysis of individual patient data for 10,801 women in 17 randomized trials. Lancet. 2011;378(9804):1707–16.
4. Hassett MJ, Hughes ME, Niland JC, et al. Selecting high priority quality measures for breast cancer quality improvement. Med Care. 2008;46:762–70.
5. Hughes KS, Schnaper LA, Berry D, et al. Lumpectomy plus Tamoxifen with or without irradiation in women 70 years of age or older with early breast cancer. N Engl J Med. 2004;351:971–7.
6. Early Breast Cancer Trialists' Collaborative Group (EBCTCG), Peto R, Davies C, Godwin J, et al. Comparisons between different polychemotherapy regimens for early breast cancer: meta-analysis of long-term outcome among 100,000 women in 123 randomized trials. Lancet. 2012;379(9814):432–44.
7. Early Breast Cancer Trialists' Collaborative Group (EBCTCG), Clarke M, Coates AS, Darby SC, et al. Adjuvant chemotherapy in estrogen-receptor-poor breast cancer: patient level meta-analysis of randomized trials. Lancet. 2008;371(9606):29–40.
8. Early Breast Cancer Trialists Collaborative Group (EBCTCG). Effects of chemotherapy and hormonal therapy for early breast cancer on recurrence and 15-year survival: an overview of the randomized trials. Lancet. 2005;365(9472):1687–717.
9. National Quality Forum: 0559 Combination chemotherapy is recommended or administered within 4 months (120 days) of diagnosis for women under 70 with AJCC T1cN0M0, or Stage IB-III hormone receptor negative breast cancer. http://www.qualityforum.org/QPS/QPSTool.aspx. Accessed 6 Feb 2018.
10. National Quality Forum: 0220 Adjuvant hormonal therapy. http://www.qualityforum.org/QPS/QPSTool.aspx. Accessed 6 Feb 2018.
11. National Quality Forum: 0223 Adjuvant chemotherapy is recommended within 4 months (120 days) of diagnosis to patients under the age of 80 with AJCC III (lymph node positive) colon cancer. http://qualityforum.org/QPS/QPSTool.aspx. Accessed 6 Feb 2018.
12. National Quality Forum: 0225 At least 12 regional lymph nodes are removed and pathologically examined for resected colon cancer. http://qualityforum.org/QPS/QPSTool.aspx. Accessed 6 Feb 2018.
13. Ludwig MS, Goodman M, Miller DL, Johnstone PA. Postoperative survival and the number of lymph nodes sampled during resection of node-negative non-small cell lung cancer. Chest. 2005;128(3):1545–50. http://www.ncbi.nlm.nih.gov/pubmed/16162756.
14. Limited thoracic lymphadenectomy worsens survival in 55,122 patients with resected Stage I non-small cell lung cancer P217 society of surgical oncology 66th Annual Symposium, March 6–9, 2013.
15. Samayoa AX, Pezzi TA, Pezzi CM, et al. Rationale for a minimum number of lymph nodes removed with non-small cell lung cancer resection: correlating the number of nodes removed with survival in 98,970 patients. Ann Surg Oncol. 2016;23(Suppl 5):1005–11.
16. Handy JR Jr, Costas K, Nisco S, et al. Regarding American College of Surgeons Commission on cancer non-small cell lung cancer quality measure 10RLN. Ann Thorac Surg. 2016;102:1040–1.
17. Krantz SB, Lutfi W, Kuchta K, et al. Improved lymph node staging in early-stage lung cancer in the National Cancer Database. Ann Thorac Surg. 2017;104:1805–14.

18. Smeltzer MP, Faris NR, Ray MA, et al. Association of pathologic nodal staging quality with survival among patients with non-small cell lung cancer after resection with curative intent. JAMA Oncol. 2018;4(1):80–7.
19. Non-small cell lung cancer Version 2.2018. In: NCCN Clinical Practice Guidelines in Oncology (NCCN Guidelines®). http://www.nccn.org. Accessed 8 Feb 2018.
20. Shulman LN, Palis BE, McCabe R, et al. Survival as a quality metric of cancer care: use of the National Cancer Data Base to assess hospital performance. J Oncol Pract. 2018;14(1):e59–72.
21. Cancer program standards: ensuring patient-centered care manual. 2016 ed. https://www.facs.org/quality-programs/cancer/coc/standards. Accessed 8 Feb 2018.

# Chapter 7
# Patient Navigation in Cancer Care Delivery

**Ted A. James and Kimberly A. Maurer**

*Navigate; from the Latin—'navis' (ship) and 'igare' (to drive); to sail over, on, or through, in safety.*

## An Introduction to Cancer Patient Navigation

The past several decades have witnessed incredible advances in oncology with ever-increasing innovations in cancer-related diagnosis and management. As a result, the overall prognosis of most cancer types has improved steadily, with more and more patients experiencing prolonged survival. However, many patients experiencing cancer struggle with the complexity of care and some do not benefit equally from the advances in cancer management. In 2013 the Institute of Medicine published a report on the quality of cancer care, describing that many patients with cancer do not receive care that adequately meets their needs [1]. Among several problems, the report cited the lack of patient-centered care, and a care delivery system that is frequently fragmented and poorly coordinated. Furthermore, the provision of care does not always meet other quality domains of being safe, effective, timely, efficient, and equitable. This is due in large part to suboptimal care processes, persistent health

T. A. James (✉)
Department of Breast Surgical Oncology, Beth Israel Deaconess Medical Center, Harvard Medical School, Boston, MA, USA

BreastCare Center, Beth Israel Deaconess Medical Center, Harvard Medical School, Boston, MA, USA
e-mail: ted.james@bidmc.harvard.edu

K. A. Maurer
BreastCare Center, Beth Israel Deaconess Medical Center, Harvard Medical School, Boston, MA, USA
e-mail: kmaurer1@bidmc.harvard.edu



P. Hopewood, M. J. Milroy (eds.), *Quality Cancer Care*,
https://doi.org/10.1007/978-3-319-78649-0_7

disparities, and barriers to access that all too often afflict our increasingly complex healthcare system. As a result, the quality of clinical outcomes diminishes. Failures in quality during the phases of cancer care can create serious consequences. Ineffective outreach programs, lack of screening, difficulty arranging appointments, or an inability to reach underserved populations can result in patients developing preventable cancer or presenting with advanced disease. Treatment delays may arise from referrals not made, or patients not understanding treatment plans. Poor adherence to treatment recommendations or poor patient experiences may predispose to inferior clinical outcomes. And finally, when end-of-life issues are not proactively addressed, palliative care is insufficient and patients may miss opportunities for early alleviation of symptoms.

Patient navigation in oncology was initially developed to address unmet needs of low income and underinsured populations; however, because cancer care is so complicated, it has become clear that all patients regardless of socioeconomic-demographic background may benefit from navigation. In addition to coordination of medical care, many nonmedical issues facing patients with cancer may need to be addressed. These issues are not just financial; they can also be logistical, emotional, and cultural. For instance, patients may not be adequately informed about their course of treatment, or may encounter practical challenges trying to accommodate treatment care plans and schedules. This may be daunting even to those with abundant support and resources. Without appropriate assistance, some patients give up.

Patients also face a myriad of treatment options where decision-making can be complicated. The need for improved patient education and tools to optimize shared decision-making are well documented [2]. For example, many women with breast cancer report not receiving adequate education regarding options for surgery and lacked information that ideally should be incorporated into their decision-making process. Studies have also demonstrated that some patients were not meaningfully engaged in treatment discussions and had decisions made without soliciting their preferences regarding the approach to treatment [3].

Within oncology, patient navigators help to address many of the challenges encountered in the management of cancer. Navigators may be nurses, social workers, nurse practitioners, or community health workers, or may not have a health profession background. To date, there is no formal professional licensing board or credentials for cancer patient navigators, although various organizations provide training and certification. Many navigators have personally faced a cancer diagnosis themselves or within their families. Navigators can work as hospital employees, independent consultants, or volunteers, or be employed by community organizations. Regardless of the background, the basic role of the navigator is to improve care coordination, address patient needs, and ultimately enhance the quality of care experienced by patients undergoing cancer treatment. Activities can include educating patients about their diagnosis, coordinating their care, serving as a patient advocate, accompanying patients on medical visits, acting as a liaison to the care team, assisting caregivers, helping with insurance issues, or managing medical paperwork. The specific role of each oncology navigator may vary based on experience, training, and practice setting. Patient navigation involves collaboration with not only patients, but also clinicians, families, and caregivers, throughout the cancer continuum, from prevention and screening through posttreatment, survivorship, and palliative and end-of-life care.

## History of Patient Navigation

Patient navigation has evolved from a strategy to improve outcomes in "vulnerable" populations by eliminating barriers to timely diagnosis and treatment of cancer and other chronic diseases. The development of the concept of patient navigation was initially related to the findings of the American Cancer Society National Hearings on Cancer in the Poor. The hearings were conducted in 1989 in seven American cities. The testimony was primarily by poor Americans of all ethnic groups who had been diagnosed with cancer [4]. In response to these findings, the nation's first patient navigation program was conceived and initiated in Harlem Hospital Center in 1990. Dr. Harold Freeman, a surgeon whom many consider to be the founding father of patient navigation, developed an approach to address the heavier burden of disease borne by the patient population that he served in Harlem. The Harlem Patient Navigation Program was designed as a system to reduce disparities in access to health care. The program predominately served patients of low economic status, many of whom did not have medical insurance. Navigation focused on breast cancer patients, specifically the "critical window of opportunity" to reduce cancer mortality by eliminating barriers to timely care from the point of a suspicious finding to further diagnosis and treatment. Commonly experienced barriers to timely care in the Harlem study were financial constraints, lack of health insurance, communication and information barriers, fear and distrust of the health system, and emotional barriers. Prior to the intervention, in a 22-year period ending in 1986, only 6% of these patients had stage 1 disease and 49% presented with either stage 3 and 4 disease. The 5-year survival rate was 39% [4, 5]. After the intervention, the results were dramatically improved. Forty-one percentage of patients presented with early-stage breast cancer (stages 0 and 1), and only 21% of patients had stage 3 or 4 disease. The 5-year survival rate increased to 70%, which was on par with the national rate at the time [6]. Based principally on the patient navigation model in Harlem, the Patient Navigator and Chronic Disease Prevention Act (HR 1812) was passed by Congress and signed into law by President Bush in 2005 [7]. The Act was a bipartisan approach to improving access to care and addressing health disparities by authorizing a $25-million demonstration program to provide patient navigator services to reduce barriers, increase cancer screening, and improve healthcare outcomes. Subsequently, the scope of patient navigation expanded across the entire cancer care continuum, including prevention, detection, diagnosis, treatment, survivorship, and end of life. Recognizing that barriers limiting or preventing access to appropriate cancer care are not unique to poor Americans, but are experienced by Americans across all socioeconomic levels, the American College of Surgeons (ACS) Commission on Cancer (CoC) in 2012 released standards that reflected the goal of "ensuring patient-centered care." One of the new standards (Standard 3.1), implemented in 2015, required all cancer programs seeking accreditation to have a patient navigation program. Pilot programs, such as the Oncology Patient Centered Medical Home and the Oncology Care Model from the Centers for Medicare and Medicaid Services, have likewise attempted to encourage oncologists to focus on navigation with coordination of care within their practice.

## Principles of Cancer Navigation

The fundamental role of a cancer navigator is to serve as an educator, advocate, and care coordinator. Each navigation program is unique and may follow a different model suited to the needs of their patient population, characteristics of the clinical practice, and available resources of the program. Some programs have disease-specific navigators, whereas others have navigators helping patients from more than one cancer type. The number of patients each navigator manages also varies based on the extent of resources, additional personnel, population needs, and cancer type. To help in the implementation of cancer navigation programs, the National Cancer Institute's Community Cancer Centers Program developed an assessment tool to help set goals and determine the progress of a navigation program. In addition, principles incorporating best practices for navigation have been developed and vetted based on experience and espoused by Dr. Freeman himself [8].

*Principle #1*: Patient navigation is a "patient-centric healthcare service delivery model." The focus of navigation is to promote the timely movement of an individual patient through an often complex cancer care continuum. An individual's journey through this continuum begins in the neighborhood where he or she lives to a medical setting where an abnormality is detected, a diagnosis is made, and then treatment is rendered. The journey continues from rehabilitation and survivorship to the end of life.

*Principle #2*: Patient navigation serves to virtually integrate a fragmented healthcare system for the individual patient. As patient care is so often delivered in a fragmented manner, particularly related to those with chronic diseases, patient navigation has the potential of creating a seamless flow for patients as they journey through the care continuum. Patient navigation can be seen as the guiding force promoting the timely movement of the patient through a complex system of care.

*Principle #3*: The core function of patient navigation is the elimination of barriers to timely care across all segments of the healthcare continuum. This function is most effectively carried out through a one-on-one relationship between the navigator and the patient.

*Principle #4*: Patient navigation should be defined with a clear scope of practice that distinguishes the role and responsibilities of the navigator from that of all other [health professionals]. Navigators should be integrated into the healthcare team to promote maximum benefit for the individual patient.

*Principle #5*: Delivery of patient navigation services should be cost effective and commensurate with the training and skills necessary to navigate an individual through a particular phase of the care continuum.

*Principle #6*: The determination of who should navigate should be determined by the level of skills required at a given phase of navigation. There is a spectrum of navigation extending from services that may be provided by trained lay navigators to services that require navigators who are professionals, such as nurses and social workers. Another consideration to take into account is that [clinicians] should ideally provide patient care that requires their level of education and experience and should not be assigned to duties that do not require their level of skills.

*Principle #7*: In a given system of care there is the need to define the point at which navigation begins and the point at which navigation ends.

*Principle #8*: There is a need to navigate patients across disconnected systems of care, such as primary care sites and tertiary care sites. Patient navigation can serve as the process that connects disconnected healthcare systems.

*Principle #9*: Patient navigation systems require coordination. In larger systems of patient care, this coordination is best carried out by assigning a navigation coordinator or champion who is responsible for overseeing all phases of navigation activity within a given healthcare site or system. It is important to distinguish a system of patient navigation from the patient navigator(s) who work within the system.

## Challenges

Despite the benefits provided by patient navigation, measuring the impact of patient navigation on the healthcare system has been challenging, and several obstacles hinder the widespread implementation and adoption of navigation in cancer programs. The lack of reimbursement for navigation services presents a potential cost barrier. Nonetheless, many institutions make the investment or partner with grantees/donors to fund these positions due to the perceived benefit in patient care. In addition, expected cost savings from the care coordination provided by patient navigators can include decreased emergency department visits, reduction in inappropriate admissions and readmissions, decreased no-show rates, reduction in unnecessary diagnostic testing, increased patient retention, and more effective patient management throughout the continuum of care [9]. Early studies on the cost-effectiveness of patient navigation have indeed demonstrated a positive financial return on investment through improved access, patient retention, treatment adherence, and clinical efficiencies [10, 11].

Another challenge is demonstrating the impact of patient navigation on subjective patient measures and objectively measured clinical outcomes in oncology.

## Outcomes of Cancer Patient Navigation

Important metrics to consider when evaluating a cancer navigation program are utilization of cancer prevention/screening services, stage at presentation, timeliness of care, treatment adherence, health service utilization, care coordination, clinical outcomes, and patient experience. Reports have demonstrated benefits in these areas; however, further studies are required to systematically determine the impact of navigation on clinical outcomes, quality, cost, and patient satisfaction in cancer care [12]. Studies are under way seeking to determine if outcomes such as tumor response, complication rates, and survival are improved with patient navigation.

## Practical Tips

When developing a patient navigation program, it is helpful to obtain commitment from top-level administration. It is beneficial to maximize patient interface (e.g., education, psychological support, needs assessment). Defining and monitoring metrics of success help in sustaining and growing patient navigation programs. For best results, navigators should be fully integrated into the clinical care team. It is also critical to provide appropriate support and training for the navigator role. Employing standardized protocols for patient interactions and developing best practices for care coordination help to ensure the navigator's success in this role.

## Case Example

The following case illustrates the role of patient navigation and highlights the influence a navigator can have on a patients' care experience.

A 51-year-old woman was recently diagnosed with right breast cancer. She had already met with a surgeon at one hospital, but wanted a second opinion. She was seen in our multidisciplinary clinic and spoke with our oncology nurse navigator a number of times prior to her appointment. The navigator helped her with obtaining her outside records and reports. The patient mentioned that there was no navigator at the first hospital she visited. She was also impressed that we had offered her an alternative treatment, and together with the benefit of having a nurse navigator she decided to stay with us for her care. She stated a number of times that having a navigator to call was a huge comfort to her. She saw genetics the same day of her multidisciplinary visit and was seen by plastics a few days later. Again, she mentioned that she was impressed by how coordinated her care was, and enjoyed having a point person that was so helpful to keep things moving forward. The navigator spoke with her again after seeing plastics, reviewed her MRI results, and together discussed her surgical plan. A few weeks later she had an oncoplastic lumpectomy with sentinel node biopsy and bilateral mastopexy. The navigator spoke with her again after surgery. Unfortunately she had positive nodes and required an axillary dissection. The navigator promptly set her up with an appointment to see a plastic surgeon to discuss lymphatic bypass. After her axillary dissection, she had insurance questions and was contemplating having her chemotherapy closer to home. When she called, she said that she had spoken with one of the practitioners, but still wanted to talk about the overall plan with the navigator because she had confidence that, "we could formulate a plan together." It was great to see this trust and rapport that had developed over several months, and to see the patient reach out to the navigator as her point person to problem-solve with her. This case exemplifies navigation at its best; a therapeutic relationship built on patient-centered care by guiding the patient through treatment, keeping things moving forward and coordinated, and supporting the patient to be empowered and truly part of the treatment process.

## Summary

Patient navigation is a healthcare delivery support system with the principal function of eliminating barriers to timely delivery of health care for individual patients across the healthcare continuum. Although initially developed to overcome barriers to care, all patients regardless of socioeconomic background may benefit for the improved care coordination, patient education, and advocacy provided by navigators. As an emerging healthcare intervention, patient navigation has the potential to significantly improve quality in cancer care delivery, including clinical outcomes and patient experience.

## References


1. Levit L, Balogh E, Nass S, Ganz PA. Delivering high-quality cancer care: charting a new course for a system in crisis. In: Institute of Medicine. Washington, DC: National Academies Press; 2013.
2. Wagner EH, Aiello Bowles EJ, Greene SM, Tuzzio L, Wiese CJ, Kirlin B, Clauser SB. The quality of cancer patient experience: perspectives of patients, family members, providers and experts. Qual Saf Health Care. 2010;19(6):484–9.
3. Lee CN, Chang Y, Adimorah N, Belkora JK, Moy B, Partridge AH, et al. Decision making about surgery for early-stage breast cancer. J Am Coll Surg. 2012;214(1):1–10. Epub 2011 Nov 6
4. Freeman HP, Rodriguez RL. History and principles of patient navigation. Cancer. 2011;117(15 0):3539–42.
5. Freeman HP, Wasfie TJ. Cancer of the breast in poor black women. Cancer. 1989;63:2562–9.
6. Oluwole SF, Ali AO, Adu A, et al. Impact of a cancer screening program on breast cancer state at diagnosis in medically underserved urban community. J Am Coll Surg. 2003;196:180–8.
7. Public Law 109-18. Patient navigator outreach and chronic disease prevention act of 2005. Washington, DC.

8. Freeman HP. The origin, evolution, and principles of patient navigation. Cancer Epidemiol Biomarkers Prev. 2012;21(10):1614–7.
9. Hopkins J, Mumber MP. Patient navigation through the cancer care continuum: an overview. J Oncol Pract. 2009;5(4):150–2.
10. Balderson D, Safavi K. How patient navigation can cut costs and save lives. Harvard Business Review. 2013. Digital article. https://hbr.org/2013/03/how-patient-navigation-brings#.
11. SG2 Health care intelligence: clinical intelligence: cancer care coordination with nurse navigators. 2006. http://www.sg2.com.
12. Ramsey S, Whitley E, Mears VW, McKoy JM, Everhart RM, Caswell RJ, et al, Patient Navigation Research Program Group. Evaluating the cost-effectiveness of cancer patient navigation programs: conceptual and practical issues. Cancer. 2009;115(23):5394–403.

# Chapter 8
# Survivorship

**Paula M. Termuhlen and Ruth E. Westra**

## Abbreviations

| | |
|---|---|
| AHRQ | Agency for Health Care Research and Quality |
| ASCO | American Society of Clinical Oncology |
| CoC | Commission on Cancer |
| FP | Family physician |
| IOM | Institute of Medicine |
| NCCN | National Comprehensive Cancer Network |
| NCI | National Cancer Institute |
| PCP | Primary care provider |
| SCP | Survivorship care plan |

## Introduction

One of the great successes of cancer care in the twenty-first century is that it has created a large cohort of cancer survivors who have unique needs as a result of the experience of cancer. In 2017, it is estimated that there will be 1,688,780 new cancer cases and the overwhelming majority will survive to add to the ever-growing cohort of cancer survivors [1]. Over the past 30 years, the 5-year relative survival rate for all cancers combined has increased for both sexes and among whites and blacks [1]. This success has translated into more than 15.5 million Americans alive with a history of cancer on January 1, 2016, and a projected 20 million-plus by January 1, 2026 [2]. This rising number of individuals who have had the personal experience of a cancer diagnosis and treatment have taught us that being a cancer patient is life

P. M. Termuhlen, MD, FACS (✉)
University of Minnesota Medical School, Duluth Campus, Duluth, MN, USA
e-mail: ptermuhl@d.umn.edu

R. E. Westra, DO, MPH
Department of Family Medicine and Community Health, University of Minnesota Medical School, Duluth Campus, Duluth, MN, USA
e-mail: rwestra@d.umn.edu



P. Hopewood, M. J. Milroy (eds.), *Quality Cancer Care*,
https://doi.org/10.1007/978-3-319-78649-0_8

changing and the effects of the experience last long beyond the active treatment phase.

As early as 1985, the renowned physician and cancer survivor, Fitzhugh Mullan, MD, described the experience of cancer as a series of seasons. He is credited with coining the term "cancer survivor" to describe his experience. In his essay published in the New England Journal of Medicine entitled "Seasons of Survival: Reflections of a Physician with Cancer," Dr. Mullan put out a call to action to "not only find therapies that will prevent or arrest the disease quickly but also to map the middle ground of survivorship and minimize its medical and social hazards" [3]. Furthermore he spoke to the need for studying survivorship as a "phenomenon in itself" that had unique characteristics separate from the traditional studies of tumor biology and treatment. In this book, we use the definition of cancer survivor as listed in the National Cancer Institute (NCI) Dictionary of Cancer Terms that considers a person to be a cancer survivor from the time of diagnosis until the end of life [4].

While this call to action simmered for many years, it exploded into life when National Academies of Science Institute of Medicine (IOM) convened the Committee on Cancer Survivorship: improving care and quality of life. The report that followed was part of a series of examinations by the IOM on the experience of cancer in the United States. This particular committee was charged with reporting on the survivors of adult cancer after primary treatment. The report published in 2005, *From Cancer Patient to Cancer Survivor: Lost in Transition*, had three aims based on an acknowledgement by the committee that the effects of cancer treatment and the experience of cancer had substantial impact on the physical and psychosocial health of survivors [5].

## *Aims of the IOM Report "From Cancer Patient to Cancer Survivor"*

- Raise awareness of the medical, functional, and psychosocial consequences of cancer and its treatment.
- Define quality health care for cancer survivors and identify strategies to achieve it.
- Improve the quality of life of cancer survivors through polices to ensure their access to psychosocial services, fair employment practices, and health insurance [5].
- In raising awareness of cancer survivorship, the committee identified four essential components: prevention, surveillance, intervention, and coordination [5]. From a medical perspective, the prevention and identification of recurrent or new cancers are essential for physical and mental health and well-being. Recognition of the late effects of cancer treatments is also necessary to promote wellness. As a partner to prevention, there is a need for the development of strategies for surveillance of cancer recurrence and new primaries and assessing the late effects of treatment on the physical and psychosocial health across the spectrum.

Interventions that holistically address the effects of cancer and its treatments on the person, their caregivers, and society are essential to supporting a cancer patient's return to wellness. Lastly, coordination and communication among patients, cancer care providers, and primary care providers are necessary to ensure that the transition from treatment to living again is overseen in a seamless fashion.

To address the aims of the Committee, ten recommendations in ten domains were offered to the stakeholders of the cancer experience, ranging from cancer patients and advocates to public and elected officials [5].

## *Areas for Recommendation in IOM Report from Cancer Patient to Cancer Survivor*

1. Raising awareness of cancer survivorship
2. Providing a care plan for survivorship
3. Developing clinical practice guidelines for survivorship care
4. Defining quality health care for cancer survivors
5. Overcoming system delivery challenges
6. Survivorship as a public health concern
7. Improving healthcare professional capacity
8. Addressing employment-related concerns
9. Improving access to adequate and affordable health insurance
10. Making investments in research

Underlying all of the recommendations was the recognition of cancer survivorship as a distinct phase of cancer care that needs to be recognized by the medical community and state and federal organizations that provide care and resources for health. There was a clear message that research into effective assessments, treatment, and support services for cancer survivorship is necessary and as important as research into the diagnosis and treatment of active cancer. Additionally, there has been an explicit call to insurers and payers of health care to ensure that evidence-based services rendered to the cancer survivor along the continuum of care are fully reimbursed to providers. The recommendations have provided a detailed list of actions to be taken on behalf of the cancer survivor. While full implementation has not been completed, much has been accomplished in the intervening years.

Following the 2005 IOM report, a number of national organizations began to implement the recommendations to improve and support cancer survivorship. Two areas of intense activity included the development of tools for use by providers of care to cancer survivors and integration of cancer survivorship into cancer program accreditation standards. Organizations such as American Society of Clinical Oncology, Journey Forward, LiveStrong, Penn Medicine OncoLink, the American Cancer Society, electronic health record providers, and others have worked to provide tools to make the delivery of survivorship care plans and treatment summaries easier for oncology teams. With the American College of Surgeons Commission on Cancer (CoC), *Cancer Program Standards 2012: Ensuring Patient-Centered Care*, accredited hospital cancer programs were required to develop an implementation plan for psychosocial distress screening and survivorship care plans [6, 7]. Recognizing the challenges associated with meeting these new patient care standards, programs were asked to have significant implementation by 2015. Even this proved daunting and based on feedback from accredited programs, additional modifications to include a broader group of health professionals who could provide patients with a survivorship care plan were integrated into the updated Standard 3.3 Survivorship Care Plan in CoC *Cancer Program Standards 2016: Ensuring Patient-Centered Care* [8].

The timing of this attention to cancer survivors also coincided with a national movement toward inter-professional and multidisciplinary health care. Thus, health providers of all types were empowered to engage in supporting cancer survivors at a heightened level. Given the key role of nurses in cancer care, the nursing profession embraced the opportunity to provide leadership and research in cancer survivorship and particularly in the areas of distress assessment and management and development of survivor-focused comprehensive programs. All cancer-related disciplines have been inspired to participate in new avenues of research into the development of effective cancer survivor programs and communication tools. In addition, how to reengage with primary care providers and navigate the transition of patients from treatment to living again have been studied to develop evidence-based approaches to providing support for the patient with cancer.

## Transition from Treatment to Living Again

While recognizing that cancer survivorship begins at diagnosis, the transition from active treatment to living again has been an area of intense exploration over the past few years. The growth of clinical practice guidelines regarding the key areas of focus for cancer survivors after active treatment has helped healthcare providers screen for issues and provide evidence-based interventions. Many clinical practice guidelines have been developed to reflect the key areas impacting quality of life for cancer survivors.

Ferrell and colleagues at the City of Hope National Medical Center are credited with adapting quality-of-life measures to a conceptual framework applied to cancer survivors [9]. The model takes into account four domains: physical well-being and symptoms, psychological well-being, social well-being, and spiritual well-being. Using a patient-centered approach, the quality-of-life model validated the key health effects of cancer and its treatment over time and provided a framework from which assessments and programs could be developed. For the cancer survivor, the physical well-being of cancer survivorship can be captured by understanding the patient's functional activities, strength and levels of fatigue, quality of sleep and rest, overall physical health, fertility, and pain. Of particular concern to patients is psychological well-being. Beyond the distress of diagnosis and being in control of treatment, overall control of one's life, anxiety, depression, and enjoyment of life are specific elements relevant to the cancer survivor. The patient moving onto life after treatment must also manage the fear of recurrence. Patients who have undergone systemic chemotherapy may have challenges with cognition and attention. The effects of chemotherapy on the brain of cancer survivors is an area of rich exploration at present. Ferrell and colleagues were also able to capture social and spiritual well-being domains of importance for cancer survivors. The impact of cancer transcends the individual and impacts family, relationships, roles, finances, and work. Appearance and sexual function may be impacted by physical changes after treatment and interplay of a diagnosis of cancer in a relationship. Spiritually, cancer survivors note reflection on the meaning of illness, dealing with uncertainty and finding inner strength and hope and engagement in religion. This understanding of the experience of life after cancer has provided a framework for the development of tools and programs to support survivors.

The National Comprehensive Cancer Network (NCCN) has taken a leadership role in producing a comprehensive evidence-based resource of clinical practice guidelines available to cancer survivor care providers at its website, www.nccn.org. Two guidelines of interest are the Survivorship and Distress Management guidelines [10, 11]. The guideline developed for survivorship provides an evidence-based approach to cancer survivor assessment and intervention. It is created and updated by a NCCN Survivorship panel which reviews key literature and provides regular updates to the guidelines. The panel is a multidisciplinary and inter-professional group of experts representing the broad range of individuals who are integral to the care of cancer patients. This group includes an oncologist, bone marrow transplant expert, urologist, gynecologist, nutritionist, cardiac specialist, infectious disease specialist, primary care provider, exercise physiologist, nurse, epidemiologist, and patient advocate. Within the Survivorship guideline, algorithms cover ten domains: cardiac toxicity; anxiety, depression, and distress; cognitive function; fatigue; menopause; pain; sexual function; sleep disorder; healthy lifestyle; and immunizations and infection. Also included is a comprehensive list of online support tools with topics ranging from physical and mental health to legal and employment issues and integrative therapies. It is important to note that inclusion of survivorship guidelines and distress management guidelines in this publically available resource adds impact to the concept that cancer survivorship is a separate but important dimension in the life of cancer patients.

Another organization which has championed the cause of cancer survivorship is the American Society of Clinical Oncology (ASCO). Similar to the NCCN, ASCO has a multidisciplinary and inter-professional Survivorship Committee. As an organization, ASCO has worked to help provide resources and define the answer to the question "Who is responsible for survivorship care?" The Survivorship Compendium available on the ASCO website at www.asco.org has multiple tools, templates, and educational products to support the provider of cancer survivorship care, including a professional education curriculum [12]. The ASCO Core Curriculum for Cancer Survivorship Education was developed after the ASCO Survivorship Committee in collaboration with the ASCO Professional Development Committee performed an environmental scan and recognized that while many resources exist, there is no single resource that prepares providers comprehensively for work with cancer survivors. Of particular emphasis is the importance of communication in care coordination for cancer survivors [13].

Many models of care exist to support the cancer survivor. However, the effectiveness of these models remains uncertain and have many challenges. Based on a technical brief prepared for the Agency for Healthcare Research and Quality (AHRQ), Halpern and colleagues analyzed the current evidence for cancer survivor health outcomes and provided a broad overview of the models of cancer survivorship care [14]. Four categories of programs were reviewed: physician-led, nurse-led, Survivorship Care Plan (SCP) development as a key component, and comparison of group versus individual counseling. The main conclusions were that additional studies were needed since limited information was available to date. Research should be based on the experiences of cancer survivors and a taxonomy should be developed to help create a common language allowing for the development of outcome metrics that are generalizable and for comparing outcomes across studies. Care coordination remains a challenge and integration across disciplines is difficult at best.

ASCO has also provided a way of considering long-term follow-up care for cancer survivors [15]. Eight different models of care with a summary of advantages and disadvantages are provided. The models are described based on the discipline taking the lead on care as well as whether a specialized setting has been created for care delivery. An emphasis on wellness versus disease management is a feature of many models. Shared models of care between oncology providers and primary care providers include a discussion of whether or not the patient transitions completely out of oncology provider care at some point (Table 8.1).

Other national cancer advocacy and education organizations have contributed to supporting the growing cancer survivor community and their care providers. This includes the LIVESTRONG organization which worked for a decade (2005–2015) in creating the Survivorship Centers of Excellence Network to advance survivorship care and improve the quality of life of cancer survivors after treatment [16]. Using the established NCI-designated comprehensive cancer centers, LIVESTRONG supported programs of a variety of types offering information, care, and services to cancer survivors, their families, and healthcare providers. Eight goals were established for the program centering on raising awareness of cancer survivorship, creating a body of evidence for survivorship care, increasing accessibility for underserved populations, and ensuring that survivor care was covered by insurance. The program successfully identified the benefits and challenges of providing survivorship care. The lessons learned have been used to create a new patient-centered effort to acknowledge and involve all cancer survivors from the beginning of their journey into more global LIVESTRONG Cancer Institutes that integrate principles of survivorship along the continuum of care.

**Table 8.1** Advantages and disadvantages of models of survivorship care

| Model | Characteristics | Advantages | Disadvantages |
|---|---|---|---|
| Oncology specialist | Follow-up with oncology team | Continuity of oncology care | Focus on illness and relapse |
| Multidisciplinary survivorship clinic | Specialized team of experts, especially good for pediatrics | Complex patients benefit most, easy to use; experts in long-term care | Not needed by all; resource intensive |
| Community generalist care | Survivor care delivered by primary care provider | Focus on wellness | Difficult to stay current on changes in cancer care |
| Shared care of survivor | Care coordinated between primary care and oncology specialist | Flexible for all patients regardless of complexity; patient may or may not transition completely out of oncology care | Requires a high level of communication; time intensive |
| Disease- or treatment-specific clinic | Homogenous patient population | Easy for guideline compliance | Only available for cancers with high incidence |
| General survivorship clinic | Provides care for all cancers | Single provider with psychosocial expert support | Difficult to develop expertise in all cancers |
| Consultative survivorship clinic | One-time visit focused on delivery of survivorship care plan and treatment summary | Empowers patients and uses fewer resources | Limits long-term evaluation of side effects |
| Integrated survivorship clinic | Survivor care delivered as part of treatment setting | Survivorship expert delivers care within oncology setting | Patient may expect primary care to be delivered in the same setting and marginalizes primary care providers |

## Distress Assessment and Management

A core component of providing care for cancer survivors is accurately assessing their needs—physical, psychosocial, and spiritual. Most care providers are comfortable with discussions of physical needs and changes after a cancer diagnosis. However, the other areas remain challenging. Patients are often reluctant to mention in a clinical care setting the concerns or issues they may have that fall outside of physical health and well-being. Thus, heightened awareness of holistic approaches to well-being while surviving cancer is needed to stimulate the development of assessment tools and intervention guidelines.

One of the ways to heighten awareness is to mandate it in accreditation settings. The American College of Surgeons CoC in its *Cancer Program Standards 2012: Ensuring Patient-Centered Care* created accreditation Standard 3.2 mandating programs to develop and implement a process to integrate and monitor on-site psychosocial distress screening and referral for care [6]. The importance of screening for distress and psychosocial health needs as part of a high-quality cancer program was emphasized in the 2007 IOM report, *Cancer Care for the Whole Patient: Meeting Psychosocial Health Needs*, which served as the impetus for expanding access to services and developing tools for assessment [17].

The 2007 IOM report was based on the work of the NCCN that quickly developed the clinical care guideline Distress Management [11]. A multidisciplinary and inter-professional panel of experts in oncology, nursing, social work and counseling, psychology, psychiatry, and clergy was convened to review psychosocial care and to make recommendations regarding integration into cancer programs. Four steps are outlined as part of the process:

1. Screening for distress and psychosocial needs, including measuring the level of distress and screening at regular intervals and at times of vulnerability
2. Making and implementing a treatment plan to address the needs
3. Referring to appropriate services for care
4. Reevaluating and adjusting the plan as needed

In support of cancer care for the whole patient, the 2012 CoC Standard 3.2 was endorsed by the American Psychosocial Oncology Society, Association of Oncology Social Work, and Oncology Nursing Society with a joint position statement [18]. In it, a call for a universal definition of distress and the use of validated instruments for assessment was added to the recommendations of the NCCN as noted above. Furthermore, a task force was created to provide assistance and recommendations for meeting the standard [19]. Inclusion of a psychosocial representative on the hospital cancer committee with documentation of distress screening discussions is necessary to ensure that the standard is fully met. Timing for screening should occur not just at the initial visit but also at clinical visits when patients are at highest risk of distress such as during transitions of care. Both clinician-administered and patient-administered assessments of distress are valid and both have their place. Because oncology providers may fail to recognize patient distress, standardized screening is necessary. Prior to implementing screening, cancer programs need to develop pathways of full evaluation and referral so that if a screened patient is identified as distressed, intervention can be offered and begun as soon as possible. Documentation of the screening tool and results is imperative for communicating with other providers and to provide information to measure outcomes.

Many types of healthcare providers are able to administer the distress scales and provide support. In particular, distress assessment and management leadership has been embraced by oncology nursing professionals.

Distress as defined by the NCCN and adopted for use by others is defined as a multifactorial, unpleasant, emotional experience of a psychological, social, and/or spiritual nature that may interfere with the ability to cope effectively with cancer, its physical symptoms, and its treatment. [11] Distress exists along a continuum. Some patients due to other physical and mental health concerns may be at higher risk for moderate-to-severe distress. High levels of distress can make decision-making difficult and at its worst can promote nonadherence to treatment [20].

Given how the CoC Cancer Program Standard has only recently been fully implemented, data is sparse about the effectiveness of distress management in cancer survivors. However, there is at least one randomized controlled clinical trial that shows some evidence of diminished distress at future screenings in lung and breast cancer patients who underwent distress management as part of a comprehensive cancer program [21]. However, barriers remain to implementation such as buy-in among cancer professionals, lack of information on how to implement the screening, and ensuring that appropriate referrals are made when elevated stress is found [22].

## Survivorship Care Plans

The road map to cancer survivorship for the patient and care providers is the survivorship care plan (SCP). It is the key document that represents communication and care coordination during the posttreatment phase. It was explicitly called for in the IOM 2005 report as Recommendation 2 and it is to have two components: a comprehensive care summary and a follow-up plan that is clearly explained [5]. Additionally, it is to be written by the principal provider of oncology treatment and should be reimbursed by third-party payers. Information needed for long-term care includes cancer type, treatments, and possible side effects; a schedule for recommended follow-up; recommendations about preventive practices and how to maintain health; and availability of psychosocial services and information about legal protections for employment and health insurance.

The CoC implemented the Survivorship Care Plan Standard 3.3 beginning with the 2012 Standards and expected full implementation by 2015. As noted earlier, additional modifications with the 2016 Standards allowed a wider variety of individuals to provide the SCP than was originally described. This modification acknowledged both the broad range of cancer professionals who work intimately with cancer patients and the challenges of creating a tool that meets the needs of most patients and providers. In accordance with the IOM 2005 report, the treating oncology provider was initially the sole person who could provide the SCP to the patient. This was modified in the CoC 2016 Standards to include a wider array of oncology health professionals who often provide support and ongoing education for patients. The current list includes physicians, registered nurses, advanced-practice nurses, nurse practitioners, physician assistants, and credentialed clinical navigators. In a partnership with the ASCO, the CoC references the data elements described by ASCO to be included in the treatment summary and SCP [23]. The key components of the SCP include the treatment summary and the follow-up care plan. The treatment summary should include contact information, diagnosis, stage, treatments received, ongoing toxicity or side effects, genetic testing results, or recommendations. The follow-up care plan should include contact information, ongoing therapy, schedule for visits, a list of future tests, symptoms of possible recurrent cancer, late or long-term treatment effects, and psychosocial concerns. Ideally the SCP is provided to the patient at the end of the active treatment but at minimum to meet CoC Standard 3.3 delivery must occur within 6 months after completion of adjuvant therapy other than long-term hormonal therapy and up to 18 months after diagnosis for patients on long-term hormonal therapy.

A wide variety of organizations have worked to create both patient-generated and oncology provider-generated SCP templates. One of the most commonly used templates is the ASCO Treatment Summary and Survivorship Care Plan template [24]. It is suitable for most cancer types. Modified disease-specific templates for the most common types of cancers are also available. It is a provider-generated document that can be used to share both with the patient and primary care providers. The OncoLife Survivorship Care Plan by Penn Medicine is an online tool that allows patients to start the process and work with their providers to complete a full treatment summary and follow-up plan [25]. The Journey Forward organization has developed a mobile app for patients to start their SCP and complete it with their oncology team. It also includes a guided assessment to help patients identify specific concerns to be brought to their cancer team [26]. The American Cancer Society has developed a mobile app related to survivorship care. This app is for oncology providers to have easy access to evidence-based follow-up, side effect/long-term effects, and recommended testing for a variety of cancers which can then be used to develop SCP for patients or used by primary care providers for ongoing care [27].

One of the goals of SCPs and survivorship care has been to improve health and quality-of-life outcomes for cancer survivors. However, to date it has been difficult to show improved outcomes. A systematic review in 2014 of ten prospective studies of 2286 cancer survivors of a variety of common malignancies failed to show a significant effect of SCPs on cancer survivor distress, satisfaction with care, cancer care coordination, or oncologic outcomes in randomized controlled trials [28]. It has been suggested that many factors may be at play making it difficult to show benefit of using a tool such as the SCP [29]. The lack of standardization of SCPs makes it difficult to assess outcomes. Current SCPs do not contain the full complement of recommendations from the 2005 IOM Report. It has been postulated that the lack of comprehensive inclusion of the 2005 IOM recommendations may contribute why it has been difficult to demonstrate improved outcomes. Lastly, there are continued challenges in the transition from the oncology team to reengagement with the primary care team and effective communication among providers.

## Implementation of the Survivorship Care Plan-A View from a Family Physician

Family physicians (FPs) and other primary care providers (PCPs) are often the initial point of contact for patients presenting with cancer and follow-up care. Thus, the primary care team is well positioned to support the cancer survivor from the time of diagnosis and across the continuum of cancer survivorship. Initial symptoms of concern may be expressed and the FP or PCP will complete a physical examination, create a differential diagnosis, and initiate a workup to determine the presence and/or absence of cancer. Educated patients through public health strategies are more prepared to look for symptoms of concern and these are commonly the presenting complaint at an office visit. Family history and patterns of heredity assist in prioritizing potential cancers of major concern for each patient. However, PCPs still need to be cognizant of the cancer potential in a differential diagnosis. Cancer treatments including surgery, chemotherapy, and radiation therapy have improved and patients with cancer may survive longer and have decreased morbidity. However, the complexity of the treatments has also increased and the rapid pace of changing treatment protocols adds to the difficulty of staying knowledgeable about the various impacts of the treatment on each patient. Thus, it is important to develop a SCP for patients that can be communicated in language that is understandable to the patient and the family who may then bring the document to their FP or PCP for further discussion.

The initial diagnosis may be made by the FP or PCP and will often require a referral to surgery and/or medical oncology for development of a treatment plan. Often patients will return to the FP or PCP and request further clarification of their treatment options. The FP (PCP) may be a trusted care giver for several years and the patients desire their opinion. To this end, it is often difficult for the FP or PCP to assist in the decision-making process as they may or may not have received the consultation information from the surgeon or the oncologist. Because of this, it is essential to make sure that all members of the potential treatment team are included regularly in communications to facilitate supportive discussions with patients and to ensure that coordination of care occurs. The care given by the FP or PCP and the supportive assistance to the patient will be much improved with a robust SCP provided to the patient as early as possible.

A comprehensive SCP is especially important in rural communities. The FP or PCP will most likely need to refer to a larger tertiary center for specialized surgical and oncology consultations. Trying to guide a family through a difficult medical diagnosis is more difficult when the medical documentation does not reach the primary care team in time. The importance of a SCP, broadly shared, fully completed, and provided early in the cancer survivorship continuum, cannot be overemphasized. A list of helpful items to provide to the primary care team in a timely fashion is noted here:

## *What Does a FP or PCP Need to Know About a Patient's Cancer Care?*

### Chemotherapy Information

1. Type of chemotherapy and the mode of delivery
2. Timing of the chemotherapy and the location of the administration
3. Important laboratory tests and reasons why the chemotherapy may be held

4. Will the surgeon/oncologist follow the patient throughout the duration of treatment?
5. Potential side effects
6. Information regarding the prognosis if appropriate and the benefit/risks of the chemotherapy strategy

### Radiation Information

1. Radiation treatment protocol, including frequency and length of treatments
2. Potential side effects of the radiation
3. Benefit/risk of the radiation therapy

### Surgery Information

1. Procedure name and whether organs or partial organs were removed
2. Possible complications—early and late
3. Potential impact on nutrition or mobility

### Follow-Up Strategies

1. Frequency of patient visits to the surgeon/oncologist
2. Recommended testing and frequency of testing to identify cancer recurrence
3. Recommended testing for potential side effects
4. Ongoing therapy such as hormonal therapy—duration and type
5. Coordination of visits to both the FP or PCP and the oncology team
6. Management strategy of chronic conditions and ongoing care plan

As the patient receives treatment for their cancer diagnosis and enters the post-treatment survivorship phase, strategies to maintain or improve overall health are important. FPs and PCPs are well skilled in establishing preventive protocols for additional diseases [30]. However, the team needs an accurate understanding of the potential disease manifestations that may occur related to the initial cancer diagnosis and treatments. The development of the SCP, and in particular the treatment summary, clarifies these elements of need for the patient and the FP or PCP as outlined earlier in this chapter. Transitioning from cancer treatment to the posttreatment survivorship phase requires thoughtful communication between the oncology team and the FP or PCP with the inclusion of the patient and their family in order for the most effective care to be provided. By including the FP or PCP, patients may receive more preventive care, targeted for their particular risks [31]. Because of the complexity of cancer diagnosis, the potential for recurrence and in some instances ongoing therapy, patients may desire to continue follow-up with the oncology team which reflects a shared model of care for the survivor.

As the patient continues to survive and thrive, there is usually less contact with the oncology specialist and the patient may return more frequently to the FP or PCP for additional concerns. If the SCP has not been shared with the primary care team, the patient may present for a new concern or symptom and the physician may not have any information. Most FPs or PCPs will ask if there have been any changes since the last appointment. However, it is difficult to allow enough time for a visit, if the past history of a cancer is unknown until the time of the visit. A lack of information from the oncology care team usually leads to record requests and a delay in further care for the patient especially if the oncology care was not in the same health system.

The transition from original diagnosis of cancer to surviving cancer is a difficult journey. The SCP can ease some of the complexities of care by creating a road map for the patient and the primary care team to work toward wellness in this new phase of cancer survivorship. However, more than likely patients will have multiple comorbidities not accounted for in the SCP [31]. Treating the cancer and looking for recurrences are essential but if chronic conditions are not continuously addressed such as hypertension or asthma, the patient may be at higher risk for other problems. Plans need to be in place for the follow-up care of preexisting conditions. The patient may suffer from inadequate management of chronic conditions if the oncology team assumes that the FP or PCP is following the condition and the FP or PCP assumes that the oncologist is following the condition. In effect, no one is following the chronic conditions. Maintaining and establishing this care with the assistance of the FP or PCP on the patient care team will enable quality of care. The hand-off from the specialist is especially critical for the follow-up of chronic conditions. It is appropriate to look for any medication changes that may have resulted during cancer treatment and to make sure that patients have regular medication refills. Chronic conditions such as diabetes, hypertension, arthritis, COPD, and hypothyroidism need to be followed and an appropriate strategy for regular appointments maintained. This can be exhausting for the patient especially under stress from the cancer diagnosis. Ultimately, the patient must be empowered to guide their SCP with the mutual and coordinated support of both the primary care team and the oncology team.

## Summary

There are over 15 million people in the United States who are alive today after completing treatment for cancer. It has been recognized that there is a continuum of experience after a diagnosis of cancer known as cancer survivorship with an impact on quality of life. The period of time after completion of active treatment has been recognized as a unique phase in cancer survivorship as patients transition from a focus on cancer to overall health and well-being. All patients with cancer have varying levels of distress which can be managed if properly assessed. Tools have been created to help patients and healthcare providers have a treatment summary and follow-up plan known as a survivorship care plan (SCP). Coordination of care between the patient, oncology team, and primary care team remains a challenging but intensely desired goal. Cancer program accreditation standards have been created to help improve outcomes of care for this ever-growing group of people. Many national organizations have become stakeholders in the health and well-being of cancer patients in the posttreatment phase of cancer survivorship. Evidence-based clinical guidelines have been developed and outcomes are being measured to demonstrate effectiveness of cancer survivorship programs.

## References

1. Siegel RL, Miller KD, Jemal A. Cancer statistics, 2017. CA Cancer J Clin. 2017;67:7–30.
2. Miller KD, Siegel RL, Lin CC, Mariotto AB, Kramer JL, Rowland JH, et al. Cancer treatment and survivorship statistics, 2016. CA Cancer J Clin. 2016;66(4):271–89.
3. Mullan F. Seasons of survival: reflections of a physician with cancer. N Engl J Med. 1985;313(4):270–3.
4. Survivor. In: The NCI dictionary of cancer terms. National Cancer Institute. 2017. https://www.cancer.gov/piblications/dictionaries/cancer-terms?edrid=450125. Accessed 28 May 2017.
5. Committee on Cancer Survivorship: Improving Care and Quality of Life, National Cancer Policy Board. Institute of Medicine and National Research Council of the National Academies. Executive summary. In: Hewitt M, Greenfield S, Stovall E, editors. From cancer patient to cancer survivor: lost in translation. Washington, DC: The National Academies Press; 2005. p. 1–15.
6. Standard 3.2 Psychosocial distress screening. In: American College of Surgeons Commission on Cancer Program Standards 2012: Ensuring patient-centered care American College of Surgeons. 2012. https://www.facs.org/~/media/files/quality%20programs/cancer/coc/programstandards2012.ash/. Accessed 28 May 2017.
7. Standard 3.3 Survivorship care plan. In: American College of Surgeons Commission on Cancer Program Standards 2012: Ensuring patient-centered care. American College of Surgeons. 2012. https://www.facs.org/~/media/files/quality%20programs/cancer/coc/programstandards2012.ashx. Accessed 28 May 2017.
8. Standard 3.3 Survivorship care plan. In: American College of Surgeons Commission on Cancer Program Standards 2016: Ensuring patient-centered care. American College of Surgeons. 2016. https://www.facs.org/~/media/files/quality%20programs/cancer/coc/2016%20coc%20standards%20manual_interactive%20pdf.ashx. Accessed 28 May 2017.
9. Ferrell BR, Hassey Dow K, Grant M. Measurement of the quality of life in cancer survivors. Qual Life Res. 1995;4(6):523–31.
10. Survivorship. Version 1.2017. National Comprehensive Cancer Network, Inc. 2017. https://www.nccn.org/professionals/physician_gls/pdf/survivorship.pdf. Accessed 29 May 2017.
11. Distress management. Version 2.2016. National Comprehensive Cancer Network, Inc. 2016. https://www.nccn.org/professionals/physician_gls/pdf/distress.pdf. Accessed 29 May 2017.
12. Survivorship compendium. In ASCO Practice & Guidelines. American Society of Clinical Oncology. 2017. https://www.asco.org/practice-guidelines/cancer-care-intitiatives/prevention-survivorship/survivorship/survivorship-compendium. Accessed 29 May 2017.
13. Shapiro CL, Jacobsen PB, Henderson T, Hurria A, Nekhlyudov L, Ng A, et al. ReCAP: ASCO core curriculum for cancer survivorship education. J Oncol Pract. 2016;12(2):145. e108-17
14. Halpern MT, Viswanathan M, Evans TS, Birken SA, Basch E, Mayer DK. Models of cancer survivorship care: overview and summary of current evidence. J Oncol Pract. 2015;11(1):e19–27.

15. Models of long-term follow-up care. In: ASCO Practice & Guidelines. American Society of Clinical Oncology. 2017. https://www.asco.org/practice-guidelines/cancer-care-initiatives/prevention-survivorship/survivorship/survivorship3. Accessed 29 May 2017.
16. LIVESTRONG Survivorship centers of excellence. In: What we do. LIVESTRONG. 2017. https://www.livestrong.org/what-we-do/program/centers-of-excellence-network. Accessed 29 May 2017.
17. Committee on Psychosocial Services to Cancer Patients/Families in a Community Setting, Board on Health Care Services. Institute of Medicine of the National Academies. In: Adler NE, Page AEK, editors. Cancer care for the whole patient: meeting psychosocial health needs. Washington, DC: The National Academies Press; 2007.
18. Implementing screening for distress: the joint position statement from the American Psychosocial Oncology Society, Association of Oncology Social Work, and Oncology Nursing Society. Oncol Nurs Forum. 2013;40(5):423–4.
19. Pirl WF, Fann JR, Greer JA, Braun I, Deshields T, Fulcher C, et al. Recommendations for the implementation of distress screening programs in cancer centers: report from the American Psychosocial Oncology Society (APOS), Association of Oncology Social Work (AOSW), and Oncology Nursing Society (ONS) joint task force. Cancer. 2014;120(19):2946–54.
20. Partridge AH, Wang PS, Avorn J. Nonadherence to adjuvant tamoxifen therapy in women with primary breast cancer. J Clin Oncol. 2003;21(4):602–6.
21. Carlson LE, Groff SL, Maciejewski O, Bultz BD. Screening for distress in lung and breast cancer outpatients: a randomized controlled trial. J Clin Oncol. 2010;28(33):4884–91.
22. Pearman T, Garcia S, Penedo F, Yanez B, Wagner L, Cella D. Implementation of distress screening in an oncology setting. J Community Support Oncol. 2015;13(12):423–8.
23. Mayer DK, Shapiro CL, Jacobson P, McCabe MS. Assuring quality cancer survivorship care: we've only just begun. Am Soc Clin Oncol Educ Book. 2015:e583–91. https://doi.org/10.14694/EdBook_AM.2015.35.e583.
24. ASCO treatment summary and survivorship care plan. In: Survivorship compendium. American Society of Clinical Oncology. 2017. https://ww.asco.org/practice-guidelines/cancer-care-initiatives/prevention-survivorship/survivorship-compendium. Accessed 29 May 2017.
25. OncoLife care plan. In: OncoLink. Penn Medicine. 2017. http://www.oncolink.org/oncolife/. Accessed 29 May 2017.
26. My care plan. In: Patient tools. Journey Forward. 2017. https://www.journeyforward.org/planning-tools/my-care-plan. Accessed 29 May 2017.
27. ACS survivorship care guidelines app. In: National cancer survivorship resource center. American Cancer Society. 2017. https://www.cancer.org/health-care-professionals/national-cancer-survivorship-resource-center/survivorship-guidelines-app-faq.html. Accessed 29 May 2017.
28. Brennan ME, Gormally JF, Butow P, Boyle FM, Spillane AJ. Survivorship care plans in cancer: a systematic review of care plan outcomes. Br J Cancer. 2014;111(10):1899–908.
29. Powel LL, Seibert SM. Cancer survivorship, models, care plans: a status update. Nurs Clin North Am. 2017;52(1):193–209.
30. Cavers D, Cunningham-Burley S, Watson E, Banks E, Campbell C. Experience of living with cancer and comorbid illness: protocol for a qualitative systematic review. BMJ Open. 2017;7(5):e013383.
31. Wilbur J. Surveillance of the adult cancer survivor. Am Fam Physician. 2015;91(1):29–36.

# Chapter 9
# Oncology Rehabilitation

**Julie K. Silver, Vishwa S. Raj, and Eric M. Wisotzky**

## Abbreviations

| | |
|---|---|
| AIMSS | Aromatase inhibitor-induced musculoskeletal symptoms |
| ALL | Acute lymphoblastic leukemia |
| ALND | Axillary lymph node dissection |
| AML | Acute myeloid leukemia |
| CDT | Complete decongestive therapy |
| CIPN | Chemotherapy-induced peripheral neuropathy |
| CLL | Chronic lymphocytic leukemia |
| CML | Chronic myeloid leukemia |
| CoC | Commission on Cancer |
| COPD | Chronic obstructive pulmonary disease |
| CT | Computed tomography |
| ES | Ewing's sarcoma |

J. K. Silver (✉)
Department of Physical Medicine and Rehabilitation, Harvard Medical School, Boston, MA, USA

Spaulding Rehabilitation, Massachusetts General and Brigham and Women's Hospitals, Boston, MA, USA
e-mail: julie_silver@hms.harvard.edu

V. S. Raj
Section of Rehabilitation, Department of Supportive Care, The Levine Cancer Institute, Charlotte, NC, USA

Department of Physical Medicine and Rehabilitation, Carolinas Rehabilitation, Carolinas Medical Center, Carolinas Healthcare System, Charlotte, NC, USA
e-mail: vishwa.raj@carolinashealthcare.org

E. M. Wisotzky
Rehabilitation Medicine, Georgetown University School of Medicine, Washington, DC, USA

Division of Rehabilitation Medicine, Cancer Rehabilitation, MedStar National Rehabilitation Network, Washington, DC, USA
e-mail: eric.m.wisotzky@medstar.net



P. Hopewood, M. J. Milroy (eds.), *Quality Cancer Care*,
https://doi.org/10.1007/978-3-319-78649-0_9

| | |
|---|---|
| FVC | Forced vital capacity |
| GVHD | Graft-versus-host disease |
| HH | Home health agencies |
| HL | Hodgkin's lymphoma |
| ICF | International Classification of Functioning, Disability and Health |
| ICU | Intensive care unit |
| IRF | Inpatient rehabilitation facilities |
| LOS | Length of stays |
| LTAC | Long-term acute care hospitals |
| LTCH | Long-term care hospitals |
| MCI | Mild cognitive impairment |
| MM | Multiple myeloma |
| MRI | Magnetic resonance imaging |
| NAPBC | National Accreditation Program for Breast Centers |
| NCI | National Cancer Institute |
| NCMMR | National Center for Medical Rehabilitation Research |
| NHL | Non-Hodgkin's lymphoma |
| NIH | National Institutes of Health |
| NSCLC | Non-small cell lung carcinoma |
| OT | Occupational therapy |
| PAC | Post-acute care |
| PSA | Prostate-specific antigen |
| PT | Physical therapists |
| QOL | Quality of life |
| RT | Radiation therapy |
| SCT | Stem cell transplantation |
| SLNB | Sentinel lymph node biopsy |
| SLP | Speech and language pathology services |
| SNF | Skilled nursing facilities |
| SNRIs | Serotonin and norepinephrine reuptake inhibitors |
| TKI | Tyrosine kinase inhibitors |
| TNS | Transcutaneous nerve stimulation |
| WHO | World Health Organization |

## Introduction

Cancer rehabilitation is defined as "medical care that should be integrated throughout the oncology care continuum and delivered by trained rehabilitation professionals who have it within their scope of practice to diagnose and treat patients' physical, psychological, and cognitive impairments in an effort to maintain or restore function, reduce symptom burden, maximize independence and improve quality of life in this medically complex population" [1]. Silver et al. described the need to focus on cancer survivors' impairments and resultant disability [2]. This review suggested that most cancer patients, perhaps 65–90%, would benefit from rehabilitation interventions but found that far fewer numbers receive this care. Although the American College of Surgeons Commission on Cancer (CoC) includes cancer rehabilitation as an eligibility requirement, a recent study found that more than 90% of National Cancer Institute (NCI)-Designated Cancer Centers providing clinical care did not have an easily identifiable patient-focused description or link to cancer rehabilitation services on their website [3]. Moreover, only 8% of websites included accurate and detailed information, including listing four core rehabilitation services (physiatry consultations and physical, occupational, and speech therapy).

Recently the Rehabilitation Medicine Department of the Clinical Center at the National Institutes of Health (NIH) with support from the National Cancer Institute (NCI) and the National Center for Medical Rehabilitation Research (NCMRR) convened a panel of subject matter experts to assess and make recommendations about cancer rehabilitation care [4]. The recommendations encouraged stronger efforts toward integrating cancer rehabilitation care models into oncology care from the point of diagnosis onward. They also supported incorporating evidence-based rehabilitation clinical assessment tools, and including rehabilitation professionals in the care continuum in order to facilitate best practice comprehensive cancer care and maximize the functional capabilities of survivors. This chapter provides an overview of how rehabilitation fits into the oncology care continuum and provides examples of cancer-related and cancer treatment-related impairments and problems that are commonly encountered in cancer populations. A comprehensive review of any of these topics is beyond the scope of this chapter and, therefore, readers are encouraged to review some of the key references cited.

## Continuum of Care

Rehabilitation interventions can be provided in several different phases of care, from the time of diagnosis to the end of life. Dietz described four stages of rehabilitation for the cancer patient: (1) preventative, (2) restorative, (3) supportive, and (4) palliative. Treatment in the preventative phase is meant to prevent functional decline of a survivor prior to and during oncological treatment. In the restorative phase, individuals are expected to experience a decline but, through rehabilitation intervention, return to their prior performance status. The supportive phase assumes that a functional decline has occurred, but employs adaptive techniques and therapeutic interventions to allow a patient to reach certain levels of improvement or independence. Finally, in the palliative phase, goals include minimizing or eliminating complications from advanced disease with the goal being to improve quality of life (QOL) [5].

## *Prehabilitation*

Prehabilitation occurs between the time of diagnosis and the beginning of acute oncological treatment to provide physical and psychological interventions that reduce the incidence and severity of future impairments [2]. In one study of individuals with non-small cell lung carcinoma (NSCLC), those who participated in prehabilitation programs showed significantly or clinically relevant improvement in physical fitness [6]. Training was performed in various settings, including at home, in the hospital, and at an outpatient therapy practice or department. Interest in prehabilitation spans several cancer diagnoses because of the potential implications that performance status may have on patient outcomes. A randomized, controlled, parallel group, open-label, multicenter trial is currently evaluating physical recovery 4 weeks postoperatively after cancer surgery in individuals participating in preoperative and postoperative physical activity [7]. Outcomes include length of sick leave, complication rate and severity, length of hospital stay, hospital readmission, and quality of life (QOL). Multimodal approaches, including exercise, nutritional assessment and intervention, and stress reduction techniques, have been shown to improve walking capacity through the perioperative period in patients with colorectal cancer, as compared to patients for whom rehabilitation started after surgery [8]. These activities can complement enhanced recovery programs and facilitate the return to baseline activities of daily living [9]. Barriers for patient access to prehabilitation care include the availability of skilled clinicians trained in cancer care delivery and insurance benefit covering therapy or exercise services.

## *Acute Care Rehabilitation*

Rehabilitation in acute care can be provided by therapy teams in collaboration with physician consultation. Physical therapists (PTs) focus on mobility and safety and help optimize plans of care and discharge settings for patients in the acute care setting [10]. Multidisciplinary discharge planning, with case management and therapy, can result in improved patient outcomes. In one study, when discharge recommendations by PTs were not implemented, patients were 2.9 times more likely to be readmitted to acute care within 30 days of discharge [11]. Outcomes of PT services in the intensive care unit (ICU) have shown improved functional mobility and reduced hospital admissions [12]. Early exercise intervention in critically ill ICU survivors improved 6-min walk test distance, isometric quadriceps strength, and subjective feelings of functional well-being [13].

## *Post-acute Care Rehabilitation*

Medicare guidelines define post-acute care (PAC) as inpatient rehabilitation facilities (IRF), skilled nursing facilities (SNF), long-term care hospitals (LTCH, also known as long-term acute care hospitals, or LTAC), and home health agencies (HH) [14].

**Table 9.1** Admission criteria for inpatient rehabilitation facility programs

| Criteria and comments |
|---|
| Requirement for active and ongoing intervention from multiple therapy disciplines<br>• Including PT, OT, SLP, or prosthetics and orthotics |
| Intensive rehabilitation program consisting of either:<br>• 3 h of therapy per day for at least 5 days per week OR<br>• 15 h of intensive rehabilitation therapy within a 7-consecutive-day period beginning with the day of admission (in certain well-documented cases) |
| Intensive rehabilitation therapy program for which the patient's condition and functional status allow for the patient to make reasonably expected and measurable improvement:<br>• Within a prescribed period of time<br>• That will be of practical value to improve the patient's functional capacity or adaptation to impairments |
| Face-to-face visits for at least 3 days per week by a rehabilitation physician to:<br>• Address medical and functional needs<br>• Modify the course of treatment as needed |
| Intensive and coordinated interdisciplinary team approach |

Although outpatient therapy is not traditionally considered PAC, it remains an additional option for rehabilitation care delivery.

Admission to an IRF must meet reasonable and necessary criteria (Table 9.1) [15]. In addition, IRFs that participate in the Medicare program are required to document that no less than 60% of patients are consistent with 1 of 13 specific conditions [16]. Although cancer is not technically included within these diagnoses, several cancer conditions can be categorized as compliant (Table 9.2) [17]. To qualify for SNF rehabilitation, individuals need a minimum 3-day hospitalization in acute care. The Medicare A benefit would cover all skilled care fees for the first 20 days of SNF rehabilitation, with partial coverage from days 21 to 100 [18]. In addition, patients require a specific set of services relevant to their care (Table 9.3) [19].

LTCHs are a specialized type of hospital that cares for patients with complex medical conditions, including oncological conditions [20]. They serve the role of acute care hospitals with average length of stays (LOS) exceeding 25 days [21]; however, they are also subject to several regulatory requirements regarding patient participation. For example, in order for discharges to be paid at the Standard Federal instead of the site-neutral payment rate, discharges must comply with the following regulations: (1) discharge principal diagnoses should not be categorized into one of the 15 "psychiatric and rehabilitation" diagnosis-related groups; (2) discharge must have been immediately preceded by a hospital discharge [LTCH admission should be within 1 day of the hospital discharge]; and (3) the patient must have either spent 3 days in the intensive care unit while in acute care or received at least 96 h of respiratory ventilation services during the LTCH stay [22]. In addition, LTCHs are subject to a 25% threshold rule, which prevents the LTCH from admitting more than 25% of their total discharges either from a host hospital for which the LTCH is collocated or from any facility that is within 250 yards of the hospital. If the LTCH exceeds the 25% rule, it is subject to financial penalty.

The primary rehabilitation focus of HH programs includes maintenance of physical functioning, mental functioning, and QOL, and slowing of the rate of decline in

**Table 9.2** Conditions compliant with the 60% rule for inpatient rehabilitation facilities

| Conditions and comments |
|---|
| Amputation |
| Arthropathies that have led to functional impairments of ambulation and ADLs, including:<br>• Active polyarticular rheumatoid arthritis<br>• Psoriatic arthritis<br>• Seronegative arthropathies |
| Brain injury |
| Burns<br>• With evidence that less intensive treatments were attempted and failed to improve the patient's condition before admission to IRF |
| Congenital deformity |
| Fracture of femur (hip) |
| Knee or hip joint replacement (or both) during an acute care hospitalization immediately preceding IRF stay and meeting one of the following criteria:<br>• Patient underwent bilateral hip or bilateral knee joint replacement surgery during the acute care hospitalization and immediately preceding IRF admission<br>• Patient is extremely obese with body mass index of at least 50 at the time of admission to IRF<br>• Patient is 85 years or older at the time of admission to IRF |
| Major multiple trauma |
| Neurological disorders including:<br>• Multiple sclerosis<br>• Motor neuron disease<br>• Polyneuropathy<br>• Muscular dystrophy<br>• Parkinson's disease |
| Severe or advanced osteoarthritis with the following conditions*:<br>• Involvement of two or more weight-bearing joints with joint deformity<br>• Atrophy of muscles surrounding the joint<br>• Significant functional impairment of ambulation and ADLs<br>*Joint cannot be counted if it has a prosthesis |
| Spinal cord injury |
| Stroke |
| Systemic vasculitides<br>• With joint inflammation leading to functional impairments of ambulation and ADLs |

order to allow the patient to remain in the home setting [23]. Therapy interventions may include PT, occupational therapy (OT), and speech and language pathology services (SLP). Individuals receiving home health services must be under the care of a physician who then certifies the need for skilled therapy services, and must meet one of the following requirements: (1) expected improvement of condition in a reasonable and generally predictable period of time, (2) need for a skilled therapist to safely and effectively design a maintenance program for the specified condition, and (3) need for a skilled therapist to safely and effectively perform a maintenance program for the specified condition. Furthermore, the patient must be certified as homebound to receive these services [24].

**Table 9.3** Items and services furnished to an inpatient of a subacute nursing facility

| Care and comments |
|---|
| Nursing care provided by or under the supervision of a registered professional nurse<br>• Bed and board in connection with furnishing of such nursing care |
| Physical or occupational therapy and/or speech-language pathology services<br>• Furnished by the skilled nursing facility or by others under arrangements with them made by the facility |
| Medical social services |
| Such drugs, biologicals, supplies, appliances, and equipment, furnished for use in the skilled nursing facility<br>• As are ordinarily furnished by such facility for the care and treatment of inpatients |
| Medical services<br>• Provided by an intern or resident-in-training of a hospital with which the facility has in effect a transfer agreement under an approved teaching program of the hospital<br>• Other diagnostic or therapeutic services provided by a hospital with which the facility has such an agreement in effect |
| Other services necessary to the health of the patients<br>• As are generally provided by skilled nursing facilities, or by others under arrangements |

Outpatient rehabilitation can be provided in three different types of organizations: rehabilitation agencies, clinics, and public health agencies [25]. Although covered by Medicare Part B, outpatient "therapy cap" limits exist. The therapy provider must provide documentation for medically reasonable and necessary services and provide this information on the claims form [26]. If outpatient therapy costs are higher than the threshold amounts, a Medicare contractor may review medical records for medical necessity [27].

## Cancer and Cancer-Related Impairments

### *Cancer-Related Pain*

Oncology-related pain may be due to the cancer itself, effects of treatment, or effects from other comorbid conditions. Determining the etiology of the pain and establishing the correct diagnosis are essential to effective treatment. Working closely with a rehabilitation team, including physiatrists who are trained in the diagnosis and treatment of neurological and musculoskeletal pain conditions, is important.

Pain symptoms in cancer survivors can be confusing and are often due to multiple factors (e.g., medication side effects, loss of range of motion due to surgery or radiation therapy, deconditioning, overuse of a "healthy" part of the body). Additionally, patients often report pain symptoms in conjunction with other symptoms—sometimes called a "cluster" [28]. For example, patients experiencing pain may also have difficulty with sleep. Sleep deprivation combined with pain may intensify symptoms of fatigue and anxiety or depression. Treating the pain as well as other associated symptoms is important to both quality of life and function.

Pain is typically divided into *nociceptive* and *neuropathic* pain. Nociceptive pain is further subdivided into *visceral* and *somatic* pain. Visceral pain is usually poorly localized, dull aching pain whereas somatic pain is often sharp and well localized to discrete anatomic regions. *Neuropathic pain* is due to injury or inflammation of nerve tissue in the central or peripheral nervous system. Chemotherapy-induced peripheral neuropathy (CIPN) is the most common neurological condition in survivors treated with chemotherapy, but other focal neuropathies may develop as well (e.g., postsurgical neuropathies from incisions, neuromas, and scar tissue). Medications which may be considered for neuropathic pain include gabapentin, pregabalin, tricyclic antidepressants, and serotonin norepinephrine reuptake inhibitors [29].

The pharmacologic treatment of cancer pain is often dealt with in a sequential stepwise approach based upon the severity and type of pain as proposed by the World Health Organization (WHO analgesic ladder, Table 9.4) [30]. When looking at the analgesic ladder, one can consider skipping steps, or starting at a higher step for times of acute/severe pain and then stepping down once the pain has been controlled. Of note, bisphosphonates (pamidronate and zoledronic acid) have analgesic properties in cases of bone pain secondary to metastasis and multiple myeloma.

Nonpharmacological approaches can also be considered. Psychological approaches such as patient education, relaxation, guided imagery, meditation, hypnosis, and group therapy have been shown to be helpful for pain in cancer survivors. In one study, hypnosis appeared to be helpful for pain in breast cancer survivors [31].

Studies that have evaluated the benefits of exercise during and after cancer treatment have demonstrated that supervised physical activity in conjunction with appropriate precautions (e.g., monitoring of blood counts, cardiopulmonary status) is usually safe and has positive benefits regarding health and QOL. Supervised exercise may confer more benefit than unsupervised exercise and safety should always be a priority in this population [32]. Exercise, including resistance, aerobic, and range of motion, can be incorporated throughout the cancer care continuum and included in prehabilitation [33]. However, even supervised exercise may cause more pain in survivors, and the risk and benefits should always be considered [34], and

**Table 9.4** Analgesic ladder

| Step | Pain level | Intervention | Comment |
|---|---|---|---|
| 1 | Mild | Non-opioid analgesics such as acetaminophen or NSAIDs | Long-term use of NSAIDs must be monitored as they can cause GI bleeding as well as platelet and renal dysfunction |
| 2 | Mild-moderate | Weak opioids (such as tramadol and codeine) | May be given in combination with non-opioid analgesics |
| 3 | Moderate-severe | Strong opioids such as morphine, oxycodone, fentanyl, hydromorphone, and methadone | – |
| 4 | Moderate-severe | Surgical procedures, such as brain stimulators, nerve blocks, and neurolysis | – |

the prescription modified based on the patient's response. Balance training, although more focused on improving balance than pain, is a specific type of intervention that has been demonstrated to be superior to cardiovascular and strengthening exercises in people with neuropathy (e.g., CIPN) [35].

Targeted exercises such as those prescribed in physical therapy may improve upper quadrant morbidity by increasing range of motion and strength and reducing pain in breast and head and neck cancer survivors [36–38]. Exercises including strength training, walking, cycling, yoga, qigong, or tai chi may improve strength and endurance as well as lessen pain in cancer survivors.

Modalities such as transcutaneous nerve stimulation (TENS) were shown in one study to improve bone pain in cancer patients [39]. Other nonpharmacological treatments can be considered such as massage and acupuncture. However, it is important to note that modalities, including but not limited to electrical stimulation, superficial heat, and massage, generally are not performed directly over a tumor site [40]. Deep heat (e.g., ultrasound and phonophoresis) is usually contraindicated, although evidence is lacking and the contraindication is based on a "standard of care" belief. Spinal traction and/or manipulation is contraindicated in those patients with spinal metastases or with significant osteoporosis.

Interventional approaches may be considered in cases of more severe pain [41]. Celiac plexus block has been shown to help pain in patients with pancreatic cancer. It also helped to decrease opioid consumption. Kyphoplasty and vertebroplasty have been shown to significantly reduce pain and reduce analgesic consumption in cancer patients with compression fractures. Intrathecal drug delivery systems have been shown to improve intractable cancer pain.

## *Fatigue*

Fatigue may lead to decreased function and significant disability in cancer survivors. Like pain, fatigue may limit function at home, at work, in the community, and in social and recreational activities. For example, in a study of gynecological cancer survivors, researchers found that fatigue was a significant problem for the women in the study, particularly on the initial return to work [42].

Fatigue is a common complaint for those without a cancer diagnosis, and so it is important to differentiate the usual fatigue symptoms that people may experience from cancer-related fatigue (CRF). By definition, CRF *is an unusual, persistent, subjective sense of tiredness related to cancer or cancer treatment that interferes with functioning* [43]. CRF becomes problematic and pathologic when it occurs during normal daily activities, persists for long periods of time, and does not respond to rest [44, 45]. CRF is a diagnosis of exclusion and other potential causes of fatigue in cancer survivors should be ruled out during evaluation, including but not limited to anemia, emotional distress (e.g., depression), deconditioning, hormonal imbalance (e.g., thyroid dysfunction), infection, malnutrition, medication side effects, and sleep disturbance (e.g., insomnia and/or sleep apnea).

Treating fatigue in cancer survivors may involve pharmacologic and nonpharmacologic approaches. An excellent review of fatigue in cancer survivors by Gerber succinctly summarized the most important interventions in this manner, “Effective treatments include correction of other medical problems, especially anemia, cognitive behavioral therapy, exercise, modafinil, and corticosteroids for short-term use” [46]. When using medications, it is important to assess the side effects and combination of all prescription and nonprescription drugs as well as any other over-the-counter supplements that a patient is taking. Treating underlying medical conditions such as thyroid dysfunction or insomnia may also require the use of medications. With regard to nonpharmacologic approaches, much of the research has focused on aerobic exercise. For example, a recent meta-analysis of exercise in breast cancer survivors found that exercise interventions improve short-term fatigue in this population [47]. However, muscle fatigue may affect physical performance and fatigue [48]. The sports medicine literature includes a considerable evidence base to support the benefits of both aerobic and resistance exercise. In contrast, resistance exercise has been less well studied in the cancer population, although it should be considered in the context of treating fatigue [49]. There are numerous other interventions, some focusing on mind-body strategies, such as meditation, that may also be beneficial in treating fatigue.

## *Lymphedema and Other Swelling Disorders*

Swelling disorders are common sequelae in patients with cancer. There can be many causes of edema including venous thromboembolism, venous compression (from tumor or radiation fibrosis), venous insufficiency, metastatic cancer to lymphatics, cellulitis, medication side effects (e.g., from chemotherapy or corticosteroids), hypoalbuminemia, postoperative edema, postradiation edema, seroma, lipedema, and lymphedema.

Lymphedema is defined as an abnormal accumulation of protein-rich fluid and chronic inflammation that results in the swelling of subcutaneous tissue because of mechanical failure of part of the lymphatic system. Lymphedema is typically a painless swelling, but associated morbidity may include discomfort. Other sequelae may include disfigurement, difficulty using the affected limb, secondary musculoskeletal disorders (which may cause pain), skin disorders, and cellulitis.

Lymphedema may occur in many types of cancer including, but not limited to, breast cancer (affecting the arm(s) and/or chest/breast), gynecological cancer (affecting the leg(s)), and head and neck cancer (affecting the neck and/or face). It is important to be aware that the risk and incidence of lymphedema depend on the cancer diagnosis and treatment. This awareness will inform patient counseling and index of suspicion for lymphedema. The risk of developing lymphedema in breast cancer patients varies depending on the study cited (Table 9.5) [50].

The definitive diagnosis of lymphedema can be challenging, and there are multiple tools to assess swelling including circumferential limb measurements, calcu-

**Table 9.5** Lymphedema risk in breast cancer patients

| Intervention | Risk |
|---|---|
| Sentinel lymph node biopsy (SLNB) | <5% |
| SLNB and radiation | Approximately 10% |
| Axillary lymph node dissection (ALND) | Approximately 20–30% |
| ALND and radiation | Approximately 30–50% |

**Table 9.6** Lymphedema staging

| Stage | Description | Comment |
|---|---|---|
| 0 | Subclinical | No visible edema, but slight limb heaviness may be noted |
| 1 | Mild | Pitting edema, reversible with elevation |
| 2 | Moderate | No relief with elevation, nonpitting, very mild skin thickening (fibrosis) possible |
| 3 | Severe | Affected limb becomes very large, misshapen, and skin is very fibrotic |

lating limb volume, water displacement, perometry, and bioimpedance spectroscopy. The gold standard of diagnosis is a nuclear medicine test called lymphoscintigraphy [51]. Many guidelines, including the CoC's National Accreditation Program for Breast Centers (NAPBC), recommend baseline measurement before lymph node dissection followed by periodic reassessment after surgery [52].

It should be noted that of breast cancer patients who at some point are diagnosed with lymphedema, approximately 80% will present within the first 2 years after surgery and 89% will present by year three after surgery [53]. In the remaining 11% of patients, lymphedema can occur at any time, including 20 years or more after lymph node dissection. Given that the late development of lymphedema is less common, other etiologies (especially cancer recurrence) should be considered. Several different staging systems exist for lymphedema in patients. One that is commonly used is that proposed by the International Society of Lymphology (Table 9.6) [54].

In terms of treatment, for lymphedema that is diagnosed subclinically (via bioimpedance) or for very mild lymphedema (<8% increase in limb volume), 1 month of wearing a compression sleeve during the day along with frequent elevation can typically reverse the condition [55]. Slowly progressing with upper extremity resistance exercises may help as well. For mild edema that does not respond to a compression sleeve or for edema with a >8% increase in volume, patients should be referred to a certified lymphedema therapist for complete decongestive therapy (CDT). CDT entails (1) manual lymphatic drainage via gentle lymphatic massage, (2) multilayer bandaging, (3) teaching of exercises, and (4) education about precautions and skin care. After discharge from CDT, patients typically wear a compression garment to prevent recurrence. Some patients may also benefit from a home pneumatic compression pump. If conservative treatment fails, other available treatments include stellate ganglion blocks or surgeries such as liposuction, lymphovenous anastomosis, or vascularized lymph node transfer.

The topic of lymphedema precautions is controversial [56] and physicians should familiarize themselves with the nuances of the available data regarding precautions so as to counsel patients in the most effective manner. Because the greatest risk factor for lymphedema is obesity [57], patients should be counseled about weight control and lifestyle modifications. Upper extremity resistance exercise has been deemed to be safe in patients with lymphedema or at risk for lymphedema [58]. However, patients should use caution to slowly build up resistance training and to not use resistance they would consider greater than "somewhat difficult." Survivors with lymphedema are typically instructed to wear a compression sleeve during resistance exercise. Those at risk for lymphedema may choose to wear a sleeve during resistance exercise. Individuals with or at risk for lymphedema are usually instructed to avoid blood pressure checks, venipuncture, tight-fitting clothes, and excessive heat to the limb. These recommendations are controversial however. Survivors are typically instructed to wear a compression sleeve with air travel as altitude may induce edema. This point is also controversial and patients should be counseled about the risks and benefits of this intervention. As survivors after lymph node dissection and/or radiation are potentially at risk for cellulitis, common sense skin precautions are advised, including avoiding trauma to the skin of the affected extremity. If the skin is broken, cleaning the skin and using a topical antibiotic are recommended, and immediate medical attention should be sought following any sign of cellulitis.

## *Cognitive Dysfunction*

Cognitive dysfunction in cancer survivors may result from the cancer itself due to primary or metastatic brain tumors. Although there is some oncology-focused rehabilitation research aimed at treating cognitive dysfunction [59, 60], there is a much larger body of literature describing cognitive interventions in noncancer conditions including but not limited to traumatic brain injury and stroke that are beyond the scope of this chapter. However, it is important to note that the cognitive issues in cancer survivors are often similar to those in noncancer populations and multidisciplinary rehabilitation care is well developed and should be the standard of care for oncology patients. Oncologists may be more familiar with the roles of neuropsychologists and physical therapists (to treat physical impairments due to brain tumors) than they are with other members of a best practice cognitive rehabilitation team including physiatrists as well as occupational and speech therapists. For more information and best practice guidelines, readers are referred to a comprehensive and excellent evidence-based review of cognitive rehabilitation published by the American Congress of Rehabilitation Medicine that elegantly describes how to translate the evidence into practice [61].

Delirium is also a common cause of cognitive problems in cancer patients, especially the elderly and/or those with advanced oncological disease. Reversing the symptoms of delirium is a priority for both oncology and rehabilitation care providers and the literature provides excellent guidelines and interventions designed to address this problem [62].

Mild cognitive impairment (MCI) is often called "chemo brain" and may result from chemotherapy as well as other oncology-directed treatments such as radiation therapy. The phenomenon is well described in the literature though the diagnosis and contributing factors remain elusive. Exercise has been a mainstay of treating MCI [63].

## *Bone Issues*

The most prevalent forms of primary bone cancer include osteosarcoma, chondrosarcoma, and Ewing's sarcoma [64].

Osteosarcoma is the most common primary bone malignancy. Incidence is greatest between the ages of 10 and 14, and in adults older than the age of 65. It is more common in males than females (5.4 vs. 4.0 per million, respectively). The most commonly affected areas are near the metaphyseal growth plate, specifically in the femur, tibia, and humerus [65]. Surgery remains the mainstay of treatment, with limb salvage serving as the first option for intervention. Wide margins and expected functional recovery are important when performing limb salvage surgery. Although no survival advantage has been shown when comparing amputation to limb salvage, there are specific situations when amputation is preferred. Neoadjuvant and adjuvant chemotherapy may also be necessary [66]. Radiation therapy (RT) can be applied in cases of unresectable tumors, intralesional resection, or palliation for symptomatic metastases [67].

Chondrosarcoma accounts for 25% of all bone tumors [68]. Cure can be achieved with complete surgical resection for nonmetastatic lesions. For low-grade chondrosarcoma, intralesional curettage followed by local adjuvant treatment can provide appropriate local control, and thus decrease morbidity associated with wide excision and reconstruction. Although slow growing, RT could be used in cases of incomplete resection, palliation, and circumstances where complete resection would not be possible or would cause significant morbidity [69].

Although Ewing's sarcoma (ES) is most commonly diagnosed in the second and third decades of life, it is the second most common malignant tumor in children and young adults [70]. Chemotherapy can be administered prior to surgery in an attempt to eradicate micrometastases, decrease tumor size preoperatively, and guide postoperative chemotherapy options. RT is effective in treating centrally located lesions and destroying all viable tumor cells; it can also be provided both preoperatively and postoperatively in cases of tumors with high risk of local relapse. Surgical resection can help improve the rate of local control [71].

Bone is a common site for metastatic disease, and the most common primary sites include breast and prostate cancers. Bone lesions exist in two forms, osteolytic and osteoblastic. Osteolytic lesions are bone destructive, promoting bone resorption in cases of primary cancers such as multiple myeloma (MM) and breast cancer. Osteoblastic lesions, such as prostate cancer, are bone forming and commonly occur adjacent to metastatic tumors. Treatment focuses on decreasing tumor

**Table 9.7** Mirels' scoring system

| Score | Site of lesion | Size of lesion (cortex involvement) | Nature of lesion | Pain |
|---|---|---|---|---|
| 1 | Upper limb | <1/3 | Blastic | Mild |
| 2 | Lower limb | 1/3–2/3 | Mixed | Moderate |
| 3 | Trochanteric region | >2/3 | Lytic | Severe |

burden, preventing progression, and reducing bone-associated complications, such as pathological fractures, hypercalcemia, and pain. RT and/or surgery are influenced by the level of tumor involvement at the time of diagnosis [72]. Mirels' classification system can be used to determine the stability for metastases of the long bone, and risk of impending pathological fracture (Table 9.7). Prophylactic fixation is recommended for scores of 9 or greater, whereas scores of 7 or less can be managed with RT and medications. Clinical judgment for fixation must be used for a score of 8 [73].

Impairments amenable to rehabilitation protocols may result from the treatment of bone tumors as well as the bone tumors themselves. Functional decline can result in further surgical intervention secondary to hematoma, wound necrosis, and dehiscence. Patients with significant muscle manipulation and resection may experience heterotopic ossification, which can lead to pain and impaired range of motion around large joints. Acute and chronic musculoskeletal issues, fibrosis, contracture, and peripheral nerve injuries are all possible after treatment with RT [74]. Endoprostheses are effective treatments for patients with bone tumors and limb salvage, although the affected limb is subject to limitations in range of motion due to loss of limb muscle mass. This may also worsen ambulation capacity and increase the need for assistance during gait [75]. Individuals with bone tumors experience several functional impairments that limit their daily lives. Leg length discrepancy and amputation are common, and cause gait abnormalities that require assistive devices, such as canes, crutches, walkers, and wheelchairs. Difficulties with ambulation surround poor balance, decreased strength, or lack of mobility after surgical resection. These impairments affect vocational work, social life, participation in leisure activities, and identity [76]. Rehabilitation can provide supportive care to address these tumor and treatment effects, improve physical performance, and reintegrate individuals within their social constructs.

## Examples of Impairments in Specific Cancer Types

### *Breast Cancer*

Functional morbidity is common in breast cancer survivors and there is a large potential role for rehabilitation specialists to play in their care. Cardiovascular and overall strengthening exercise regimens have been studied fairly extensively and with impressive results that include improving QOL and function and potentially reducing the risk of cancer recurrence [77].

Less commonly studied, yet very important with respect to pain and disability in the breast cancer population, is upper quadrant impairment. Breast and arm pain are strongly associated with sick leave and disability [78]. Notably, general cardiovascular exercise may confer QOL benefits and potentially reduce the risk of cancer recurrence, but would not address the upper quadrant functional morbidity issues that are common in this population. Musculoskeletal disorders, regardless of where on the body they present, can typically be treated with conventional rehabilitation approaches including, but not limited to, PT, OT, medications, and/or injections.

Postmastectomy pain syndrome is a nondescript diagnosis that encompasses a variety of anatomic diagnoses which may cause pain in breast cancer survivors. In one study, nearly half the women developed myofascial pain irrespective of the type of breast and axillary surgery performed [79]. Shoulder dysfunction is common in breast cancer survivors with a 2016 study showing that 10% of survivors developed adhesive capsulitis [80]. Multiple studies have demonstrated altered mechanics in the shoulder on the side of the breast cancer as well as on the contralateral side [81]. These findings can be associated with rotator cuff tendinopathy, myofascial pain, cervical radiculopathy, and other upper quadrant functional impairments [82]. Intercostobrachial neuralgia is anecdotally a common cause of postmastectomy pain, although true incidence has not been established. This condition can be treated similar to other neuropathic pain disorders. For example, medications that treat neuropathic pain or ultrasound-guided intercostobrachial nerve block can be considered [83].

Pre-reconstruction pain syndrome may be seen in patients who have had mastectomy with either implant or autologous tissue reconstruction. It may present as tightness, pain, and/or spasm of chest wall muscles. Treatment can include stretching and myofascial release (with caution regarding mobilization of a tissue expander or implant), muscle relaxants, nerve-stabilizing medications, serotonin and norepinephrine reuptake inhibitors (SNRIs), or botulinum toxin injections (for which image guidance may be warranted in order to avoid implant puncture). Ultrasound-guided serratus plane block is another procedure that can be considered for diffuse chest wall pain or tightness [84].

Chest wall neuromas may occur and typically present as lateral chest wall pain at the nipple line (T4) or below the breast (T5) [85]. Treatment considerations include manual release, neuropathic pain medications, or local corticosteroid injection. Incisional pain presents along the surgical incision which may be hypomobile and adhered to the underlying chest wall. Treatments include scar massage, topical medications, or local corticosteroid injection.

Axillary cording, often called axillary web syndrome, is a common condition that typically occurs shortly after lymph node dissection and may spontaneously resolve. The patient may feel a "pop" which is usually not a concern. Resolution can be hastened by manual release and stretching exercises performed by a PT or OT.

Chemotherapy-induced peripheral neuropathy is a common cause of pain in all cancer survivors treated with chemotherapeutic agents and is a well-described complication of taxane-based therapy in the breast cancer population [86]. Whether to discontinue chemotherapy midcourse is an oncological decision that may benefit from a prospective surveillance approach [87]. From a rehabilitation perspective, the focus is on treating associated pain, proprioception, and balance issues. Importantly balance training, a unique type of prescribed exercise, likely will improve the latter symptoms more than cardiovascular or strengthening exercises [35].

Women who are postmenopausal with estrogen receptor-positive breast tumors (up to 80% of those with breast cancer) are often given aromatase inhibitors. This class of medications has been demonstrated to decrease the risk of breast cancer recurrence as much as 40% [88]. Aromatase inhibitor-induced musculoskeletal symptoms (AIMSS) occur in up to 50% of patients [89]. Arthralgias are common and well-known side effects associated with these drugs, typically affecting the wrist/hand, knee, spine, ankle/foot, and hip. Tendinopathies are less well known, but aromatase inhibitors are one of the four classes of drugs that have been documented to cause tendon problems. These may include de Quervain's tenosynovitis (first dorsal compartment of the wrist), trigger fingers, and finger flexor tenosynovitis at the wrist (contributing to pressure on the median nerve in the carpal tunnel and leading to carpal tunnel syndrome) [90].

There is a lack of high-quality evidence for interventions to treat AIMSS. Cardiovascular exercise likely has the highest level of evidence and the typical 150 min of moderate-intensity cardiovascular exercise is recommended [91]. Acupuncture has been studied but results have been mixed [92]. Duloxetine has shown promise but studies have been small, single-arm noncontrolled trials [93]. The same can be said for glucosamine/chondroitin sulfate which some patients will use [94]. Oral corticosteroids were used in one noncontrolled trial (prednisolone 5 mg daily for 5 days) with some short-term and long-term relief [95]. Trials of vitamin D supplementation have had mixed results [96]. Those with positive results have recommended keeping 25-hydroxyvitamin D levels at about 40 ng/mL. Clinicians can consider typical rehabilitation approaches including the use of NSAIDs, other medications (gabapentin, pregabalin, and opioids), physical/occupational therapy, bracing, and corticosteroid injections depending on the specific symptom.

Aromatase inhibitors also cause bone loss and, while osteopenia and osteoporosis are generally silent conditions, they may predispose patients to significant pain and disability. For example, a breast cancer survivor, who is now on an aromatase inhibitor but was previously treated with chemotherapy, may have some chemotherapy-induced peripheral neuropathy and problems with balance which might predispose her to falls that may result in a hip fracture. Therefore, even someone who does not complain of pain while on an aromatase inhibitor may benefit from balance training to reduce the potential for future pain and disability.

## *Lung Cancer*

Lung cancer rehabilitation is challenging for a variety of reasons including that most people are diagnosed later in life with advanced-stage disease and often have comorbidities such as chronic obstructive pulmonary disease (COPD). Lung cancer treatment, in both early and advanced disease, often causes or contributes to pain, dyspnea, fatigue, cognitive deficits, impaired balance, and mood disorders—all of which tend to negatively impact health-related QOL [97, 98].

A recent review by Bayly and Lloyd-Williams focused on rehabilitation in advanced disease [99]. They noted that studies mostly utilizing patient self-report measures have demonstrated functional impairments, limitations, and restrictions across all domains in the International Classification of Functioning, Disability and Health (ICF). Rehabilitation research that provides an evidence base to direct interventions in this population is sparse. However, the implementation of low-dose chest computed tomography (CT) screening will support earlier diagnosis and surgical treatment options for this patient population.

A recent systematic review highlighted the value of prehabilitation in lung cancer treatment and noted that interventions were likely most effective if they were appropriately prescribed by knowledgeable healthcare professionals (e.g., the patients were supervised and/or had personalized interventions) [6]. A 2017 Cochrane database systematic review in surgical non-small cell lung cancer patients found that preoperative exercise training may reduce the risk of developing a postoperative pulmonary complication, duration of intercostal catheter use, and postoperative length of hospital stay, and improve both exercise capacity and forced vital capacity (FVC) in people undergoing lung resection [100]. In the surgical population, a panel of experts convened by Silver and Carli described multimodal lung cancer prehabilitation opportunities that included general cardiovascular exercise, targeted respiratory muscle exercise, smoking cessation, stress reduction, and nutritional support [33].

Although conventional pulmonary rehabilitation programs may benefit patients diagnosed with lung cancer, it's important to recognize the special needs of the oncology population and ensure that they are addressed. For example, in a conventional pulmonary rehabilitation program, the wait list to get in may take weeks or months. Furthermore, these programs do not prepare patients for upcoming surgery and typically wouldn't address the associated issues of increased protein intake and glycemic control. Smoking cessation efforts may be less aggressive and take longer as they are often targeted at improving symptoms of COPD and not postoperative morbidity such as wound and pulmonary infections. Conventional pulmonary rehabilitation programs don't necessarily have experience with the various lung cancer surgical procedures or other oncology-directed treatment and clinicians may not be familiar with how to treat post-thoracotomy pain syndromes or other problems. The opportunity for conventional pulmonary rehabilitation programs to address the unique needs of cancer patients is evolving [101].

Studies have generally demonstrated benefits of rehabilitation in the lung cancer population, especially with regard to exercise tolerance and walking distance. High-intensity aerobic exercise, if tolerated by patients, may have the greatest effect on pulmonary and physical function [102]. However, one study in post-thoracotomy patients demonstrated that functional gains came at the cost of increased pain [34]. Therefore, it is important to carefully prescribe rehabilitation interventions, including therapeutic exercise, in this vulnerable population.

## Prostate Cancer

Prostate cancer is the most common malignancy in men [103]. For low-grade localized cancers, active surveillance using serum prostate-specific antigen (PSA), biopsy, and MRI is recommended. If intervention is pursued, several options exist for local treatment. Specifically, patients may receive surgical intervention with radical prostatectomy, external beam RT, brachytherapy, cryotherapy, high-intensity focal ultrasound, and photodynamic therapy. Long-term androgen deprivation combined with radical RT is the standard of care for high-risk and locally advanced disease, and is used as an adjuvant to external beam RT for higher risk disease. Metastatic disease can be treated with surgical castration or antiandrogen medications. If the metastatic disease is castration resistant, several treatment options exist, including single-drug steroids, hormonal treatments, and cytotoxic chemotherapy. Bone metastases are common in castration-resistant prostate cancer that can be treated with agents that inhibit osteoclastic activity, such as bisphosphonate therapy or denosumab [104].

For individuals receiving androgen deprivation therapy, bone mineral density can decrease significantly and increase the risk of fracture. Fractures may also be secondary to bone metastases and RT to the bone. In the case of metastases to the spine, spinal cord compression could cause generalized weakness below the level of the lesion, and bowel and bladder dysfunction. Several complications can occur during surgical intervention, including thrombosis and peripheral nerve injury due to positioning [105]. RT and hormonal therapy can result in urinary complications and gastrointestinal toxicity leading to further surgical intervention and functional decline [106]. Prostatectomy is associated with higher risk of urinary incontinence [107]. For individuals who receive RT combined with hormonal therapy, fatigue can influence QOL, general activity levels, concentration, and mood [108]. Many of these conditions and impairments can be treated by rehabilitation professionals and managed with medical, therapy, and nursing interventions.

## Colorectal Cancer

Several risk factors have led to increasing incidence in the rate of colorectal cancer worldwide, including unhealthy diet, obesity, physical inactivity, and smoking [109]. However, rates continue to decrease in the United States secondary to risk factor modifications [110]. Worldwide annual incidence for colorectal cancer in 2012 was 1,360,000 [111]. Surgical resection and total mesorectal excision are standard approaches for operative intervention, with emphasis on removal of the cancer and corresponding lymph nodes. Laparoscopy is commonly used in place of open surgery, and results in fewer blood transfusions, improved return of bowel function, and shorter duration of hospital stay. Neoadjuvant treatment with chemotherapy and RT may be needed for more diffuse disease or higher risk of recurrence.

For stage III disease after curative resection, and stage II disease with high risk of relapse, adjuvant chemotherapy is recommended. Surgical resection at the site of metastases and palliative chemotherapy should be offered when possible for progressive disease [112].

Morbidity is still a concern, despite the improved survival rates for all stages of colorectal cancer [113]. Long-term survivors experience fatigue and health effects attributed to the cancer and its treatment, including physical discomfort and activity limitations [114]. Complications from surgery are more common in the elderly, such as urinary, respiratory, and surgical wound infections. They also had higher rates of cardiovascular and respiratory complications [115]. Surgical nerve damage in rectal cancer can lead to chronic urinary incontinence and difficulty with bladder emptying [116]. Treatment with oxaliplatin can result in peripheral neuropathy with sensory impairment in a stocking-glove distribution. This in turn may cause difficulty with fine motor skills, urinary retention, and neuropathic discomfort in the spine (Lhermitte's sign). Also, rectal cancer can result in chronic diarrhea and bowel dysfunction. Neoadjuvant and adjuvant RT can increase bowel frequency [117]. The incidence of pelvic fractures in women who underwent pelvic RT for rectal cancer is higher [118]. Cognitive deficits have been noted in processing speed, verbal memory, attention, and working memory 2 years after intervention [119]. With appropriate medical, nursing, and therapeutic rehabilitation interventions, several of these comorbidities can be addressed and treated to improve overall functionality and QOL.

## *Head and Neck Cancer*

Head and neck cancers often lead to significant functional morbidity requiring multidisciplinary rehabilitation. This morbidity must be screened and addressed as recent studies have pointed to a relatively high suicide rate in head and neck cancer survivors [120] given the poor quality of life associated with altered speech and swallowing, pain, and physical disfigurement. The rehabilitation team will often include physiatry, PT, OT, SLP, dieticians, social workers, and psychologists. The morbidity is typically related to cancer treatments.

Surgery for head and neck cancer can be a source of morbidity. Modified radical neck dissection (what is typically performed today) spares the sternocleidomastoid and spinal accessory nerve. However, clinically there is still often morbidity related to traction/inflammation of the spinal accessory nerve leading to shoulder dysfunction. In addition, many lymph nodes are often dissected, which (in combination with radiation) can lead to disfiguring and uncomfortable head and neck lymphedema. Glossectomy may lead to tongue pain, dysphagia, and dysarthria.

Radiation can lead to fibrosis with subsequent shortening and contracture of soft tissues. This can result in clinical syndromes of cervical dystonia and trismus (impaired jaw opening). In addition, atrophy of neck extensor muscles may lead to dropped head syndrome which can anecdotally be treated with a Headmaster™ Cervical Collar to support neck extension.

Dysgeusia (altered taste) is another common side effect of chemotherapy and/or radiation in head and neck cancer patients. This symptom can lead to poor nutrition due to difficulty eating. Dieticians and SLPs may be helpful in managing this symptom. There are some studies demonstrating benefit from acupuncture as well as zinc gluconate (140 mg/day) supplementation [121].

Trismus is typically defined as jaw opening (incisor to incisor) of <25 mm [122]. It is due to tonic contractions of muscles of mastication and/or fibrosis/shortening of ligaments of the jaw. Treatment can include jaw-opening exercises with a PT and/or SLP, muscle relaxants and/or nerve-stabilizing medications, jaw-opening splints (such as Dynasplint® or TheraBite®) [123], or botulinum toxin injections to masseter, medial pterygoid, and temporalis muscles. Notably, because they induce weakness, botulinum toxin injections are often controversial and should be carefully considered and monitored.

Head and neck lymphedema is common after radiation and neck dissection surgeries. The morbidity of head and neck lymphedema is high and includes pain, decreased range of motion, dysphagia, difficulty with voice production, disfigurement, and potential for cellulitis. Like lymphedema in other body regions, head and neck lymphedema can be treated by a certified lymphedema therapist with complete decongestive. Compression garments for the face and neck are available for day- and nightwear. Pneumatic compression pumps for head and neck lymphedema are newly available and further study will be needed to confirm their effectiveness.

## *Hematological Cancer*

### Lymphoma

The annual incidence of Hodgkin's lymphoma (HL, 2010–2014) was 3 cases per 100,000 [124]. Although it is commonly found in peripheral lymph nodes, it can affect other organ systems such as liver, lung, and bone marrow. Early-stage HL is treated with combination chemotherapy, followed by involved-field RT, whereas more intensive chemotherapy combinations are appropriate for advanced-staged HL. Consolidative RT may also be an option for treatment. Allogeneic stem cell transplantation (SCT) may be appropriate for early-relapsed or refractory HL [125]. Non-Hodgkin's lymphoma (NHL) accounts for 90% of all lymphoma diagnoses [126]. Risk factors include immunosuppression, organ transplantation, previous chemotherapy administration with SCT, inherited immunodeficiency syndromes, or autoimmune disease. Early-stage disease is treated with RT. However, chemotherapy without RT may also be used. Systemic chemotherapy followed by consolidative radiation is appropriate for localized aggressive lymphomas [127].

Patients with HL may develop noncoronary atherosclerotic disease, pulmonary disease, and endocrine dysfunction as long-term complications from treatment. Individuals with NHL may experience secondary cancers, including myelodysplasia, acute myeloid leukemia (AML), and solid tumors. Other conditions associated with NHL include cardiovascular disease, infertility, neuropathy, renal insufficiency, gastrointestinal toxicity, and lung fibrosis [128]. Post-chemotherapy cognitive impairments were found in patients who received rituximab and bendamustine [129]. For patients with HL, cognitive changes occur in the ability to learn and remember, speed of reactions, attention, and executive functions [130]. Functional deficits associated with these complications should be evaluated by trained clinical professionals that can prescribe appropriate medical and therapeutic exercise programs that improve performance status and functionality in daily life.

## Leukemia

Acute lymphoblastic leukemia (ALL) is a common disorder in both children and adults, but most often diagnosed between the ages of 2 and 5 years with an incidence of 1 in 2000 for children between the ages of 0 and 15 [131]. Treatment comprises three phases: (1) remission-induction, which eliminates leukemic cell burden and restores normal hematopoiesis in a majority of patients; (2) intensification (consolidation), which eradicates residual leukemic cells; and (3) continuation (maintenance) therapy, which lasts 2 years or longer [131]. Allogeneic SCT should be considered for high-risk patients [131]. For AML, outcomes vary according to age, performance status, and chromosomal and molecular aberrations. Chemotherapy follows an induction and consolidation program (with or without hematopoietic SCT). The most effective long-term therapy for AML is allogeneic hematopoietic SCT [132].

Chronic lymphocytic leukemia (CLL) is the most common leukemia diagnosed in the Western world [133]. Treatment for CLL is not recommended until it is symptomatic or there is disease progression and, when appropriate, the primary recommended treatment is combined immunochemotherapy. Combination therapy with alkylating agents and purine analogues allows for better overall response rate, complete response, and progression-free survival, and allogeneic hematopoietic SCT is supported in individuals with poor-risk disease [133]. Chronic myeloid leukemia (CML) affects 1 individual per 100,000 per year, and accounts for 15% of all new cases of leukemia in the Western hemisphere [134]. When not treated, increased instability is noted during the acceleration phase; and then transition occurs to a terminal transformation (blast crisis) [134]. Tyrosine kinase inhibitors (TKI) are the mainstay of treatment. Allogeneic SCT is recommended in specific cases where TKI are not effective [135].

Tumor lysis syndrome can occur in the treatment of leukemia. Chemistry abnormalities can ensue, which may lead to renal failure. Patients are also at high risk for infection as well as longer term effects, such as decreased cardiac ejection fraction. Childhood survivors may experience osteonecrosis of various joints, and subsequent orthopedic interventions [136]. Cognitive impairments have been noted in pediatric survivors of ALL treated with chemotherapy only, specifically regarding processing speed, executive functioning, and working memory [137]. In addition, adult survivors of childhood ALL also experience sensory and motor deficits from previous chemotherapeutic intervention, which can lead to limitation in balance, mobility, and walking efficiency [138]. These issues can often lead to functional decline, and require aggressive rehabilitation services to allow patients the opportunity to improve.

### Multiple Myeloma

MM accounts for 10% of all hematological malignancies, with an age-adjusted annual incidence of 4.3 per 100,000 in the United States [139]. Treatment phases for MM include initial therapy, autologous SCT, consolidation/maintenance therapy, and treatment of relapse [139]. Lytic lesions are common in MM, and evaluation using Mirels' criteria can help determine whether surgical intervention is necessary. Bisphosphonates are used to prevent the progression of bony disease and to treat hypercalcemia, but can also cause renal toxicity and osteonecrosis of the jaw. Patients are at high risk for thrombosis and infection. Other potential complications include anemia, cord compression, peripheral neuropathy, hyperviscosity syndrome, and hyperuricemia and tumor lysis syndrome [140]. Given the potential for orthopedic and spine intervention, as well as decline due to medical comorbidities associated with the cancer and its treatment, rehabilitation principles could be applied to improve mobility and functionality.

### Complications from Stem Cell Transplantation

Stem cell transplantation may result in several complications for the hematological patient. Initial concerns may revolve around rejection of the marrow graft or relapse of malignancy. Cytoreductive chemotherapy can place the patient at high risk for infection. Cardiac toxicities, peripheral neuropathy, and Guillain-Barré syndrome may also occur. Graft-versus-host disease (GVHD) can be both acute and chronic, and lead to fibrosis and collagen vascular disease-like symptoms [141]. Physical losses have also been noted after autologous and allogeneic hematopoietic SCT, as demonstrated by lower values for the 2-min walking test, grip strength of both hands, and the Schober's test [142]. Many of these conditions and associated impairments are amenable to rehabilitation intervention.

## Conclusion

Cancer rehabilitation is a crucial, yet underutilized, part of oncology care. First and foremost, care should be focused on what is best for the patient as rehabilitation clearly helps people live better lives—functioning at higher levels with less pain, fatigue, and disability. From a policy and healthcare delivery perspective, as oncology shifts toward value-based care paradigms, it will be increasingly important to consider the role that rehabilitation and prehabilitation may have in reducing hospital lengths of stay, unanticipated readmissions, and even survival. There is no doubt that most cancer survivors would benefit from cancer rehabilitation interventions, and this care should be provided by experts and recommended to all patients who need it.

## References

1. Silver JK, Raj VS, Fu JB, Wisotzky EM, Smith SR, Kirch RA. Cancer rehabilitation and palliative care: critical components in the delivery of high-quality oncology services. Support Care Cancer. 2015;23:3633–43.
2. Silver JK, Baima J, Mayer RS. Impairment-driven cancer rehabilitation: an essential component of quality care and survivorship. CA Cancer J Clin. 2013;63:295–317.
3. Silver JK, Raj VS, Fu JB, Wisotzky EM, Smith SR, Knowlton SE, et al. Most national cancer institute-designated cancer center websites do not provide survivors with information about cancer rehabilitation services. J Cancer Educ. 2017. https://www-ncbi-nlm-nih-gov.ezp-prod1.hul.harvard.edu/pubmed/28064402. Accessed 20 June 2017.
4. Stout NL, Silver JK, Raj VS, Rowland J, Gerber L, Cheville A, et al. Toward a national initiative in cancer rehabilitation: recommendations from a subject matter expert group. Arch Phys Med Rehabil. 2016;97:2006–15.
5. Broadwell DC. Rehabilitation needs of the patient with cancer. Cancer. 1987;60:563–8.
6. Driessen EJ, Peeters ME, Bongers BC, Maas HA, Bootsma GP, van Meeteren NL, et al. Effects of prehabilitation and rehabilitation including a home-based component on physical fitness, adherence, treatment tolerance, and recovery in patients with non-small cell lung cancer: a systematic review. Crit Rev Oncol Hematol. 2017;114:63–76.
7. Onerup A, Angenete E, Bock D, Borjesson M, Fagevik Olsen M, Gryback Gillheimer E, et al. The effect of pre- and post-operative physical activity on recovery after colorectal cancer surgery (physsurg-c): study protocol for a randomised controlled trial. Trials. 2017;18:212.
8. Minnella EM, Bousquet-Dion G, Awasthi R, Scheede-Bergdahl C, Carli F. Multimodal prehabilitation improves functional capacity before and after colorectal surgery for cancer: a five-year research experience. Acta Oncol. 2017;56:295–300.
9. Carli F, Gillis C, Scheede-Bergdahl C. Promoting a culture of prehabilitation for the surgical cancer patient. Acta Oncol. 2017;56:128–33.
10. Masley PM, Havrilko CL, Mahnensmith MR, Aubert M, Jette DU. Physical therapist practice in the acute care setting: a qualitative study. Phys Ther. 2011;91:906–19.
11. Smith BA, Fields CJ, Fernandez N. Physical therapists make accurate and appropriate discharge recommendations for patients who are acutely ill. Phys Ther. 2010;90:693–703.
12. Malone D, Ridgeway K, Nordon-Craft A, Moss P, Schenkman M, Moss M. Physical therapist practice in the intensive care unit: results of a national survey. Phys Ther. 2015;95:1335–44.
13. Burtin C, Clerckx B, Robbeets C, Ferdinande P, Langer D, Troosters T, et al. Early exercise in critically ill patients enhances short-term functional recovery. Crit Care Med. 2009;37:2499–505.
14. Mechanic R. Post-acute care--the next frontier for controlling medicare spending. N Engl J Med. 2014;370:692–4.
15. Inpatient rehabilitation therapy services: Complying with documentation requirements. Department Of Health and Human Services, Centers for Medicare & Medicaid Services. 2012. https://www.cms.gov/Outreach-and-Education/Medicare-Learning-Network-MLN/MLNProducts/downloads/inpatient_rehab_fact_sheet_icn905643.pdf. Accessed 30 Apr 2017.
16. Shay PD, Ozcan YA. Freestanding inpatient rehabilitation facility performance following the 60 percent rule: a matter of fit. Med Care Res Rev. 2013;70:46–67.

17. Inpatient rehabilitation facility prospective payment system. Department of Health and Human Services, Center for Medicare & Medicaid Services. 2017. https://www.cms.gov/Outreach-and-Education/Medicare-Learning-Network-MLN/MLNProducts/downloads/InpatRehabPaymtfctsht09-508.pdf. Accessed 30 April 2017.
18. Goldberg TH. The long-term and post-acute care continuum. W V Med J. 2016;112:68–74.
19. Coverage of extended care (snf) services under hospital insurance. Medicare Benefit Policy Manual. Rev 228, 10–13-16. Centers for Medicare & Medicaid Services. 2016. https://www.cms.gov/Regulations-and-Guidance/Guidance/Manuals/downloads/bp102c08.pdf. Accessed 24 April 2017.
20. Eskildsen MA. Long-term acute care: a review of the literature. J Am Geriatr Soc. 2007;55:775–9.
21. Kahn JM, Werner RM, David G, Ten Have TR, Benson NM, Asch DA. Effectiveness of long-term acute care hospitalization in elderly patients with chronic critical illness. Med Care. 2013;51:4–10.
22. Long term care hospital prospective payment system. Department Of Health and Human Services, Centers for Medicare & Medicaid Services. 2016. https://www.cms.gov/Outreach-and-Education/Medicare-Learning-Network-MLN/MLNProducts/Downloads/Long-Term-Care-Hospital-PPS-Fact-Sheet-ICN006956.pdf. Accessed 28 April 2017.
23. Ellenbecker CH, Samia L, Cushman MJ, Alster K. Patient safety and quality in home health care. In: Hughes R, editor. Patient safety and quality: an evidence-based handbook for nurses. Rockville, MD: Agency for Healthcare Research and Quality, U.S. Department of Health and Human Services; 2008. https://archive.ahrq.gov/professionals/clinicians-providers/resources/nursing/resources/nurseshdbk/nurseshdbk.pdf. Accessed 12 Jun 2017.
24. U.S. Centers for Medicare & Medicaid Services. Your medicare coverage - home health services. https://www.medicare.gov/coverage/home-health-services.html. Accessed 26 April 2017.
25. U.S. Centers for Medicare & Medicaid Services. Outpatient rehabilitation providers. 2013. https://www.cms.gov/Medicare/Provider-Enrollment-and-Certification/CertificationandComplianc/OutpatientRehab.html. Accessed 1 May 2017.
26. U.S. Centers for Medicare & Medicaid Services. Your medicare coverage - physical therapy/occupational therapy/speech-language pathology services. https://www.medicare.gov/coverage/pt-and-ot-and-speech-language-pathology.html. Accessed 1 May 2017.
27. U.S. Centers for Medicare & Medicaid Services. Medicare limits on therapy services. 2017. https://www.medicare.gov/Pubs/pdf/10988-Medicare-Limits-Therapy-Services.pdf. Accessed 1 May 2017.
28. Silver JK. Cancer rehabilitation and prehabilitation may reduce disability and early retirement. Cancer. 2014;120:2072–6.
29. Silver J, Mayer RS. Barriers to pain management in the rehabilitation of the surgical oncology patient. J Surg Oncol. 2007;95:427–35.
30. Cancer pain relief: With a guide to opioid availability. 2nd ed. Geneva, Switzerland: World Health Organization; 1996.
31. Spiegel D, Bloom JR. Group therapy and hypnosis reduce metastatic breast carcinoma pain. Psychosom Med. 1983;45:333–9.
32. Buffart LM, Kalter J, Sweegers MG, Courneya KS, Newton RU, Aaronson NK, et al. Effects and moderators of exercise on quality of life and physical function in patients with cancer: an individual patient data meta-analysis of 34 rcts. Cancer Treat Rev. 2017;52:91–104.
33. Carli F, Silver JK, Feldman LS, McKee A, Gilman S, Gillis C, et al. Surgical prehabilitation in patients with cancer: state-of-the-science and recommendations for future research from a panel of subject matter experts. Phys Med Rehabil Clin N Am. 2017;28:49–64.
34. Stigt JA, Uil SM, van Riesen SJ, Simons FJ, Denekamp M, Shahin GM, et al. A randomized controlled trial of postthoracotomy pulmonary rehabilitation in patients with resectable lung cancer. J Thorac Oncol. 2013;8:214–21.
35. Streckmann F, Zopf EM, Lehmann HC, May K, Rizza J, Zimmer P, et al. Exercise intervention studies in patients with peripheral neuropathy: a systematic review. Sports Med. 2014;44:1289–304.

36. Takamura Y, Miyauchi A, Tomoda C, Uruno T, Ito Y, Miya A, et al. Stretching exercises to reduce symptoms of postoperative neck discomfort after thyroid surgery: prospective randomized study. World J Surg. 2005;29:775–9.
37. McNeely ML, Parliament M, Courneya KS, Seikaly H, Jha N, Scrimger R, et al. A pilot study of a randomized controlled trial to evaluate the effects of progressive resistance exercise training on shoulder dysfunction caused by spinal accessory neurapraxia/neurectomy in head and neck cancer survivors. Head Neck. 2004;26:518–30.
38. Hase K, Kamisako M, Fujiwara T, Tsuji T, Liu M. The effect of zaltoprofen on physiotherapy for limited shoulder movement in breast cancer patients: a single-blinded before-after trial. Arch Phys Med Rehabil. 2006;87:1618–22.
39. Searle RD, Bennett MI, Johnson MI, Callin S, Radford H. Transcutaneous electrical nerve stimulation (tens) for cancer bone pain. J Pain Symptom Manag. 2009;37:424–8.
40. Cristian A, Tran A, Patel K. Patient safety in cancer rehabilitation. Phys Med Rehabil Clin N Am. 2012;23:441–56.
41. Paice JA, Portenoy R, Lacchetti C, Campbell T, Cheville A, Citron M, et al. Management of chronic pain in survivors of adult cancers: American Society of Clinical Oncology Clinical Practice Guideline. J Clin Oncol. 2016;34:3325–45.
42. Grunfeld EA, Cooper AF. A longitudinal qualitative study of the experience of working following treatment for gynaecological cancer. Psychooncology. 2012;21:82–9.
43. Nccn clinical practice guidelines in oncology: Cancer-related fatigue. Version 1.2009. Rockledge, PA: National Comprehensive Cancer Network; 2009.
44. Dimeo FC. Effects of exercise on cancer-related fatigue. Cancer. 2001;92:1689–93.
45. Fukuda K, Straus SE, Hickie I, Sharpe MC, Dobbins JG, Komaroff A. The chronic fatigue syndrome: a comprehensive approach to its definition and study. International chronic fatigue syndrome study group. Ann Intern Med. 1994;121:953–9.
46. Gerber LH. Cancer-related fatigue: persistent, pervasive, and problematic. Phys Med Rehabil Clin N Am. 2017;28:65–88.
47. Juvet LK, Thune I, Elvsaas IKO, Fors EA, Lundgren S, Bertheussen G, et al. The effect of exercise on fatigue and physical functioning in breast cancer patients during and after treatment and at 6 months follow-up: a meta-analysis. Breast. 2017;33:166–77.
48. Twomey R, Aboodarda SJ, Kruger R, Culos-Reed SN, Temesi J, Millet GY. Neuromuscular fatigue during exercise: methodological considerations, etiology and potential role in chronic fatigue. Neurophysiol Clin. 2017;47:95–110.
49. Keilani M, Hasenoehrl T, Baumann L, Ristl R, Schwarz M, Marhold M, et al. Effects of resistance exercise in prostate cancer patients: a meta-analysis. Support Care Cancer. 2017 Sep;25(9):2953–68.
50. Miller CL, Specht MC, Skolny MN, Horick N, Jammallo LS, O'Toole J, et al. Risk of lymphedema after mastectomy: potential benefit of applying acosog z0011 protocol to mastectomy patients. Breast Cancer Res Treat. 2014;144:71–7.
51. Jensen MR, Simonsen L, Karlsmark T, Bulow J. Lymphoedema of the lower extremities--background, pathophysiology and diagnostic considerations. Clin Physiol Funct Imaging. 2010;30:389–98.
52. NABPC Standards Manual. 2014 ed. Chicago, IL: American College of Surgeons; 2014.
53. Norman SA, Localio AR, Potashnik SL, Simoes Torpey HA, Kallan MJ, Weber AL, et al. Lymphedema in breast cancer survivors: incidence, degree, time course, treatment, and symptoms. J Clin Oncol. 2009;27:390–7.
54. Cheville AL, McGarvey CL, Petrek JA, Russo SA, Thiadens SR, Taylor ME. The grading of lymphedema in oncology clinical trials. Semin Radiat Oncol. 2003;13:214–25.
55. Stout NL, Pfalzer LA, Springer B, Levy E, McGarvey CL, Danoff JV, et al. Breast cancer-related lymphedema: comparing direct costs of a prospective surveillance model and a traditional model of care. Phys Ther. 2012;92:152–63.
56. Ferguson CM, Swaroop MN, Horick N, Skolny MN, Miller CL, Jammallo LS, et al. Impact of ipsilateral blood draws, injections, blood pressure measurements, and air travel on the risk of lymphedema for patients treated for breast cancer. J Clin Oncol. 2016;34:691–8.

57. Cemal Y, Pusic A, Mehrara BJ. Preventative measures for lymphedema: separating fact from fiction. J Am Coll Surg. 2011;213:543–51.
58. Schmitz KH, Ahmed RL, Troxel A, Cheville A, Smith R, Lewis-Grant L, et al. Weight lifting in women with breast-cancer-related lymphedema. N Engl J Med. 2009;361:664–73.
59. Bergo E, Lombardi G, Pambuku A, Della Puppa A, Bellu L, D'Avella D, et al. Cognitive rehabilitation in patients with gliomas and other brain tumors: state of the art. Biomed Res Int. 2016;2016:3041824.
60. Vargo M, Henriksson R, Salander P. Rehabilitation of patients with glioma. Handb Clin Neurol. 2016;134:287–304.
61. Haskins EC. Cognitive rehabilitation manual: translating evidence-based recommendations into practice. 1st ed. Reston, VA: American Congress of Rehabilitation Medicine; 2012.
62. Bush SH, Kanji S, Pereira JL, Davis DH, Currow DC, Meagher DJ, et al. Treating an established episode of delirium in palliative care: expert opinion and review of the current evidence base with recommendations for future development. J Pain Symptom Manag. 2014;48:231–48.
63. Zimmer P, Baumann FT, Oberste M, Wright P, Garthe A, Schenk A, et al. Effects of exercise interventions and physical activity behavior on cancer related cognitive impairments: a systematic review. Biomed Res Int. 2016;2016:1820954.
64. Dai X, Ma W, He X, Jha RK. Review of therapeutic strategies for osteosarcoma, chondrosarcoma, and ewing's sarcoma. Med Sci Monit. 2011;17:RA177–90.
65. Ottaviani G, Jaffe N. The epidemiology of osteosarcoma. Cancer Treat Res. 2009;152:3–13.
66. Tiwari A. Current concepts in surgical treatment of osteosarcoma. J Clin Ortho Trauma. 2012;3:4–9.
67. Schwarz R, Bruland O, Cassoni A, Schomberg P, Bielack S. The role of radiotherapy in oseosarcoma. Cancer Treat Res. 2009;152:147–64.
68. Andreou D, Ruppin S, Fehlberg S, Pink D, Werner M, Tunn PU. Survival and prognostic factors in chondrosarcoma: results in 115 patients with long-term follow-up. Acta Orthop. 2011;82:749–55.
69. Gelderblom H, Hogendoorn PC, Dijkstra SD, van Rijswijk CS, Krol AD, Taminiau AH, et al. The clinical approach towards chondrosarcoma. Oncologist. 2008;13:320–9.
70. Rani PS, Shyamala K, Girish HC, Murgod S. Pathogenesis of Ewing sarcoma: a review. J Adv Clin Res Insights. 2015;2:164–8.
71. Ozaki T. Diagnosis and treatment of Ewing sarcoma of the bone: a review article. J Orthop Sci. 2015;20:250–63.
72. Suva LJ, Washam C, Nicholas RW, Griffin RJ. Bone metastasis: mechanisms and therapeutic opportunities. Nat Rev Endocrinol. 2011;7:208–18.
73. Jawad MU, Scully SP. In brief: classifications in brief: Mirels' classification: metastatic disease in long bones and impending pathologic fracture. Clin Orthop Relat Res. 2010;468:2825–7.
74. Shapeero LG, Poffyn B, De Visschere PJ, Sys G, Uyttendaele D, Vanel D, et al. Complications of bone tumors after multimodal therapy. Eur J Radiol. 2011;77:51–67.
75. Fukumothi DK, Pupo H, Reganin LA, Matte SR, Lima BS, Mattos CA. Functional assessment of endoprosthesis in the treatment of bone tumors. Rev Bras Ortop. 2016;51:569–73.
76. Fauske L, Bruland OS, Grov EK, Bondevik H. Cured of primary bone cancer, but at what cost: a qualitative study of functional impairment and lost opportunities. Sarcoma. 2015;2015:484196.
77. Dieli-Conwright CM, Lee K, Kiwata JL. Reducing the risk of breast cancer recurrence: an evaluation of the effects and mechanisms of diet and exercise. Curr Breast Cancer Rep. 2016;8:139–50.
78. Wennman-Larsen A, Alexanderson K, Olsson M, Nilsson MI, Petersson LM. Sickness absence in relation to breast and arm symptoms shortly after breast cancer surgery. Breast. 2013;22:767–72.
79. Torres Lacomba M, Mayoral del Moral O, Coperias Zazo JL, Gerwin RD, Goni AZ. Incidence of myofascial pain syndrome in breast cancer surgery: a prospective study. Clin J Pain. 2010;26:320–5.
80. Yang S, Park DH, Ahn SH, Kim J, Lee JW, Han JY, et al. Prevalence and risk factors of adhesive capsulitis of the shoulder after breast cancer treatment. Support Care Cancer. 2017;25:1317–22.

81. Crosbie J, Kilbreath SL, Dylke E, Refshauge KM, Nicholson LL, Beith JM, et al. Effects of mastectomy on shoulder and spinal kinematics during bilateral upper-limb movement. Phys Ther. 2010;90:679–92.
82. Stubblefield MD, Keole N. Upper body pain and functional disorders in patients with breast cancer. PM R. 2014;6:170–83.
83. Wisotzky EM, Saini V, Kao C. Ultrasound-guided intercostobrachial nerve block for intercostobrachial neuralgia in breast cancer patients: a case series. PM R. 2016;8:273–7.
84. Zocca JA, Chen GH, Puttanniah VG, Hung JC, Gulati A. Ultrasound-guided serratus plane block for treatment of postmastectomy pain syndromes in breast cancer patients: a case series. Pain Pract. 2017;17:141–6.
85. Tang C, Eder S, Lee D, Rabow M, Esserman L. Abstract p3-10-03: a simple intervention to relieve chronic neuropathic post-mastectomy pain. Cancer Res 2013;73.
86. Kudlowitz D, Muggia F. Clinical features of taxane neuropathy. Anti-Cancer Drugs. 2014;25:495–501.
87. Stubblefield MD, McNeely ML, Alfano CM, Mayer DK. A prospective surveillance model for physical rehabilitation of women with breast cancer: chemotherapy-induced peripheral neuropathy. Cancer. 2012;118:2250–60.
88. Gaillard S, Stearns V. Aromatase inhibitor-associated bone and musculoskeletal effects: new evidence defining etiology and strategies for management. Breast Cancer Res. 2011;13:205.
89. Crew KD, Greenlee H, Capodice J, Raptis G, Brafman L, Fuentes D, et al. Prevalence of joint symptoms in postmenopausal women taking aromatase inhibitors for early-stage breast cancer. J Clin Oncol. 2007;25:3877–83.
90. Kirchgesner T, Larbi A, Omoumi P, Malghem J, Zamali N, Manelfe J, et al. Drug-induced tendinopathy: from physiology to clinical applications. Joint Bone Spine. 2014;81:485–92.
91. Irwin ML, Cartmel B, Gross CP, Ercolano E, Li F, Yao X, et al. Randomized exercise trial of aromatase inhibitor-induced arthralgia in breast cancer survivors. J Clin Oncol. 2015;33:1104–11.
92. Crew KD, Capodice JL, Greenlee H, Brafman L, Fuentes D, Awad D, et al. Randomized, blinded, sham-controlled trial of acupuncture for the management of aromatase inhibitor-associated joint symptoms in women with early-stage breast cancer. J Clin Oncol. 2010;28:1154–60.
93. Henry NL, Banerjee M, Wicha M, Van Poznak C, Smerage JB, Schott AF, et al. Pilot study of duloxetine for treatment of aromatase inhibitor-associated musculoskeletal symptoms. Cancer. 2011;117:5469–75.
94. Greenlee H, Crew KD, Shao T, Kranwinkel G, Kalinsky K, Maurer M, et al. Phase ii study of glucosamine with chondroitin on aromatase inhibitor-associated joint symptoms in women with breast cancer. Support Care Cancer. 2013;21:1077–87.
95. Kubo M, Onishi H, Kuroki S, Okido M, Shimada K, Yokohata K, et al. Short-term and low-dose prednisolone administration reduces aromatase inhibitor-induced arthralgia in patients with breast cancer. Anticancer Res. 2012;32:2331–6.
96. Singer O, Cigler T, Moore AB, Levine AB, Do HT, Mandl LA. Hypovitaminosis d is a predictor of aromatase inhibitor musculoskeletal symptoms. Breast J. 2014;20:174–9.
97. Hung R, Krebs P, Coups EJ, Feinstein MB, Park BJ, Burkhalter J, et al. Fatigue and functional impairment in early-stage non-small cell lung cancer survivors. J Pain Symptom Manag. 2011;41:426–35.
98. Shannon VR. Role of pulmonary rehabilitation in the management of patients with lung cancer. Curr Opin Pulm Med. 2010;16:334–9.
99. Bayly JL, Lloyd-Williams M. Identifying functional impairment and rehabilitation needs in patients newly diagnosed with inoperable lung cancer: a structured literature review. Support Care Cancer. 2016;24:2359–79.
100. Cavalheri V, Granger C. Preoperative exercise training for patients with non-small cell lung cancer. Cochrane Database Syst Rev. 2017;6:CD012020.
101. Wang H, Liu X, Rice SJ, Belani CP. Pulmonary rehabilitation in lung cancer. PM R. 2016;8:990–6.

102. Edvardsen E, Skjonsberg OH, Holme I, Nordsletten L, Borchsenius F, Anderssen SA. High-intensity training following lung cancer surgery: a randomised controlled trial. Thorax. 2015;70:244–50.
103. Centers for Disease Control and Prevention. Cancer among men. 2016. https://www.cdc.gov/cancer/dcpc/data/men.htm. Accessed 18 June 2017.
104. Attard G, Parker C, Eeles RA, Schroder F, Tomlins SA, Tannock I, et al. Prostate cancer. Lancet. 2016;387:70–82.
105. Michaelson MD, Cotter SE, Gargollo PC, Zietman AL, Dahl DM, Smith MR. Management of complications of prostate cancer treatment. CA Cancer J Clin. 2008;58:196–213.
106. Simoneau AR. Treatment- and disease-related complications of prostate cancer. Rev Urol. 2006;8(Suppl 2):S56–67.
107. Chen RC, Hamstra DA, Sandler HM, Zietman AL. Complications of prostate cancer treatment. Lancet Oncol. 2014;15:e150.
108. Luo HC, Lei Y, Cheng HH, Fu ZC, Liao SG, Feng J, et al. Long-term cancer-related fatigue outcomes in patients with locally advanced prostate cancer after intensity-modulated radiotherapy combined with hormonal therapy. Medicine. 2016;95:e3948.
109. Center MM, Jemal A, Smith RA, Ward E. Worldwide variations in colorectal cancer. CA Cancer J Clin. 2009;59:366–78.
110. Edwards BK, Ward E, Kohler BA, Eheman C, Zauber AG, Anderson RN, et al. Annual report to the nation on the status of cancer, 1975-2006, featuring colorectal cancer trends and impact of interventions (risk factors, screening, and treatment) to reduce future rates. Cancer. 2010;116:544–73.
111. Torre LA, Bray F, Siegel RL, Ferlay J, Lortet-Tieulent J, Jemal A. Global cancer statistics, 2012. CA Cancer J Clin. 2015;65:87–108.
112. Brenner H, Kloor M, Pox CP. Colorectal cancer. Lancet. 2014;383:1490–502.
113. Jemal A, Clegg LX, Ward E, Ries LA, Wu X, Jamison PM, et al. Annual report to the nation on the status of cancer, 1975-2001, with a special feature regarding survival. Cancer. 2004;101:3–27.
114. Schneider EC, Malin JL, Kahn KL, Ko CY, Adams J, Epstein AM. Surviving colorectal cancer: patient-reported symptoms 4 years after diagnosis. Cancer. 2007;110:2075–82.
115. Grosso G, Biondi A, Marventano S, Mistretta A, Calabrese G, Basile F. Major postoperative complications and survival for colon cancer elderly patients. BMC Surg. 2012;12(Suppl 1):S20.
116. Lange MM, Maas CP, Marijnen CA, Wiggers T, Rutten HJ, Kranenbarg EK, et al. Urinary dysfunction after rectal cancer treatment is mainly caused by surgery. Br J Surg. 2008;95:1020–8.
117. Denlinger CS, Barsevick AM. The challenges of colorectal cancer survivorship. J Natl Compr Cancer Netw. 2009;7:883–93; quiz 94
118. Baxter NN, Habermann EB, Tepper JE, Durham SB, Virnig BA. Risk of pelvic fractures in older women following pelvic irradiation. JAMA. 2005;294:2587–93.
119. Vardy JL, Dhillon HM, Pond GR, Rourke SB, Bekele T, Renton C, et al. Cognitive function in patients with colorectal cancer who do and do not receive chemotherapy: a prospective, longitudinal, controlled study. J Clin Oncol. 2015;33:4085–92.
120. Henry M, Rosberger Z, Bertrand L, Klassen C, Hier M, Zeitouni A, et al. Suicidal ideations are prevalent in head and neck cancer patients and predate diagnosis: longitudinal study indicating the need for suicide prevention and collaborative care in ent clinics. Psychooncology. 2017;26:46.
121. Heckmann SM, Hujoel P, Habiger S, Friess W, Wichmann M, Heckmann JG, et al. Zinc gluconate in the treatment of dysgeusia--a randomized clinical trial. J Dent Res. 2005;84:35–8.
122. Dijkstra PU, Huisman PM, Roodenburg JL. Criteria for trismus in head and neck oncology. Int J Oral Maxillofac Surg. 2006;35:337–42.
123. Stubblefield MD, Manfield L, Riedel ER. A preliminary report on the efficacy of a dynamic jaw opening device (dynasplint trismus system) as part of the multimodal treatment of trismus in patients with head and neck cancer. Arch Phys Med Rehabil. 2010;91:1278–82.

124. National Cancer Institute Surveillance, Epidemiology, and End Results Program. Cancer stat facts: Hodgkin lymphoma. https://seer.cancer.gov/statfacts/html/hodg.html. Accessed 18 June 2017.
125. Gobbi PG, Ferreri AJ, Ponzoni M, Levis A. Hodgkin lymphoma. Crit Rev Oncol Hematol. 2013;85:216–37.
126. Shankland KR, Armitage JO, Hancock BW. Non-hodgkin lymphoma. Lancet. 2012;380:848–57.
127. Zimmermann M, Oehler C, Mey U, Ghadjar P, Zwahlen DR. Radiotherapy for non-hodgkin's lymphoma: still standard practice and not an outdated treatment option. Radiat Oncol. 2016;11:110.
128. Ng AK, LaCasce A, Travis LB. Long-term complications of lymphoma and its treatment. J Clin Oncol. 2011;29:1885–92.
129. Zimmer P, Mierau A, Bloch W, Struder HK, Hulsdunker T, Schenk A, et al. Post-chemotherapy cognitive impairment in patients with b-cell non-hodgkin lymphoma: a first comprehensive approach to determine cognitive impairments after treatment with rituximab, cyclophosphamide, doxorubicin, vincristine and prednisone or rituximab and bendamustine. Leuk Lymphoma. 2015;56:347–52.
130. Fayette D, Gaherova L, Mocikova H, Markova J, Kozak T, Horacek J. Chemotherapy-related cognitive impairment in patients with hodgkin lymphoma - pathophysiology and risk factors. Klin Onkol. 2017;30:93–9.
131. Inaba H, Greaves M, Mullighan CG. Acute lymphoblastic leukaemia. Lancet. 2013;381:1943–55.
132. Saultz JN, Garzon R. Acute myeloid leukemia: a concise review. J Clin Med. 2016;5.
133. Nabhan C, Rosen ST. Chronic lymphocytic leukemia: a clinical review. JAMA. 2014;312:2265–76.
134. Apperley JF. Chronic myeloid leukaemia. Lancet. 2015;385:1447–59.
135. Baccarani M, Castagnetti F, Gugliotta G, Palandri F, Rosti G. Treatment recommendations for chronic myeloid leukemia. Mediterr J Hematol Infect Dis. 2014;6:e2014005.
136. Davis AS, Viera AJ, Mead MD. Leukemia: an overview for primary care. Am Fam Physician. 2014;89:731–8.
137. Kanellopoulos A, Andersson S, Zeller B, Tamnes CK, Fjell AM, Walhovd KB, et al. Neurocognitive outcome in very long-term survivors of childhood acute lymphoblastic leukemia after treatment with chemotherapy only. Pediatr Blood Cancer. 2016;63:133–8.
138. Ness KK, Hudson MM, Pui CH, Green DM, Krull KR, Huang TT, et al. Neuromuscular impairments in adult survivors of childhood acute lymphoblastic leukemia: associations with physical performance and chemotherapy doses. Cancer. 2012;118:828–38.
139. Rajkumar SV, Kumar S. Multiple myeloma: diagnosis and treatment. Mayo Clin Proc. 2016;91:101–19.
140. Al-Farsi K. Multiple myeloma: an update. Oman Med J. 2013;28:3–11.
141. Jaing TH. Complications of haematopoietic stem cell transplantation. ISBT Sci Ser. 2011;6:332–6.
142. de Souza CV, Miranda EC, Garcia C Jr, Aranha FJ, de Souza CA, Vigorito AC. Functional evaluation indicates physical losses after hematopoietic stem cell transplantation. Rev Bras Hematol Hemoter. 2012;34:345–51.

# Chapter 10
# Building a Team to Improve Cancer Survivorship: Integrative Care's Increasing Role

**Susan Hedlund**

## Introduction to the Four Major Domains for Survivors

Numerous breakthroughs in cancer treatment, and greater understanding of the biology of the numerous diseases that fall under the diagnosis of "cancer," have led to improved rates of survival, from what was once considered a terminal diagnosis. While progress in the treatment of some cancers (i.e., breast, prostate, colon) is greater than in others (i.e., pancreatic, lung) the statistics of survival after a cancer diagnosis are improving. According to the National Cancer Institute, the number of people living beyond a cancer diagnosis in the United States reached 14.5 million in 2016. That number is expected to reach 19 million by 2024 [1, 2]. The term "survivorship" describes the patient's experience of moving beyond the diagnosis of cancer and treatment toward health maintenance and wellness.

The definitions of a "cancer survivor" vary, but most sources rely on the definition provided by the National Coalition of Cancer Survivors, which describes a person as a survivor from the diagnosis going forward. While most cancer programs consider cancer survivors as those treated with curative intent or those who have transitioned to maintenance therapy, not all patient advocacy groups define cancer survivorship in that way. Additionally, not all people who have had a cancer diagnosis identify with or like the term "survivor."

The Institute of Medicine published an important text, *From Cancer Patient to Cancer Survivor: Lost in Transition* (2006) [3], and it highlighted the breadth of survivor needs, including support across psychological, physical, social, and spiritual domains. Many survivors report feeling lost following the completion of active treatment. They no longer have the structure of regular treatment visits and the support that comes from frequent interaction with their care team, but they live in fear

S. Hedlund, LCSW, OSW-c
Department of Patient and Family Support Services, Knight Cancer Institute,
School of Medicine, Oregon Health and Science University, Portland, OR, USA
e-mail: hedlunds@ohsu.edu



P. Hopewood, M. J. Milroy (eds.), *Quality Cancer Care*,
https://doi.org/10.1007/978-3-319-78649-0_10

of a recurrence. Meeting the needs in any one of these domains for each patient can be difficult. Trying to meet them across a growing population of survivors requires a new model of care delivery that extends into the survivorship period.

The Institute of Medicine outlined a quality-of-life model that addressed the four domains of most concern to cancer survivors.

## *Physical*

Many cancer survivors report lingering side effects long after the completion of active treatment. Among the most common are fatigue, and issues related to strength. For others, pain or peripheral neuropathies, lymphedema, and other lingering side effects may persist. Problems with sleep and concerns about overall physical health may remain. Returning to normal functional activities may prove difficult. For patients of childbearing age, fertility issues may be highlighted. Sexual functioning is often altered as a result of treatment as well.

## *Psychological*

It is not uncommon for cancer survivors to experience distress at diagnosis and throughout the course of treatment. This distress may extend into the survivorship period, and may involve fear of recurrence, feelings of lack of control, and may at times be experienced as anxiety or depression. For others, employment may have been interrupted by diagnosis and treatment, and the financial burdens incurred as a result of treatment may be extreme.

In a systematic review of studies on financial hardship in cancer survivors, 47–49% of cancer survivors report financial distress. Financial distress due to out-of-pocket costs related to cancer treatment is associated with increased risk of death by 79% [4]. Additionally a 2016 study by CancerCare revealed that patients alter care to reduce costs: 29% skipped doctors' appointments, 38% postponed or did not fill medication prescriptions, 34% skipped medication doses, and 31% cut oral medications in half [5, 6].

## *Social*

Cancer impacts both the individual with the disease and those who care about him/her. Families also experience high levels of distress throughout the cancer experience, and may be eager for the cancer survivor to get back "to normal." The survivor, on the other hand, may no longer feel able or willing to resume all of the old roles and activities, having been changed by the cancer experience. This dynamic can challenge even the healthiest of relationships. The cancer survivor may have both body image concerns and changes in sexual functioning. Roles and relationships may be challenged, and may lead to isolation for the cancer survivor.

## *Spiritual*

It is not uncommon for cancer survivors to search for a sense of meaning in the experience. Some may find their faith strengthened, and others find their faith shaken as a result. Many survivors report a new sense of purpose and/or priorities and hope. Others may find their sense of self shaken. It is possible to discover one's inner strength and resilience after the cancer experience, but may require assistance in doing so.

Given the breadth and depth of survivor needs, it is not surprising that most cancer providers are not able to provide comprehensive support.

A 2013 survey found that 60–75% of survivors reported unmet needs [7]. Another recent study found that more than 50% of survivors reported receiving no psychosocial support from either support groups or professional counseling [8].

This lack of support is concerning on multiple levels. One concern is that unaddressed psychosocial needs can have implications for survivor's health. A 2013 population-based study found that depressed cancer survivors were twice as likely to die prematurely compared to non-distressed survivors [9].

Cancer survivors are at especially high risk for anxiety, depression, and other forms of psychosocial distress because of the multiple stressors, vulnerabilities, and challenges they face. According to the NCCN Guidelines for Distress Management risk factors for psychosocial distress include cognitive impairment, severe comorbid illnesses, uncontrolled symptoms, communication barriers, or a history of psychiatric disorder, depression, or substance abuse. Social issues such as living alone, having young children, being of younger age or female, and prior physical or sexual abuse are also risk factors for psychosocial distress [10].

## Surveillance

Another area of concern is that of surveillance. Cancer surveillance involves using physical exams, imaging, blood tests, and other strategies to monitor patients for recurrence and development of secondary cancers. Cancer providers find surveillance challenging for a number of reasons: they may lack evidence-based guidelines, patients do not always prioritize follow-up care, and it is not always clear which clinicians should deliver which services. As a result, US providers vary significantly in their clinical practice. The American Society of Clinical Oncology (ASCO) surveyed its 3400 members who identified breast cancer as a major part of their work. Using four idealized patient vignettes, the survey found significant variations in surveillance patterns, despite evidence from well-designed, randomized clinical trials. "There was marked variation in surveillance intensity" [11].

Recognizing this relatively new "stage" along the treatment continuum, ASCO issued suggested guidelines for follow-up and surveillance specific to disease sites and types. They also developed a Survivorship Care Plan (SCP) template intended to assist with this need. The SCP includes a summary of the patient's diagnosis, all treatments received, a list of providers, and where treatment was received. This first part of the document is intended to be the "looking back" part of the care plan. Additionally, the document includes follow-up and surveillance guidelines, including healthy living recommendations (e.g.: smoking cessation, weight management, psychosocial support). This represents the "looking ahead" part of the document. The document is to be given to the patient following completion of treatment, and forwarded to the patient's primary care provider as well.

In 2015, the Commission on Cancer program of the College of Surgeon, which accredits most cancer centers nationally, issued three new "patient-centered" standards as a part of the accreditation standards [12]. The three standards, patient navigation, distress screening, and survivorship, are being rolled out and cancer centers are being evaluated to determine their compliance in addressing these needs. While cancer centers vary widely in scope, size, and number of patients treated, the survivorship standard is the one proving most difficult to implement. The standard mandates that any patient treated with curative intent receive a completed Survivorship Care Plan (SCP) at the end of active treatment that includes treatment summary, surveillance guidelines, and recommendation for health lifestyle behaviors. The Commission on Cancer's original survivorship standard required that by 2015, 10% of eligible patients receive the SCP, and the percentage increased annually so that by 2019 100% of patients would receive the care plan. This standard has recently been revised to require cancer programs accredited by the CoC meet a threshold of 50% of patients treated with curative intent to receive a Survivorship Care Plan. This will be implemented beginning January 1, 2018.

There are a number of barriers that cancer centers have experienced in meeting this standard as previously written. For large, often academic medical centers with multiple providers and clinical settings, it is difficult to identify all of those treated with curative intent. While working with the institution's cancer registry is very helpful, there exists great variation in how providers document and practice, extending the challenge in identifying who is eligible.

A major barrier is that in many centers using electronic health records, the system does not auto-populate the care plan, thus requiring someone to "mine" the data in the medical record to complete the summaries. Additionally, many cancer centers use multiple electronic health records that do not communicate with one another. Thus, creating a SCP requires mining data from multiple systems. For example, surgery reports may exist in one system, whereas chemotherapy and radiation medicine exist in other systems. Completion of the SCP is time consuming, with many providers reporting the time it takes to complete the document as anywhere from

30 min to 2 h, and this is not reimbursable. Reimbursement is available for survivorship visits if provided by an MD, nurse practitioner, or physician assistant. There is little reimbursement for social workers or dietitians. The final barrier that has been raised is the lack of evidence that receiving the SCP makes a difference in patient behavior or follow-up. This has made it a particularly hard "sell" to providers and cancer programs already stretched to meet patient needs. This unfunded mandate, with little evidence to support patient compliance, coupled with the time it takes to complete the document, and limited reimbursement, has been met with frustration and resistance in some cancer centers. As noted, the Commission on Cancer has reevaluated and rewritten this standard [12].

The spirit of the mandate, however, goes well beyond the document itself. Ideally, survivorship care improves patient outcomes and patient satisfaction, and may reduce costs of care by supporting the overall physical and psychological well-being of survivors. Providers should monitor patients for cancer recurrence and educate patients about late and long-term effects. Psychosocial needs should be addressed by referrals to support services, social workers, or other counselors to meet their emotional needs. Referral to rehabilitation and nutritional support is important throughout the cancer continuum, beginning at diagnosis, and well into the survivorship period. Diet, smoking cessation, and exercise are also important aspects of recovery and health maintenance. Assessing a patient's readiness to make lifestyle changes can be helpful through the use of motivational interviewing techniques. Motivational interviewing is being increasingly used in healthcare settings to determine the best strategies to assist patients in making lifestyle changes [13]. There is evidence that today's young adults may be the first generation in modern history to be less healthy than their parents. Respiratory diseases and cancers, diabetes and obesity, heart and liver disease, and some psychological problems such as depression are all strongly linked to health behavior and lifestyles. Many of the maladies that cause people to consult healthcare professionals are largely preventable or remedial through health behavior change.

Motivational interviewing is a counseling approach developed by William Miller and Stephen Rollnick, originally evolved from the experience of working with "problem drinkers." Miller and Rollnick described a more detailed description of the motivational procedures. Motivational interviewing is a goal-oriented, client-centered counseling style for eliciting behavior change by helping clients explore and resolve their ambivalence toward change. It is a focus- and goal-directed approach in which the therapist or physician attempts to influence clients/patients to consider making change. For patients considering healthier lifestyle changes, exploring and acknowledging ambivalence is central to the conversation. Change can be very difficult, and acknowledging this, vs. judging it is central to the purpose of motivational interviewing. The intention is to elicit client awareness of the issues and consequences of the continued behavior, and to help them see more about the future. It is essential that the practitioner be nonjudgmental, nonconfrontational, and nondirective, but rather curious and supportive [14].

## Integrative Care

Many cancer survivors reevaluate their lives and lifestyles following the diagnosis and treatment of cancer. In an effort to keep cancer at bay, and to exert some control over one's health, an increasing number of cancer patients are choosing to use integrative approaches to aid in their recovery. Previously referred to as "alternative" or "complementary" therapies, an estimated 50% of Americans are increasingly utilizing integrative approaches to maintain health. An estimated 90% of cancer patients and survivors are said to use such approaches [15]. These approaches fall under several categories: healing touch, mind-body approaches, creative arts, nutrition, and fitness. Many integrative approaches are highly effective in managing the symptoms and side effects of cancer. Additionally, it gives cancer patients a sense of efficacy and control by taking an active approach to their health.

Integrative medicine addresses a patient's body, mind, and spirit, and encourages patients to be partners in their treatment [16]. Integrative medicine includes support groups, therapeutic massage, acupuncture, meditation, yoga, art, and music therapy, among others. It is important to note that some integrative therapies have not been studied. Others have been shown to be effective for symptom relief (e.g., to alleviate nausea, vomiting, and fatigue). To date, there is not consistently proven scientific evidence that integrative medicine will slow cancer progression.

As noted, the use of integrative medicine has grown partly in response to efforts by patients to take a more active role in their health care and use therapies that focus on overall health and healing. By integrating integrative medicine into conventional allopathic treatment, healthcare providers are better able to address the physical, emotional, spiritual, and quality of life needs of patients (Table 10.1).

In 1998, the National Institutes of Health (NIH) expanded its efforts to evaluate integrative medicine (then referred to as complementary medicine-CAM) by founding the National Center for Complementary and Alternative Medicine (NCCAM). NIH has invested in research to study how integrative therapies work, where they are effective, and which patients might benefit from specific therapies (e.g., people living with cancer, HIV/AIDs, heart disease, diabetes, or chronic illnesses). The National Cancer Institute Office of Cancer Complementary and Alternative Therapy is charged with holding integrative medicine therapies to the same rigorous scientific investigation used to evaluate standard cancer treatments.

**Table 10.1** Basic principles of integrative medicine [17]

| |
|---|
| • Reaffirms importance of the relationship between health providers and patients |
| • Encourages patient-centered care, empowering patients as partners in their treatment |
| • Focuses on the whole person—the body, mind, and spirit |
| • Uses evidence-based therapies (conventional and integrative medicine) to support and achieve optimal health and healing |

A growing number of hospitals, cancer centers, and individual healthcare providers are offering integrative medicine options and increasingly they are important for survivorship care. When used in addition to other standard cancer treatments, certain integrative therapies can play an important role in enhancing the quality of a person's overall care and peace of mind. Some techniques are "passive," requiring limited participation (e.g., massage, Reiki) while others are "active" (yoga, tai chi, support groups).

Integrative therapies can help manage symptoms, reduce treatment side effects (e.g., fatigue, depression, nausea), and enhance feelings of well-being and quality of life. The following describes some of the integrative medicine offerings available in many cancer centers.

## Alternative Medical Systems

Alternative medical systems include Chinese medicine, Ayurveda, homeopathic, and naturopathic medicine. Chinese medicine emphasizes the balance of qu ("chee") or vital energy. Within this system, illness is described as a disturbance of vital energy. Ayurveda is a system of healing which evolved from the teachings of ancient India. It stresses the use of body, mind, and spirit in disease prevention and treatment and strives to achieve harmony within the individuals. Integrative approaches include acupuncture, herbal medicine, restorative physical exercise, and controlled breathing.

### *Mind-Body Interventions*

Mind-body interventions use strategies to enhance the mind's impact on the body's function and physical symptoms. Interventions are used to help patients relax, reduce stress, and relieve symptoms associated with cancer treatments. Examples include meditation, support groups, hypnosis, yoga, tai chi, expressive arts (music, art, writing), and prayer.

Examples of touch therapies are massage and Reiki. Massage offers the benefit of maintaining energy, relieving stress and tension, and decreasing anxiety [18]. Reiki promotes healing through gentle hands-on touch for restoring harmony and relaxation.

Examples of mind-body therapies include yoga, meditation, and mindfulness-based stress reduction (MBSR). MBSR has experienced growing popularity in healthcare settings for both patients and healthcare providers alike. Mindfulness refers to open, nonjudgmental, moment-to-moment awareness of what is present. Randomized controlled trials demonstrate beneficial changes in psychosocial quality of life, anxiety, depression, fatigue, sleep disturbances, pain, sexual dysfunction, physiological arousal (e.g., blood pressure), immune function, and cortisol levels [19, 20].

Acupuncture is a safe, painless, and effective form of traditional Chinese medicine. Acupuncture is used to reopen the normal flow of energy, thereby relieving symptoms associated with the specific points of needle placement. Acupuncture can be very helpful as adjunctive care for treatment in cancer. Many of the side effects from cancer therapies can be minimized if not avoided by utilizing alternative measures to support the body during the continuum from diagnosis through survivorship. Research supports using acupuncture to treat chemotherapy-induced nausea and vomiting, poor appetite, constipation or diarrhea, insomnia and fatigue, hot flashes, xerostomia, anxiety and depression, peripheral neuropathy, and pain [21, 22].

The creative arts can offer a useful outlet for cancer survivors that may allow them to work through some of the changes and emotions that accompany the cancer journey. While many people take advantage of the benefits of counseling and/or support groups, others find that writing, creating art work, or music can offer a different opportunity for expression [23]. The expressive arts allow individuals to use art as a means of self-expression to reconcile emotional conflicts and to foster self-awareness and personal growth. Thus, through the creative process, individuals under physical, emotional, and/or spiritual stress can work though and integrate their situations to facilitate healing. The creative process is naturally healing: therefore the benefits and possibilities with people under stress can be profound.

Nutrition and fitness are also areas in which cancer survivors can influence their healing. Numerous studies have shown the benefits of physical activity on the reduction of fatigue and improved strength and physical functioning [24, 25], and others find that modifying diet becomes important [26].

## *Support Groups*

Cancer support groups became popular, particularly in the 1980s as the “silence” around a cancer diagnosis began to change. Prior to that time, many people were reluctant to talk about cancer, in part because of the fear associated with the diagnosis, compounded by the lack of understanding of the disease itself, and limited treatment options.

Support groups began as a way to offer mutual support with others going through a similar experience. It helped to reduce the isolation and loneliness of the cancer journey.

In 2000, Dr. David Spiegel and Dr. Catherine Classen published a seminal work about the value of support groups, Group Therapy for Cancer Patients: A Research-based Handbook of Psychosocial Care [27]. In one study Spiegel matched demographically women with metastatic breast cancer. He randomly assigned one group of women to support groups, and another to traditional psychosocial support offered through the cancer center. The underlying assumption was that women in the support group arm would report higher levels of support than women assigned to traditional support, which proved to be true. What was not expected was the finding that the women assigned to the support group arm lived an additional 18 months longer than the women not in the support group [27]. Support groups gained great popularity during that time. Further research has suggested that the longer survival time is not directly linked to being in a cancer support group per se, but rather that having high levels of good psychosocial support in one's life aids in recovery and quality of life.

Since that time, support groups have evolved and changed. Support groups may be disease specific, general cancer support, and/or support groups for families and caregivers. Most groups are facilitated by trained oncology professionals including oncology social workers, psychologists, and/or oncology nurses. Most are open ended, and often include psycho-education as a part of the support. Family groups may offer the opportunity for couples, children, and other family members to give and receive support.

Based on the principle of *mutual aid*, support groups offer reassurance and support by coming together with others who share similar experiences. Support groups can greatly reduce a sense of isolation that can come with the cancer experience.

Other sources of support can include weekend retreats, classes on specific topics, and peer volunteer outreach. More recently, online support groups have become increasingly popular. When offered through credible sites (e.g., CancerCare, Cancer Support Community, and others), online groups are accessible to those who have difficulty traveling, are impaired by side effects or other symptoms, and are available at times when traditional support groups may not be.

Some oncology practices are offering education and support groups specific to survivors, and offering topics of interest after treatment. These groups are often facilitated by a nurse, social worker, physician, or nurse practitioner, and may include topics related to recovery or side effects. Such topics may include dealing with neuropathies, fatigue, insomnia, sexual challenges, relationship issues, and financial concerns.

Many cancer survivors discover that they need assistance in navigating life post-cancer diagnosis and treatment. Groups and retreats can offer the opportunity to examine how life and priorities have, and have not, changed, as a result of a cancer diagnosis. Being able to examine fears, discoveries, and opportunities in safe settings with others who understand these dynamics can be very helpful to cancer survivors.

Retreats are another option for people who are recovering from cancer. Offered at a number of sites across the United States, they provide an opportunity for people recovering from cancer to step apart from their daily lives and to consider how the cancer experience has impacted them. Often the retreats include a combination of group support and examination of the cancer experience, as well as wellness activities such as yoga, massage, cooking classes, and other activities. The intention is to help cancer survivors further integrate the experience and identify new or renewed life priorities.

## Caregiver Support

Family members of cancer survivors and other caregivers may find value in meeting with others providing support and care to the person with cancer. Particularly if the treatment and recovery process is long, such as with bone marrow transplant, or if the disease itself creates disability or cognitive change for the person with cancer (e.g., brain tumors), additional support is indicated. Caregivers may tend to minimize their own need for care, deferring to the needs of the person with cancer. However, caregivers often experience high levels of depression and anxiety, exhaustion, and social isolation. In these situations, services can be tailored with this special population in mind, and may include education, support, and referral to community resources for additional support.

### *A Word About Professional Caregivers (Healthcare Providers)*

Working as a healthcare professional in oncology is highly rewarding and the advances in treatment options and increased rates of survival are deeply gratifying. However, working in oncology can also be emotionally and physically exhausting, as well as at times very difficult. Despite the numerous steps forward in the field, people still can and do die of cancer. Over a career it is not uncommon for an oncology professional to have experienced numerous losses. It is imperative for oncology professionals to find ways to renew and restore one's self, and to be cognizant of signs of burnout, compassion fatigue, and moral distress. Fortunately, many cancer centers have created opportunities for their teams to receive support both formally and informally. Some teams have created memorial rituals to acknowledge the loss of patients. Other programs offer mindfulness-based stress reduction programs for the healthcare professional and/or opportunities for support groups for the professionals.

## Conclusions

As the number of cancer survivors continues to increase, the demand and need for ongoing programs of support will continue to grow. Cancer centers are challenged to develop such programs. Some services are billable and reimbursable, while others may be supported through philanthropy.

Given the profound impact that cancer has on the lives of patients, comprehensive survivorship programs should include attention to the whole person and a range of services to support ongoing recovery. These should include integrative medicine approaches as well as psychosocial support. This will help the person with cancer and their loved ones to feel more fully supported while also enhancing patient satisfaction, and may give individual cancer programs a competitive edge. Ongoing research regarding the efficacy of integrative therapies is also indicated as well as ongoing evaluation of the best approaches to survivorship.

## References

1. National Cancer Institute. Cancer statistics. cancer.gov/about-cancer/what-is-cancer/statistic. Accessed 28 May 2017.
2. McCabe MS, Bhatia S, Oeffinger KC, Reaman GH, Tyne C, et al. American Society of Clinical Oncology statement: achieving high-quality cancer survivorship care. J Clin Oncol. 2013;31(5):631–40.
3. Committee on Cancer Survivorship. Improving care and quality of life, national cancer policy board. In: Hewitt M, Greenfield S, Stovall E, Institute of Medicine and National Research Council of the National Academies, editors. From cancer patient to cancer survivor: lost in transition. Washington DC: The National Academies Press; 2005.
4. American Society of Clinical Oncology. cancer.net/survivorship/follow-care-after-cancer-treatment/asco-cancer-treatment-summaries-and-survivorship-care-plans; 2015.
5. Cancercare. Patient access & engagement report; 2016.
6. Altice CK, Banegas MP, Tucker-Seeley RD, Yabroff KR. Financial hardship experienced by cancer survivors. J Natl Cancer Inst. 2016;109(2). pii: djw205. Print 2017 Feb.
7. Forsythe LP, Parry C, Alfano CM, Kent EE, Leach CR, Haggstrom DA, et al. Use of survivorship care plans in the United States, associations with survivorship care. J Natl Cancer Inst. 2013;105(20):1579–87.
8. Kent EE, Arora NK, Rowland JH, Bellizzi KM, Forsythe LP, Hamilton AS, et al. Health information needs and health-related quality of life in a diverse population of long-term cancer survivors. Patient Educ Couns. 2012;89(2):345–52.
9. Mols F, Husson O, Roukema JA, van de Poll-Franse LV. Depressive symptoms are a risk factor for all-cause mortality. J Cancer Surviv. 2013;7(3):484–92.
10. Jacobsen PB, Ransom S. Implementation of NCCN distress management guidelines by member institutions. J Natl Compr Cancer Netw. 2007;5(1):99–103.
11. Margenthaler JA, Allam E, Chen L, Virgo KS, Kulkarni UM. Surveillance of patients with breast cancer after curative-intent primary treatment: current practice patterns. J Oncol Pract. 2012;8(2):79–83.
12. Commission on Cancer, Cancer Program Standards. Ensuring patient-centered care; 2016 Edition.
13. Rollnick S, Miller W, Butler CC. Motivational interviewing in health care: helping patients change behavior. New York: Guilford Press; 2008.
14. Rosengren DB. Building motivational interviewing skills: a practioner workbook. New York: Guilford Press; 2009.
15. Yates JS, Mustian KM, Morrow GR, Gillies LJ, Padmanaban D, Atkins JN, et al. Prevalence of complementary and alternative medicine use in cancer patients during treatment. Support Care Cancer. 2005;13(10):806–11.
16. Chan CLW, Dickens R. Oncology social work practice in integrative medicine. In: Christ G, Messner C, Bhear L, editors. Handbook of oncology social work: psychosocial care for people with cancer. New York: Oxford University Press; 2015. p. 872.
17. Consortium of Academic Health Centers for Integrative Medicine. imconsortium.org. Accessed 20 May 2017.
18. MacDonald G. Medicine hands: massage therapy for people with cancer. Scotland: Findhorn Press; 2014.

19. Würtzen H, Dalton SO, Christensen J, Andersen KK, Elsass P, Flyger HL, et al. Effect of mindfulness-based stress reduction on somatic symptoms, distress, mindfulness and spiritual well-being in women with breast cancer. A randomized controlled trial. Acta Oncol. 2015;54(5):712–9.
20. Bower JE, Crosswell AD, Stanton AL, Crespi CM, Winston D, et al. Mindfulness meditation for younger breast cancer survivors: a randomized controlled trial. Cancer. 2015;121(8):1231–40.
21. Chin HY, Shyu YK, Chang PC, Tsai PC. Effects of acupuncture on menopause-related symptoms in breast cancer survivors: a meta-analysis of randomized controlled trials. Cancer Nurs. 2016;39(3):228–37.
22. Mao JJ, Bowman MA, Xie SX, Bruner D, De Micele A, Farriar JT. Electroacupuncture vs. gabapentin for hot flashes among breast cancer survivors: a randomized placebo-controlled trial. J Clin Oncol. 2015;33(31):3615–20.
23. Pennebaker JW. Opening up: the healing power of expressing emotions. New York: Guilford Press; 1990.
24. Winters-Stone KM, Dobek J, Bennett JA, Nail LM, Leo MC, Schwartz A. The effect of resistance training on muscle strength and physical functioning in older post-menopausal breast cancer survivors: a randomized controlled trial. J Cancer Surviv. 2012;6(2):189–99.
25. Davis C. Oncology social work practice in the care of breast and ovarian cancer survivors. New York: Nova Science Publishers; 2009.
26. Davies NJ, Batchup L, Thomas R. The role of diet and physical activity in breast, colorectal, and prostate cancer survivorship; a review of the literature. Br J Cancer. 2011;105 (Suppl 1):S52–73.
27. Spiegel D, Classen C. Group therapy for cancer patients: a research-based handbook of psychosocial care. New York: Basic Books Publishers; 2000.

# Chapter 11
# Medical-Legal Partnerships in Cancer Care

**Tomas Bednar and Domna Antoniadis**

## Abbreviations

| | |
|---|---|
| ACA | Patient Protection and Affordable Care Act |
| ACP | Advance care planning |
| ADA | Americans with Disabilities Act |
| ALJ | Administrative law judge |
| BCCPTA | Breast and Cervical Cancer Prevention and Treatment Act |
| CAL | Compassionate allowance |
| CHIP | Child health insurance program |
| FDCPA | Fair Debt Collection Practices Act |
| FHA | Fair Housing Act |
| FMLA | Family Medical Leave Act |
| FPL | Federal poverty level |
| HCPOA | Healthcare power of attorney |
| IEP | Initial enrollment period |
| I-HELP | Income, housing and utilities, education and employment, legal status, personal and familial stability |
| LPR | Legal permanent resident |
| MA | Medicare advantage |
| MAGI | Modified adjusted gross income |
| MLP | Medical-legal partnership |
| National Center | National Center for Medical-Legal Partnerships |
| OOP | Out-of-pocket expenses |
| POA | Financial power of attorney |
| PRUCOL | Permanent residence under color of law |
| PRWORA | Personal responsibility and work opportunity reconciliation action |

T. Bednar (✉)
Philadelphia, PA, USA

D. Antoniadis
New York Legal Assistance Group, New York, NY, USA
e-mail: dantoniadis@nylag.org

 
P. Hopewood, M. J. Milroy (eds.), *Quality Cancer Care*,
https://doi.org/10.1007/978-3-319-78649-0_11

| | |
|---|---|
| SDH | Social determinants of health |
| SGA | Substantial gainful activity |
| SSA | Social security administration |
| SSDI | Social security disability |
| SSI | Supplemental security income |
| TANF | Temporary assistance for needy families |
| TERI | Terminal illness cases |
| TWP | Trial work period |

## Introduction to the Medical-Legal Partnership (MLP) Model

Medical-legal partnerships (MLP) are a service delivery model that integrates legal services into the daily functions of healthcare institutions and practices in order to address the health-harming legal needs of low-income individuals and improve outcomes at the patient, institutional, and population levels [1]. The model is both a result and driver of health care's broader shift towards addressing the overall social determinants of health (SDH) [2]. At their core, MLPs seek to (1) provide patients direct legal intervention and advocacy, such as assistance with public benefits and representation in court hearing; (2) implement institutional-level changes, such as creating hospital-wide legal need screening protocols; and (3) affect broader policy changes, such as advocating for increased enforcement of lead laws in identified at-risk communities [3].

The MLP model formally began in the Department of Pediatrics at Boston Medical School in 1993. Since then MLPs have spread to 294 healthcare institutions in 41 states [4]. The National Center for Medical-Legal Partnerships (National Center) develops tools and resources for stakeholders interested in establishing a MLP. Among these resources is the "MLP Toolkit," which offers an in-depth stepwise guide for healthcare and legal providers that seek to collaborate on a new MLP initiative.

Typically, MLPs consist of a partnership between a healthcare institution or practice and a nonprofit legal aid clinic with the goal of incorporating legal aid services directly into the regular practice of the healthcare partner. However, one of the key strengths of the model is its flexibility in adapting to the particular circumstances of each partnership and community. As a result, there is a wide variety of MLP types and an even broader variety of potential clinical partners such as acute care hospitals, hospice centers, federally qualified health centers, cancer centers, pediatric primary care offices, and community-based health clinics [5]. Legal partners can be pro-bono attorneys offering free services, local nonprofit legal aid organizations, and law schools providing student support. Other MLP partners can range from state departments of health and aging, nonprofit service organizations, and local community organizations to large corporate sponsors. MLPs cultivate and reward creative approaches and seemingly unlikely partnerships.

## *Clinical and Legal Models That Incorporate Medical-Legal Partnership Services into Cancer Care*

The practical realities of resource allocation and funding that providers and MLP advocates often face require partners to implement innovative approaches when integrating legal services into a cancer setting.

From a clinical practice perspective, the flexibility of the MLP model allows it to be introduced into most cancer treatment venues. One particularly fruitful area of integration is introducing MLP services into a patient navigation model. Patient navigation is generally understood to mean the "individualized assistance offered to patients, families and caregivers to overcome health care system barriers and facilitate timely access to quality medical and psycho-social care from pre-diagnosis through all phases of the cancer experience" [6]. Despite the recent growth and success of the model, providers that operate in a patient navigation system have expressed frustration with their inability to handle certain legal and system needs of patients [7]. The MLP model can integrate legal services within the patient navigation process, using tools and services that most effectively assist this distinct populations [8].

From a legal practice perspective, the types of legal resources that can be utilized in a cancer MLP can vary widely and are dependent on the resources available in the particular community. Some of the common cancer MLP delivery models include the following:

### Hotline

A legal hotline is a service designed to provide legal advice and information by telephone [9]. This includes programs that provide answers to clients' legal questions, analysis of their legal problems, and advice on solving those problems. Some hotlines may perform brief services such as making phone calls, writing letters, or preparing documents on behalf of clients. Hotlines may also provide referrals to other programs or serve as an intake for a full-service program. Hotline call handlers may be attorneys, paralegals, or law students, working under an attorney's direct supervision. The Cancer Legal Line of Minnesota is a strong example of an organization leveraging limited resources to best assist their community needs.

### Law School Partnerships

Oncology practices with access to law schools can create a partnership that incorporates law students. Often, this is done by developing a clinical practice course within the law school that provides specialized training to the law students on practicing in this type of environment. Prime examples of legal needs that lend themselves to this type of model are advance care planning documents and social security disability benefit cases. The students must be supervised by licensed attorneys, which are usually faculty members of the law school, or local legal aid attorneys. Incorporating law students provides for a more didactic and interactive approach to the treatment of legal needs in a cancer setting.

### Pro-Bono Partnerships

Many medical-legal partnerships (MLPs) rely on local pro-bono attorneys to partner with them and assist with caseloads and specialized case types. For example, an MLP that primarily focuses on public benefits and housing may nevertheless require assistance with family law and immigration issues. Local attorneys that are willing to partner with the MLP and take on these cases provide an invaluable resource at filling the gaps that typical MLP services cannot fill. Alternatively, in locations where other legal services are limited, cancer centers can consider partnering with local attorneys to provide limited services, such as monthly advance care planning document clinics or general "know-your-rights" education sessions.

### On-Site Integration

The ideal cancer MLP incorporates an attorney on-site into the practice of a cancer center. The attorney, usually an employee of a legal aid agency, sees patients referred to them by the providers and works collaboratively to address their legal needs. They also train providers on how to identify those legal needs and work to implement institutional- and population-level interventions. Just as any provider on the healthcare team, an MLP attorney's efficacy is directly connected to the degree of integration into the practice, so healthcare providers are encouraged to consider the attorneys as an essential part of the care team.

Deciding on the type of appropriate delivery model for a particular treatment environment requires, in large part, an assessment of (1) the unique legal needs of the patient population and (2) the institutional and community resources available to address those needs. While the process of developing these assessments is outside the scope of this chapter, providers or entities interested in starting a cancer MLP should refer to the National Center's MLP toolkit for further assistance, which is available on their website [4].

## *Medical-Legal Partnership: Addressing Social and Legal Determinants of Health*

The primary goal of MLPs is to improve patient well-being by addressing social determinants of health and eliminating legal and regulatory barriers to care. An MLP's ability to address the legal needs of its patient population relies upon a comprehensive understanding of the types of unique legal barriers that the population faces and how those barriers relate to the overall social determinants of patient health.

A combination of factors impacts the health of individuals and communities. Social determinants of health are structural constructs and conditions in which people are born, grow, live, work, and age that have an impact on the overall well-being and quality of life of individuals [10]. There is growing consensus on the negative impact that SDH can have on health equity, particularly as they relate to the poor and underserved as well as those suffering from chronic health conditions.

The "law," which in this context is a broad term referring to local, state, and federal statutes and codes, judicial case law, administrative regulations, and relevant institutional policies and procedures, can often serve as both an intentional architect and indirect agent of SDH. The law interacts with SDH by "(1) helping structure and perpetuate the social conditions that we describe as 'social determinants' and (2) as a mechanism or mediator through which social structures are transformed into levels and distributions of health" [11]. As an example, adjustments in eligibility criteria for the Supplemental Nutrition Assistance Program (SNAP—previously known as food stamps) or other public benefits can have direct consequences on the overall well-being of individuals [3]. A more distal example is child education laws, which can be considered to impact population-level health when you consider the link between health and education level [1]. In both cases the underlying legal frameworks mold much of the health-related social and environmental realities of the individuals' lives.

Generally, the types of legal issues that impact the well-being of low-income individuals can be separated into five categories using the National Center's acronym "I-HELP" [12]. These categories include income, housing and utilities, education and employment, legal status, and personal and family stability. Figure 11.1 outlines the five categories and highlights how MLPs can assist providers in addressing the legal needs associated with them.

Within the context of individual MLPs, the five I-HELP categories are likely to present themselves through idiosyncratic sets of legal needs. For example, the legal needs of young families in an outpatient pediatric setting tend to focus on special education issues and denials of public benefits [14], whereas the needs of individuals in an outpatient oncology setting, as discussed further below, usually focus on advance planning documents and financial security [15]. For the former group, the primary I-HELP categories are "education and employment" as well as "income." For the oncology group, the emphasized I-HELP categories are "personal and family stability" and "income." While there is commonality between the groups' overall categorical needs, each patient population expresses those needs in a distinct fashion. This unique expression of overall legal needs can be understood as the "legal determinants" of that population's health.

Each MLP partnership must adjust their services and practice flow to match their patient populations' particular needs. This general principle also applies to cancer-focused MLPs, which must come to understand how the particular legal needs of their patients can exacerbate the physical, mental, and emotional impact of a cancer

| I-HELP® ISSUE | Common Social Determinant of Health | Civil Legal Aid Interventions That Help | Impact of Civil Legal Aid Intervention on Health / Health Care |
|---|---|---|---|
| Income | Availability of resources to meet daily basic needs | **Benefits Unit**: Appeal denials of food stamps, health insurance, cash benefits, and disability benefits | 1. Increasing someone's income means s/he makes fewer trade-offs between affording food and health care, including medications.<br>2. Being able to afford enough healthy food helps people manage chronic diseases and helps children grow and develop. |
| Housing & utilities | Healthy physical environments | **Housing Unit**: Secure, housing subsidies; Improve substandard conditions; Prevent eviction; Protect against utility shut-off | 1. A stable, decent, affordable home helps a person avoid costly emergency room visits related to homelessness.<br>2. Consistent housing, heat and electricity helps people follow their medical treatment plans. |
| Education & Employment | Access to the opportunity to learn and work | **Education & Employment Units**: Secure specialized education services; Prevent and remedy employment discrimination and enforce workplace rights | 1. A quality education is the single greatest predictor of a person's adult health.<br>2. Consistent employment helps provide money for food and safe housing, which also helps avoid costly emergency health care services.<br>3. Access to health insurance is often linked to employment. |
| Legal Status | Access to the opportunity to work | **Veterans & Immigration Units**: Resolve veteran discharge status; Clear criminal / credit histories; Assist with asylum applications | 1. Clearing a person's criminal history or helping a veteran change their discharge status helps make consistent employment and access to public benefits possible.<br>2. Consistent employment provides money for food and safe housing, which helps people avoid costly emergency health care services. |
| Personal & family stability | Exposure to violence | **Family Law Unit**: Secure restraining orders for domestic violence; Secure adoption, custody and guardianship for children | 1. Less violence at home means less need for costly emergency health care services.<br>2. Stable family relationships significantly reduce stress and allow for better decision-making, including decisions related to health care. |

**Fig. 11.1** Five categories of legal issues that impact the well-being of low-income individuals [13]. Chart was recreated with permission from Marple, Kate. Framing Legal Care as Health Care. Washington, DC: The National Center for Medical-Legal Partnership, January 2015

diagnosis. By understanding the distinct legal needs of cancer patients, MLP teams can work to accomplish their goal of improving the overall health of cancer patients.

## Legal Needs of Cancer Patients

A 2007 study that drew on responses from 50 mixed-site cancer patients showed that the patients reported cancer-specific legal needs as having a significant impact on their quality of life and that despite this impact those needs were not being met through the course of their treatment [15]. The patients identified and rated 30 medically related legal needs on their impact on quality of life and the degree to which patients felt those needs were being addressed in their care. The researchers grouped the legal needs into broad categories based on initial groupings provided by patients. The resulting four categories were health care related (healthcare proxies, advance directives, etc.), employment related (FMLA, insurance rights, disability issues, etc.), financial related (social security, pensions, IRS, financial planning, etc.), and estate planning (wills, inheritance, probate, custody issues, etc.). Almost uniformly, each category of need had a perceived significant impact on quality of life and was viewed as largely unaddressed in care.

Comparing the National Center's I-HELP categories in Fig. 11.1 to the four cancer-specific categories from the Zevon et al. study further shows how patient populations tend to retain the general themes of the I-HELP categories, albeit in their own unique fashions. Both sets of categories include express concerns around financial, familial, and personal stability. However, the cancer study's highest ranked category with respect to impact on quality life, the "health-related" category, focused almost exclusively on advance care planning matters, including advance directives, do-not-resuscitate orders, and powers of attorney. These are legal needs that would only be a small part of the broader "personal and family stability" I-HELP category. Yet for cancer patients, the need for advance care planning is the primary manifestation of patients' concerns around personal and familial stability, and is subsequently perceived as having a significant impact on quality of life.

In this section we provide specific insights into the most common health-harming legal issues that cancer patients face. These issues should be the starting point of any cancer MLP's legal needs assessment and can reasonably be expected to make up a significant portion of its practice. Each main section represents one of the I-HELP categories and its cancer-specific component legal needs. The legal needs snapshots include an introduction to the basic underlying legal principles, how those principles apply to cancer patients, and practice tips for cancer MLP advocates.

## *Income, Insurance, and Debt Maintenance*

Representing the first of the I-HELP categories, the legal needs below focus on the overall financial stability of low-income cancer patients. The primary factors involved in this category include stable and consistent income streams, access to sufficient medical coverage, and management of medical and consumer debt.

For income maintenance, we consider the legal needs associated with the disability benefit programs operated by the Social Security Administration (SSA), which are two of the main sources of income for individuals with cancer. For medical coverage, we discuss the primary sources of coverage for most cancer patients, which are Medicaid, Medicare, and private insurance. For debt maintenance, we outline the approach that providers and MLP advocates should take in stabilizing and mitigating the impact of medical and consumer debt.

## Social Security Disability and Supplemental Security Income

The Social Security Administration (SSA) manages two programs that pay monthly disability benefits to people under age 65 who cannot work for at least a year because of a severe disability: Social Security Disability Insurance (SSDI) and Supplemental Security Income (SSI) [16]. The requirements for medical proof of disability are the same for both programs.

SSDI benefits are an insurance program and are paid to people who have worked long enough and recently enough to be eligible for the program. Those who receive SSDI benefits for at least 24 months also qualify for Medicare. SSI disability payments are for adults with limited income, resources, and work histories. No prior work is needed. SSI recipients generally qualify for Medicaid.

Since SSDI is fundamentally an insurance program paid for by taxes on a worker's wage whereas SSI is a welfare program for the needy, SSDI benefit amounts are usually higher than SSI payments. In certain circumstances, individuals can be eligible for both programs. Disability benefits are also available for children who have severe impairments and are intended to assist parents with the cost of caring for a child with disabilities. For the purpose of this chapter, we limit our scope to adult SSI and SSDI programs, which cover the majority of cancer patients.

### SSA's Definition of Disability

All jurisdictions use the same federal criteria and laws for determining disability eligibility for SSDI and SSI. One of the first starting points of any Social Security Application is the definition of disability. Disability is:

> "the inability to engage in any substantial gainful activity (SGA) by reason of any medically determinable physical or mental impairment which can be expected to result in death or which has lasted or can be expected to last for a continuous period of not less than 12 months [17]."

Practically, there are many regulations and rules that govern the application of the definition of disability in each individual's case. The complicated nuances of this process are a major contributor to the fact that only 34% of initial adult applicants receive disability benefits [18]. However, the overall framework can be reduced to five sequential steps.

### The Five-Step Sequential Evaluation Process

SSA uses a five-step process to determine if a claimant is too disabled to work [19]. The five-step process as applied to cancer patients is broken down in Table 11.1.

**Table 11.1** The five-step disability process applied to cancer patients

| |
|---|
| **1. Is the person currently working?** |
| The initial step is to determine if the applicant is working. Step 1 can cause challenges for many cancer patients since a diagnosis does not preclude the ability to work. However, patients can still be eligible for benefits if they show that their disability-related work expenses ultimately put their income below a certain threshold [20]. |
| **2. Is the medical condition "severe" and likely to prevent work for at least 12 months?** |
| In this step SSA considers the severity of your impairments and how they impact functional work activities such as standing, sitting, laying, and bending. Most applicants, including cancer patients, will not fail at this step so long as they have sufficient medical evidence of their disability. |
| **3. Does the diagnosis(s) meet or medically equal the qualifications under SSA's disability listings?** |
| The third step is to see if the patient's medical condition satisfies a particular disability listing on SSA's list of disabilities [21]. If a listing is met, the person is automatically deemed to satisfy the definition of eligibility, and the rest of their application will depend on non-disability requirements. One of SSA's disability categories includes "malignant neoplastic diseases." In that category there are 14 types of cancer diagnoses that qualify. |
| 4. **Can the person do past work?** |
| If a patient does not satisfy one of the step 3 listings, SSA will then assess whether the individual can perform any of their past work dating back 15 years. This step can require an applicant to fill out a "residual functional capacity assessment" and meet with an independent medical reviewer. Many cancer patients will not meet a listing in step 3 and will therefore be asked to complete the documents associated with step 4. |
| 5. **Can the person do any other type of work?** |
| If an individual is assessed as not being able to perform any of their previous work in step 4, SSA will then consider if they can perform any work in the general economy. This will depend heavily on the proof of the patient's functional limitations as well as the patient's age and education. For cancer patients, this step will again depend on the robustness of their medical documentation. |

## Critical Cases

The process of applying for SSI and SSDI benefits can be quite lengthy, with cases often taking up to 2 years to reach a final decision. For many cancer patients, waiting 2 years for a necessary income source is simply not an option. Fortunately, there are several circumstances in which the SSA will expedite an application. These are called "critical cases" [22]. The three most relevant to cancer patients are terminal diagnoses (**TERI cases**), compassionate allowance (**CAL**), and **dire need**.

### *Terminal Illness: TERI*

The SSA will expedite claims based on a terminal illness [23]. Terminal illness means the impairment cannot be reversed and is expected to end in death. Social Security will prioritize these cases and strive to expedite them every step. For cancer

**Table 11.2** SSA indicators of terminal illness—cancer

| Any malignant neoplasm (cancer) which is: | An allegation or diagnosis of: |
|---|---|
| • Metastatic (has spread)<br>• Defined as stage IV<br>• Persistent or recurrent following initial therapy<br>• Inoperable or unresectable<br>• Awaiting a heart, heart and lung, lung, liver, or bone marrow transplant (excludes kidney and corneal transplants) | • Cancer of the esophagus<br>• Cancer of the liver<br>• Cancer of the pancreas<br>• Cancer of the gallbladder<br>• Mesothelioma<br>• Small cell or oat cell lung cancer<br>• Cancer of the brain<br>• Acute myelogenous leukemia (AML) or acute lymphocytic leukemia (ALL) |

patients, the relevant TERI indicators are shown in Table 11.2. While these indicators do not guarantee eligibility, their presence does suggest to the SSA that the patient's case needs expedited review.

*Compassionate Allowances*

Some medical conditions may qualify for what the SSA calls a "compassionate allowance" (CAL) [24]. CAL conditions are severe enough that they are very likely to be approved under the SSA's Listing of Impairments (step 3 in the five-step disability process). For many of the CAL conditions, SSA will only require minimal objective medical evidence and will sometimes grant approval on the diagnosis alone. This makes it easier to approve claims quickly, sometimes in as little as 10 days. There are currently 165 CAL conditions currently recognized by the SSA. Examples of some of the cancer diagnoses that qualify as a CAL include certain types of bladder cancer, breast cancer, pancreatic cancer, ovarian cancer, and esophageal cancer.

*Dire Need*

Unlike TERI and CAL cases, dire need cases are based on the patient's financial need [25]. If a claimant does not have the resources to get food, medicine, or shelter, the SSA will treat the claim as a dire need case and will expedite the application process. Expediting a dire need case still requires the individual to satisfy the definition of disability. Nevertheless, this designation can shorten application wait times and allow patients to obtain much-needed income.

## Working While Disabled or Returning to Work

In certain circumstances, a cancer patient who is getting social security disability benefits has the option to try to return to work and retain their benefits for a period of time [26]. A person who attempts to work may continue to receive up to 4 years of support and services involving cash payments and/or healthcare coverage.

**Table 11.3** Working while disabled—continuation of benefits

| | |
|---|---|
| Nine months of trial work, called a "**trial work period**" (TWP) (not necessarily consecutive) during which a person may continue to receive benefits regardless of the amount of earnings | Continuation of Medicare for at least 39 months after the trial work period |
| A 36-month extended period of eligibility following the end of the 9-month TWP during which benefits may be paid for any month if earnings fall below the SGA level | Deduction from gross earnings of impairment-related work expenses in deciding if earnings constitute SGA. These include wheelchairs and seeing-eye dogs |
| Continuation of monthly payments and insurance coverage for a person whose impairment has shown medical improvement related to the ability to work so long as the person is participating in an approved vocational rehabilitation program that is expected to result in allowing the individual to work and become self-supporting | |

Table 11.3 is a summary of some of the potential work benefits that SSI/SSDI recipients may be eligible for:

If a patient is able to fully return to work but becomes disabled again within 5 years after a previous period of disability, he or she will not have to serve a new 5-month waiting period before disability benefits may resume. In addition, if the person was previously entitled to Medicare, that coverage will resume immediately.

## Appeal

If an applicant is denied, SSA is required to give clear and timely notice explaining the reason for the denial and how to request an appeal of the decision [27]. In order to file an appeal, a claimant must make the request in writing within 60 days from the date they receive the letter. SSA assumes receipt 5 days after the date on the letter, unless the applicant can show they received it later.

During an appeal, SSA will reconsider the entire initial decision, including all of the submitted evidence. Applicants will have the opportunity to submit new evidence and medical records as well as appear before an administrative law judge to argue their case in person. If the judge determines that the initial decision was wrong, they can reverse that decision and award any back benefits. Unfortunately, standard appeal times can be as long as 1–2 years. Although these times can be expedited using the critical case circumstances discussed above (TERI, CAL, dire need), there will inevitably be processing delays, which is why it is important that MLPs try to ensure that a patient's initial application is as strong as it can be.

## SSI/SSDI Advocacy Tips

SSA's requirement that a patient's condition be "medically determinable" highlights how a cancer patient's successful disability benefit application often relies on effective coordination between MLP team members. When a person is diagnosed with a condition that meets one of SSA's disability listings, their chances of obtaining benefits increase if the MLP team is able to quickly identify the qualifying condition and work together to translate the relevant medical data into useful evidence. Letters from healthcare providers drafted with the assistance of attorneys can prevent the long delays of the appeal process. Furthermore, training by legal providers on the basics of SSI and SSDI allows healthcare providers to understand the importance of recording their notes from a functional perspective. Providers should ask themselves: In what way does the diagnosis currently impact my patient's abilities to perform work-related activities such as sitting, walking, lifting, concentrating, speaking, or remembering?

## Medicaid

Since its initial enactment in 1965 as a humble program designed to provide medical assistance to individuals and families receiving cash assistance, Medicaid has grown to become the largest single insurer in the United States, providing coverage to 70 million individuals, accounting for one in five Americans [28]. The most recent growth came with the implementation of the Patient Protection and Affordable Care Act (ACA), which allowed states to expand Medicaid coverage to individuals earning 138% of the Federal Poverty Level (FPL) [29]. Of the newly expanded population, approximately 160,000 are believed to have an ongoing cancer diagnosis, although that figure is likely underestimated [30].

### Medicaid Administration

Medicaid is funded through a partnership between the federal and state governments that requires states to put money towards the cost of their Medicaid programs and in return receive a matching percentage of the total dollars spent from the federal government [31]. While states are required to provide certain basic services to all members, they maintain a large degree of latitude in the administration of their individual Medicaid programs. As a result, there are fundamental differences between states as to the services and delivery systems they employ.

### Categories of Coverage: Breast and Cervical Cancer and Medicaid Buy-In

Federal law requires that all states with a Medicaid program provide coverage to a list of mandatory coverage populations, such as low-income family, qualified pregnant women and children, and individuals receiving SSI [32]. States can also choose to provide coverage to other optional categories, one of which targets women who need treatment for breast or cervical cancer [33]. This category was created by Congress in 2000 under the Breast and Cervical Cancer Prevention and Treatment Act (BCCPTA) [34]. It allows states to provide full Medicaid coverage to uninsured women, regardless of income or resources, who screen positive for breast and cervical cancer under the Center for Disease Control's National Breast and Cervical Cancer Early Detection Program [35]. By 2009, every state had an established BCCPTA program [36]. Assisting patients and providers in navigating a state's BCCPTA program is a great opportunity for MLP attorneys to augment access to care.

Another important category of coverage for cancer patients is the optional Medicaid buy-in program. This program allows employed individuals with disabilities to retain their Medicaid coverage by raising the standard income and resource requirements and requiring individuals to pay small income-based premiums [37]. For cancer patients, Medicaid buy-in is an opportunity to retain necessary employment income and medical coverage while receiving treatment. However, many states require individuals to submit regular proofs of employment and disability status for continued eligibility. To address this, MLPs can help patients draft a letter clearly explaining the patient's illness, symptoms, and expected length of the treatment.

### Eligibility Requirements

Medicaid is an "entitlement" program, which means that anyone that satisfies its eligibility requirements is guaranteed to receive benefits. Eligibility for Medicaid is based on financial factors, such as income and resources, and nonfinancial factors, such as state residency and immigration status [38]. Each state is able to set certain income and resource limits for the covered populations within federal guidelines [39].

Income eligibility is determined using the "Modified Adjusted Gross Income" (MAGI) guidelines [40]. A person's MAGI is set through a three-step process: (1) their total gross income is established, (2) their adjusted gross income is calculated by subtracting tax deductions from their gross income, and (3) their MAGI is set by adding back certain deductions to their adjusted gross income. With respect to resources, states have the freedom to set resource requirements and guidelines for certain categories. For example, Medicaid buy-in programs often have resource requirements. With the passage of the ACA, many of the resource limits that previously stood as a barrier to eligibility were eliminated. Regarding nonfinancial eligibility factors, the most relevant for many cancer patients is immigration status. This is discussed in greater detail in the "Legal Status" portion of this chapter.

### Medicaid Appeals

The Medicaid Act requires states to provide a "fair hearing" for patients who have been denied eligibility or services, or who suffer from unreasonable delays [41]. More broadly, when the government takes an action that could potentially harm an individual and the reason for that action is based on a finding of fact, then "the evidence used to prove the Government's case must be disclosed to the individual so that he has an opportunity to show that it is untrue" [42]. Medicaid enrollees have several constitutional rights when states try to deny, reduce, or terminate Medicaid coverage or services [43]:

1. A meaningful notice stating the basis for the action and, when coverage is to be reduced or terminated, a pre-termination notice informing the claimant of the right to continue benefits pending a final administrative decision
2. The opportunity for a "fair hearing" during which the claimant can confront and cross-examine the witnesses and evidence relied on by the agency
3. The right of the claimant to be represented by counsel
4. An impartial decision maker
5. A reasoned decision, based solely on evidence adduced at the hearing

These are the foundational legal principles that MLP attorneys rely on when advocating with state Medicaid agencies. While legal in nature, these principles are not limited to an attorney's scope of practice, and are equally useful to any patient or advocate.

#### Medicaid Advocacy Tips

Assisting cancer practices with Medicaid applications and eligibility requirements is often an essential component of an integrated cancer MLP. MLP attorneys can intervene with states to ensure that applications are processed in a timely, accurate, and legal fashion. With the healthcare providers' assistance, MLP attorneys can also challenge unfavorable eligibility determinations or treatment denials. In order to succeed in these functions, MLPs should develop procedures that allow providers to directly refer lapses in coverage or services to their legal partner. Many of these lapses can be prevented through periodic training of healthcare staff on the basics of Medicaid eligibility, application process, and coverage appeals. This "upstream" mentality can prevent damaging delays in patient treatment and mitigate patients' stress around continued coverage.

### Medicare

Medicare is a federally funded and administered health insurance program that provides health insurance coverage to individuals aged 65 and older, to the disabled, and to those with end-stage renal disease and amyotrophic lateral sclerosis. It was established in 1965 under Title XVIII of the Social Security Act as a way to provide insurance to people aged 65 and older regardless of income or medical history [44]. In 1972 it was expanded to include people under age 65 with physical and mental disabilities eligible for SSDI payments and people with end-stage renal disease [45]. Since its introduction, it has grown to cover more than 56 million beneficiaries [46].

Although Medicare is a government-subsidized program, maintaining coverage often requires significant out-of-pocket (OOP) expenses. For cancer patients, these costs rise significantly throughout the course of treatment and beyond. A recent study assessing the OOP costs of cancer patients on Medicare found that patients with no supplemental or secondary insurance could expect to pay an average of $8115 a year [47]. This expense amounted to nearly 24% of their income. Some individuals in the study paid up to 63%. Even those with "Medigap" supplementary coverage and those on Medicare Advantage plans paid an average of $5500–$6000 in annual OOP costs. "Dual eligibles," who are low-income individuals eligible for both Medicare and Medicaid, still paid an average of $2116.

For low-income cancer patients, OOP costs represent one of the largest barriers to better health and increased quality life. The OOP costs are, in large part, a result of the structure of Medicare and how it pays for medical services. By understanding this structure, MLP teams can work together to limit debilitating OOP costs.

### Medicare Coverage as Applied to Cancer Patients

The coverage provided by Medicare is generally separated into four "parts" along with supplemental coverage through Medigap plans. Each part covers a unique set of services:

**Part A: Hospital Insurance Program**. Part A covers hospital care, skilled nursing facility care, nursing home care, hospice, and home health services [48]. With respect to cancer patients, Part A covers the expenses of inpatient stays and services, including inpatient chemotherapy and surgery. Generally, beneficiaries do not have to pay premiums for Part A services so long as they paid sufficient payroll taxes throughout their lifetimes (roughly 10 years of full-time work) [49]. However, beneficiaries are responsible for an annual deductible and coinsurance for time spent in the hospital outside of the "hospital benefit period." Part A coverage is automatically provided when a beneficiary enrolls in Medicare.

**Part B: Supplementary Medical Insurance Program**. Part B provides broad outpatient coverage for a range of services including, but not limited to, doctor visits, home health care, medical equipment, diagnostic procedures, and preventative care [50]. For cancer patients, Part B is responsible for outpatient visits as well as certain chemotherapy medications including intravenous and oral medications provided in an outpatient setting [51]. Part B has monthly premiums, an annual deductible ($183 in 2017), and an 80/20% insurer-patient coinsurance after deductible [52]. The 80/20% split means that Medicare patients are responsible for 20% of all costs of Part B coverage after paying an initial deductible. Furthermore, although Part B is technically voluntary, it is strongly recommended that beneficiaries enroll into it when they become eligible for Medicare unless they remain covered through an employer's insurance. There are significant penalties for late enrollment.

**Part C: Medicare Advantage (MA) Program**. MA Plans are healthcare plans that are run by private managed care companies that receive a fixed amount per beneficiary from the federal government to oversee beneficiaries' health care [53].

These plans are required to meet minimum federal guidelines and usually include at least Part A and Part B services as well as Part D drug coverage. Beyond the minimum federal requirements, Part C plans are free to structure services into various products to meet the needs of their beneficiaries in an effective and efficient fashion. The variety in plan type is matched by a variety in patient costs, which can include monthly premiums, deductibles, copayments, and coinsurance. Generally, Medicare Advantage plans charge the Part B premium as well as an additional premium paid directly to the plan.

**Part D: Outpatient Prescription Drug Benefit**. Part D plans cover outpatient prescription drugs and are offered by federally regulated private insurance companies. For cancer patients, Part D generally covers chemotherapy and anti-nausea drugs that cannot otherwise be provided intravenously [51]. The costs for prescription drug plans vary, but nearly all include monthly premiums as well as various coinsurance rates, including increased coinsurance during the "donut hole" in coverage [54]. Although the ACA has implemented measures to reduce the donut hole's impact and will eliminate it altogether by 2020, currently it still remains a significant source of OOP costs [55]. Individuals are eligible for Part D prescription drug coverage if they are enrolled in Part A, Part B, or both.

**Medigap: Medicare Supplemental Insurance**. Medigap policies are not a "part" of traditional Medicare but are instead plans offered through private companies to help pay some of the costs that traditional Medicare does not cover [56]. These costs include copayments, coinsurance, and deductibles. They can also offer extended service coverage outside of the scope of the traditional Medicare. Medigap plans differ from MA plans in that they are purely a supplement to full coverage, whereas MA plans are a way to obtain full Medicare coverage.

### Medicare Advocacy Tips

For cancer patients on Medicare, a large portion of their OOP costs will come from the expenses associated with prescription drug coverage under Parts B and D. The combination of Part B's 80/20% coinsurance and Part D's donut hole in coverage in addition to other copayments and deductibles can create serious financial hardships for cancer patients. Those patients that cannot afford their prescription drugs should be guided to seek "Extra Help." "Extra Help" is a program offered through the SSA that assists individuals who have low resources with their Medicare prescription drug costs [57]. Advocates should also check to see if a patient's low-income status makes them "dual eligible" for both Medicare and Medicaid. Although Medicare is the primary payer for most beneficiaries, supplementary Medicaid coverage will significantly decrease OOP costs.

If patients do not enroll into Medicare during their Initial Enrollment Period (IEP), then they run the risk of incurring significant late enrollment penalties and potentially complicating their supplemental Medicaid coverage. MLP teams should implement systems that help patients enroll in Medicare and, if needed, help patients seek "equitable relief" if there are any errors caused by Medicare in the enrollment process. In the context of Medicare, equitable relief is a request made to the federal government to correct or eliminate the effects of an "error, misrepresentation, or inaction" by federal employees [58]. It allows MLP team members to argue on the patients' behalf and correct any administrative errors.

## Private Insurance

The ability to understand the particulars of health coverage and advocate for timely, affordable, and clinically appropriate treatment is a challenge for many cancer patients. Further complicating matters are the differences between the various types of private insurance available to patients (group plans, individual plans, union plans, plans from federal and state health exchanges, etc.) as well as the patchwork of state laws that regulate them. However, there are general rights and protections available to nearly all patients on private insurance. These protections are most effective when they are combined with an interdisciplinary MLP care team.

### Protections Under the Affordable Care Act

As a result of the ACA, insurers are barred from refusing to sell or renew health insurance coverage on the basis of a patient's health status [59]. This is called "guaranteed issue." Insurers are also barred from implementing annual or lifetime limits on medical costs. In addition, many insurers can no longer refuse coverage of preexisting conditions.

Plans that are sold on the individual and small group markets must include a list of ten "Essential Health Benefits," which create a minimum floor of coverage services. These services include outpatient and emergency services, prescriptions, hospitalization, mental health and preventive care, and more. Although there are ongoing efforts to repeal and replace the ACA, the current political landscape suggests that many of these protections may remain in place.

### Private Insurance Advocacy Tips: Protections Against Denied Services

Similar to Medicare and Medicaid, cancer patients that are denied care by their private insurer are often told that the requested treatment does not satisfy the plan's definition of "medical necessity" (Table 11.4). While each plan is free to define the term in their own unique fashion, medical necessity can generally be understood as the following.

Providers should frame any initial engagement with an insurance company using the concepts in the definition of medical necessity. They should rely on their clinical judgment and use objective guidelines and evidence wherever possible. MLP attorneys can assist providers to better hone their arguments in light of the insurer's particular definition of the term.

**Table 11.4** Definition of medical necessity

| |
|---|
| Medical necessity is often seen as healthcare services that a physician exercising prudent clinical judgment would provide to a patient for the purpose of evaluating, diagnosing, or treating an illness, injury, disease, or its symptoms, and that are: |
| • In accordance with the generally accepted standards of medical practice |
| • Clinically appropriate, in terms of type, frequency, extent, site, and duration, and considered effective for the patient's illness, injury, or disease |
| • Not primarily for the convenience of the patient of physician, and not more costly than an alternative service or sequence of service at least as likely to produce equivalent therapeutic or diagnostic results as to the diagnosis or treatment of that patient's illness, injury, or disease |
| For these purposes, "generally accepted standards of medical practice" means: |
| • Standards that are based on credible scientific evidence published in peer-reviewed medical literature generally recognized by the relevant medical community |
| • Physician specialty society recommendations |
| • The views of physicians practicing in the relevant clinical area |
| • Any other relevant factors |
| • Preventative care may be medically necessary but coverage for medically necessary preventative care is governed by terms of the applicable plan documents. |

**Table 11.5** Important information for insurer treatment appeals

| Medical information | Legal information |
|---|---|
| What is the patient's diagnosis, prognosis, and current symptoms? | What is the date of the denial and the date that the patient received the denial? |
| What will happen if the patient does not obtain care? | What level of appeal is being filed (first, second, external review)? |
| What medical documentation exists (letters from providers, imaging, charts, etc.)? | What is the deadline for filing the appeal/review? |
| Has a peer review been conducted? If so, has any documentation been provided? | What are the elements of the plan's definition of medical necessity? |
| Is this experimental/investigational treatment? If so, is there any data to support it yet? | What parts of the denial need to be challenged/disproven? |
| Is there medical support showing that the recommended course of treatment is necessary given the patient's circumstances? | What are the relevant state law protections? |

If the matter cannot be resolved by speaking with the insurance company, patients retain the right to file an appeal directly to their insurance company. As a result of protections passed by the ACA, the insurance company must conduct a full and fair review of its decision. If the case is urgent, the insurance company must speed up this process. MLP attorneys can draft the appeal and work with providers to craft an argument on the patient's behalf. Table 11.5 highlights some of the relevant medical and legal questions that need to be answered before filing an effective service denial appeal.

If the insurance company denies the appeal, then the patient has the right to request an external review, which is an outside, objective, and independent panel.

The members of the panel can have no financial relationship to the insurer and therefore should have no bias in making a decision. If the external reviewer overturns the insurer's denial, the insurer must give the patient the payments or services requested.

## Medical and Consumer Debt

A cancer diagnosis can be exceedingly expensive for any patient and can become prohibitively so for many low-income individuals. When compared to other healthcare costs, cancer costs are increasing two to three times faster, and are projected to continue increasing [60]. The average out-of-pocket expenses for an individual are $1107 in the first year of a cancer diagnosis and $747 annually thereafter [61]. These estimates do not take into account the consequences of lost income for patients and their caregivers. Research has shown that about 30% of cancer patients report financial hardship and that they are 2.5 times more likely to enter bankruptcy than those without a history of cancer [62]. Cancer patients that file for bankruptcy are more likely to be younger, have lower annual household income, be unemployed, have public insurance, and have two or more cancer diagnoses [63].

The debt that cancer patients develop throughout the course of treatment can exist in several different forms. It can stem from unpaid medical bills; from unpaid mortgage, rent, or car bills; from unpaid credit card bills that were used as a temporary stopgap for other costs; from unpaid personal loans such as student loans; or even from unpaid utility bills. This myriad of possibilities highlights the underlying fact that cancer can completely disrupt an individual's income stream and their subsequent ability to pay for their normal obligations.

Although it is difficult to rid a patient of the burden of debt entirely, there are interventions that MLP teams can use to help abate some common debt-related issues. First, the MLP team should focus on reestablishing a continuous stream of income, which can include assisting the patient with applications for public benefit programs such as cash assistance or SNAP benefits (food stamps), applications for disability coverage under the SSI and SSDI programs (discussed above), and assistance with obtaining short- and long-term disability through a patient's employer.

Next, the team needs to determine the nature of the debts and rank them based on priority. Those costs associated with basic needs must be focused on first. This includes housing costs, food costs, and utility payments. MLP advocates should look into low-income utility payment programs through energy suppliers, which limit the amount that a supplier can charge qualified individuals. Furthermore, in many parts of the country that experience extreme seasonal temperatures, utility companies are often barred from turning off services during a specific range of months. With respect to housing costs, MLP lawyers can work to enter into adjusted payment terms with a bank or landlord. They can also represent clients in landlord-tenant hearings.

Once the patient's priority debts and needs are stabilized, the team can then shift its attention to other debts such as credit card debts, medical bills, and student loans.

An initial approach is to have the MLP lawyer negotiate lower payment terms with the patient's debt collectors. This can delay more drastic actions like bankruptcy and create more time for further interventions. They can also leverage state and federal consumer protection laws, such as the Fair Debt Collection Practices Act (FDCPA), which is a federal law that protects consumers from abusive, coercive, and unfair debt collection practices [64]. The FDCPA covers the collection of mortgages, credit cards, medical debts, and other debts for personal, family, and household purposes [65]. MLP lawyers may be able to use the FDCPA's protections to limit the frequency and time of day of collection calls, prevent collectors from contacting other family members regarding the debt, and perhaps even lower or discharge the debt if the collector does not adhere to the statute's (and relevant state law's) notice and collection requirements [66].

## *Housing*

Low-income families frequently face chronic housing problems that have known health risks and legal remedies [67]. These include such risks as lead paint, unsafe housing conditions, and mold proliferation. In other healthcare contexts, MLPs have proven themselves effective at not only addressing individual housing-related needs, but also implementing systemic change in targeting at-risk neighborhoods and negligent landlords [68]. A cancer diagnosis, with all of its attendant costs, can further destabilize a low-income individual's ability to maintain housing [69]. This, in turn, can cause lapses in treatment adherence and provider visits, as patients search for a new home. A diagnosis can also lead to discrimination in housing availability and accommodation. Due to the close ties between health, housing, and legal remedies, introducing legal providers into a cancer setting can be an effective way to directly impact low-income cancer patients' overall health.

### Tenant Protections

Patients that live in unsafe rental housing conditions often have a number of legal recourses available to them. They can contact their local code enforcement agency and ask for a housing inspection. This can lead to landlords receiving fines until they repair the property. They can also refer to the terms of their lease, which often outline the landlord's responsibility to maintain the functional and structural components of the property. If they live in public housing, such as the section 8 voucher program run by the US Department of Housing and Urban Development, then they are protected by even more rigorous federal regulations and lease agreements [70]. Most jurisdictions also have laws that prevent landlords from retaliating against tenants that exercise their housing rights.

Another powerful protection available to almost all tenants is the implied warranty of habitability. This warranty requires landlords to maintain their properties in a habitable condition and is read into nearly all residential leases [71]. This means that leases cannot waive the implied warranty and tenants will always be able to bring legal action under the warranty against landlords that do not appropriately maintain the property. Exactly what is required of the landlord will differ by jurisdiction, but generally it requires the landlord to maintain the property according to local housing codes and in a condition that does not preclude the ability of the tenant to live in the property.

If a patient does face the threat of eviction, then most jurisdictions will require that their landlord provide the individual notice prior to any legal action. There will also be the opportunity to appear before a judge to hear the merits of the claim. Landlords are typically barred from preemptively evicting their tenants prior to the completion of the legal action. Some jurisdictions are pushing to instate right-to-attorney laws for eviction cases [72].

### Fair Housing Act

The Fair Housing Act (FHA) was originally passed as Title VIII of the of the Civil Rights Act of 1968 and has since that time expanded to protect against the refusal to sell or rent a dwelling on the basis of race, color, religion, national origin, sex, or disability [73]. The act also prevents housing providers from refusing housing to persons with disabilities, or placing conditions on their residency, because they require reasonable accommodations for their disability [74]. The FHA therefore protects cancer patients seeking housing during or after treatment by preventing housing providers from refusing to rent or sell to the person simply because the provider is uncomfortable with that person's diagnosis.

Another type of disability discrimination specifically prohibited by the Act is the "refusal to make reasonable accommodations in rules, policies, practices, or services when such accommodations are necessary to afford such person equal opportunity to use and enjoy a dwelling" [75]. Housing providers must do everything they can to assist the individual with the disability without fundamentally altering the housing program or creating an undue financial or administrative burden. Reasonable accommodations may be necessary at all stages of the housing process, including application, tenancy, or prevention of eviction. For cancer patients who have mobility issues, the right to reasonable accommodations is a strong consumer protection. For example, a housing provider would likely need to make a reasonable accommodation for a tenant with mobility impairment caused by their cancer if that tenant requested the provider to install grab bars in their shower.

### Housing Advocacy Tips

Healthcare providers are essential allies in MLP attorneys' attempts to protect cancer patients from health -harming housing conditions and discrimination. From a preventative perspective, patient conversations with healthcare providers can lead to identification of the early stages of income insecurity and landlord-tenant troubles, which can be addressed through legal intervention. Healthcare providers can also offer medically verifiable reasons for why a patient's poor housing conditions are having a negative impact on their health, which allows MLP attorneys to better advocate with a patient's housing provider to repair the issues or move them to a different unit. The same information can also help MLP attorneys utilize the protections of the FHA to acquire reasonable accommodations for a patient's diagnosis or contest a refusal to rent or sell a property made on the basis of the patient's diagnosis.

To accomplish these goals, MLPs should ensure that healthcare providers are asking patients about their housing status and should include questions on housing on any internal MLP referral tools. MLPs can also begin to track geographic areas and individual landlords that are more commonly associated with poor housing. This data collection can potentially lead to broader legal efforts that have a population-level impact on health.

## *Employment and Disability Issues*

The ability to maintain steady employment or minimize employment-related stress is an important goal for many cancer patients. Unfortunately, when a person in the workplace is diagnosed with cancer, many unanticipated consequences can arise that threaten a patient's ability to continue to work. These consequences may lead to an individual taking a large consecutive portion of time off from work or requesting an accommodation from their employer so that they can continue to work throughout treatment. They may also face discrimination stemming from their diagnosis such as demotion in seniority status or deliberately unfavorable working conditions. Federal, state, and local laws all address the rights and protections afforded to persons with a disability who are employed, seeking employment, or were unlawfully discharged from employment.

MLP advocates should understand how these laws apply to cancer patients and what role an MLP team can play in assisting patients with their cancer-related employment and disability issues. Below is an introduction to two of the most commonly cited sources of protection for workers with cancer: the Americans with Disabilities Act (ADA) and the Family Medical Leave Act (FMLA).

### Americans with Disabilities Act

The primary federal law that protects the rights of individuals with disabilities is the Americans with Disabilities Act (ADA). The ADA was passed in 1990 in order "to provide a clear and comprehensive national mandate for the elimination of discrimination against individuals with disabilities" [76]. With respect to employment, the ADA prevents employers from discriminating against job applicants or employees on the basis of disability. This includes protections in a wide range of employer actions including recruitment, hiring, firing, promoting, and job assignments.

Since 2008, when Congress significantly expanded the definition of "disability" under the ADA, the majority of cancer patients have been protected by the law. The Equal Employment Opportunity Commission, which is the federal agency in charge of administering and enforcing the ADA, has even developed an in-depth Q&A for employers and employees about cancer in the workplace [77]. In it they state outright that cancer patients are very likely to be considered disabled under the law. They also point out that common discriminatory actions against cancer patients are founded in misperceptions of an individual's ability to work with a cancer diagnosis.

In general, the ADA applies to an employee with a disability who, with or without reasonable accommodations, can perform the essential functions of their job [78]. A person can have a disability in one of the three ways: (1) they can have a physical or mental impairment that substantially limits a major life activity, (2) they can have a record of such an impairment (important for cancer patients in remission), or (3) they can be regarded as having an actual or a perceived impairment by an employer [79]. This means that a person cannot be discriminated against if they currently have a disability, if they have a history of disability, or simply if their employer *believes* that they have a disability, even if they do not.

The ADA also has certain employer requirements. It applies only to employers that are engaged in an "industry-affecting commerce" and have 15 or more employees for at least 20 weeks [78]. Fortunately, the term "industry-affecting commerce" is construed broadly and tends not to be an issue in ADA litigation [80].

Employees protected by the ADA are entitled to request a reasonable accommodation for their disability so long as they are able to do the essential functions of their job. There is no limitation or criteria on what the accommodation can be as long as it is "reasonable" for the employer to implement [78]. An accommodation is reasonable if it does not cause "an undue burden" on the employer [78]. Generally, the accommodations cannot be unduly costly, extensive, substantial, and disruptive or fundamentally alter the nature or operation of the business.

## Family Medical Leave Act

Another key employment-related protection available to many cancer patients is medical leave under the Family Medical Leave Act (FMLA). FMLA was passed in 1993 with the primary intention of providing pregnant woman protected medical leave for the birth of their child [81]. However, FMLA leave is not limited to pregnancy, and can be taken because of any "serious health condition" that makes the employee unable to perform the functions of their job [82]. A serious health condition includes an illness, injury, impairment, or physical or mental condition that involves inpatient care or continuing treatment by a healthcare provider [83]. Cancer treatment is specifically identified as a likely qualifying condition under federal regulations [84].

FMLA provides job preservation during 12 weeks of leave in a 12-month period for the same or equivalent position [85]. This leave can be taken intermittently if needed. It also requires employers to continue covering an employee's health insurance coverage and other benefits. Not all employers are required to provide FMLA coverage to all of their employees. Coverage is only required if (1) the employer employs at least 50 workers within 75 miles of the worksite, (2) the employee worked for the employer for at least 12 months (need not be consecutive, but must occur before a 7-year break in service), and (3) the employee must have worked at least 1250 h in the previous 12 months [86].

If a cancer patient is covered under FMLA, they should speak with their human resources department to begin the process of applying for leave. The process can vary based on the internal policies of each employer and on the availability of paid leave through short- or long-term disability. However, most employees must go through some version of the following four steps: (1) notice must be given to the employer within 30 days if the leave is foreseeable [87]. If it is not foreseeable then the employee must give notice as soon as practicable. (2) After notice, the employer must notify the employee within five business days of the employee's eligibility to take FMLA and must inform the worker what documentation is needed to proceed (e.g., medical certification). (3) If required, the employee submits the necessary forms, including medical certification. (4) The employer must then provide a designation notice that identifies the leave as qualifying for FMLA.

## Employment-Related Advocacy Tips

Navigating the form-and-procedure heavy processes associated with the ADA and FMLA can be a daunting task. With an MLP attorney's help, the necessary documentation, especially medical certification forms, can be collected quickly and more efficiently. Attorneys can also assist by directly advocating with the patient's employer. For reasonable accommodations under the ADA, MLP lawyers can work with providers to craft letters that advocate for a patient's continued ability to work [88]. These letters should identify the treating provider, identify the patient's diagnosis, outline the symptoms or impairments that the diagnosis causes including symptoms from treatment, and request a specific reasonable accommodation in light of the foregoing. Examples of these accommodations include using didactic programs to avoid typing pain caused by neuropathy, being able to work remotely, sitting closer to a bathroom, being allowed to sit during shifts, having a more flexible attendance notification policy, and getting more time to complete projects. MLP lawyers can work directly with a patient's employer and providers to facilitate the creation of these accommodations.

## *Legal Status*

Legal status has a direct impact on the health of immigrant cancer patients by serving as a primary barrier to public benefits, including health coverage. Cancer providers should be aware of the basics of immigration law as it pertains to low-income cancer patients and how an MLP can help overcome immigration-related hurdles.

### Basic Rights

Since the early twentieth century, the US Supreme Court has recognized that immigrants within America are entitled to due process under the US Constitution. The Fifth and Fourteenth Amendments provide all "persons" the protection from being deprived "of life, liberty, or property, without due process of law." As articulated by the Supreme Court, even unlawful immigrants "have long been recognized as 'persons' guaranteed due process of law by the Fifth and Fourteenth Amendments" [89].

Due process under the US Constitution requires that immigrants be notified of the grounds for their removal, of their right to an attorney, and of their right to a fair hearing [90]. At that hearing the individual must be provided a reasonable opportunity to examine the evidence against them and to present evidence on their behalf. As a further protection, the Immigration Judge who oversees the hearing must inform immigrants of their eligibility for relief from deportation on such grounds as fear of ill treatment or hardship upon removal. If a judge orders an immigrant deported, the individual still has the right to appeal to the Board of Immigration Appeals as well as to federal court. In each stage of this process the individual must be informed of all of his rights in a language he or she understands or the deportation order will be considered invalid.

### Benefit Access

Over the past several decades, Congress has made significant changes in immigration and welfare policy in order to restrict the eligibility of legal permanent residents (LPRs), refugees, asylees, and other noncitizens from accessing means-tested public aid [91]. In 1996, Congress passed the Personal Responsibility and Work Opportunity Reconciliation Action (PRWORA), which created many of these restrictions and continues to serve as the source of subsequent limiting amendments [92]. Generally, access to the benefits depends on an individual's immigration status, whether they arrived (or were on a program's rolls) before August 22, 1996 (when PRWORA was enacted), and how long they have lived and worked in the United States. Table 11.6 breaks down the eligibility of lawful and unlawful immigrants for six of the most important public benefits.

**Table 11.6** Federal benefit access for various aliens

| Class of alien | SNAP (food stamps | SSI | TANF (temporary assistance for needy families) | Medicaid[a] | PPACA—exchange access |
|---|---|---|---|---|---|
| Lawful permanent alien (LPR, green card) | Ineligible for first 5 years from entry | Lf green card before August 1996 | Ineligible for first 5 years from entry, then eligible based on state option | Ineligible for first 5 years from entry | Eligible |
| LPR with 10+ years of work history | Eligible | Eligible | Eligible | Eligible | Eligible |
| Humanitarian cases—asylees, refugees, special Iraqi and Afghan immigrants, etc. | Eligible after grant of status | Eligible for first 7 years after grant of status then ineligible unless naturalizes | Eligible for first 5 years then eligible at state option | Eligible for first 7 years after grant | Eligible |
| Trafficking victims | Eligible | Eligibility depends on class of status | Eligible if resident as of August 22, 1996. Ineligible for 5 years after entry, if entry is post-August 22, 1996. Otherwise eligible at state option | Eligible at state option | Eligible |
| Temporary protected status of extended voluntary departure | Eligible | Eligible for 7 years after entry/grant of such status. Ineligible after 7 years unless naturalized | Eligible for 5 years after entry. Eligible at state option after 5 years | Eligible for 7 years after entry. Eligible at state option after 7 years | Eligible |
| Nonimmigrant visa holders | Ineligible | Ineligible | Ineligible | Ineligible | Eligible |
| Undocumented immigrants | Ineligible | Ineligible | Ineligible | Ineligible (except emergency MA) | Eligible if meet state residency requirements |

[a]States may use their own funds to expand eligibility for Medicaid beyond what is allowed by federal law

## Healthcare Benefits: Undocumented Immigrants

Undocumented immigrants who receive a cancer diagnosis are often faced with the challenge of not having meaningful access to healthcare services. With the exception of emergency medical care, undocumented immigrants are not eligible for federally funded public health insurance programs, including Medicare, Medicaid, and the Child Health Insurance Program (CHIP). Additionally, undocumented immigrants cannot purchase insurance through marketplaces created under the ACA [93]. Some states and local governments use their own funds to expand coverage to PRUCOL (Permanent Residence Under Color of Law) immigrants, which refers to individuals who are in the United States with the knowledge of immigration services and are not likely to be deported [94].

Emergency Medicaid is often the only source of medical coverage for undocumented immigrants. Generally, coverage under emergency Medicaid requires a "medical condition manifesting itself by acute symptoms of sufficient severity such that the absence of immediate medical attention could reasonably be expected to result in (1) placing the health of the individual … in serious jeopardy; (2) serious impairment to bodily functions; or (3) serious dysfunction of any bodily organ part" [95]. In practice, states often deny cancer patients that seek treatment through emergency Medicaid because their symptoms are not "acute" or because the length of their treatment regimens is undefined. For example, states usually cover the surgery and chemotherapy treatments associated with breast cancer, but are more hesitant to cover a 5-year prescription for tamoxifen.

## Immigration Advocacy Tips

MLPs can be particularly helpful for immigrant patients when it comes to access to healthcare services, visa assistance for family caregivers or related donors seeking to visit the United States, explaining and assisting immigrants with "Know Your Rights" discussions, and representing immigrants in humanitarian or immigrant applications. Providers can support MLP attorneys by medical documentation for immigration cases, especially in situations where access to health coverage relies heavily on the severity of the diagnosis. However, access to translational services is paramount for an effective immigration referral, especially in situations where the patient is already wary of potential repercussions of accessing health care. Ideally, MLPs will translate any informational forms into the most common languages represented in their patient populations so as to ensure that immigrant patients have a clear sense of their privacy rights under relevant professional codes of conduct.

## *Advance Care Planning (Personal and Familial Stability)*

Advance care planning (ACP) can broadly be understood as the framework that helps patients express their treatment goals and preferences so that those wishes can be protected and realized when patients are unable to make decisions for themselves. Many oncology patients believe that it is important to address end-of-life issues in the ACP process [96, 97]. Completing advance planning documents is an effective way to increase the likelihood that a patient's wishes are adhered to in moments of incapacity [98, 99]. Although ACP is not unique to cancer patients, its prevalence in the population combined with its frequent reliance on legal documents makes it an ideal target for MLP intervention.

This section briefly summarizes five common types of advance planning documents that MLPs are well suited to assist with: the financial power of attorney (POA), the healthcare power of attorney (HCPOA), the living will, the will of estate, and the standby guardianship. While there are a variety of other documents that can be useful in the ACP process, such as do-not-resuscitate orders and physician orders for life-sustaining treatment, these five are inherently legal documents with statutorily defined execution requirements. As a result, familiarity with their legal underpinning is important for their effective use in a cancer setting.

### Advance Care Planning Documents

The documents addressed below are intended to safeguard an individual's ability to control the broader social, financial, and medical aspects of their lives regardless of their capacity status. While each of these documents plays a different role in the ACP process, all are grounded in the legal and bioethical principle of patient autonomy and individual decision-making [100]. Due to the state-specific laws governing the execution of these documents, it is advisable that providers become familiar with their own state's requirements and, ideally, include a lawyer in their cancer care team [101]. With a lawyer's assistance, these documents can be drafted properly while also guaranteeing their legal, and therefore enforceable, status.

#### Financial Power of Attorney

A power of attorney (POA) is a written document through which an individual (the principal) assigns another person (the agent) the concurrent authority (meaning both the principal and agent retain the power simultaneously) to make financial decisions on behalf of the principal [102]. POAs are only focused on financial matters and do not overlap with healthcare decisions. For cancer patients, a POA allows an agent to assist with common financial matters like paying for everyday expenses as well as negotiating with insurance companies or assisting with the sale of a home. POAs generally become active the moment they are signed, unless they are contingent upon the principal's incapacity, in which case they are sometimes referred to as a "springing" power of attorney. The documents become void upon the death of the principal and therefore cannot be used as a substitute for a patient's will.

### Healthcare Power of Attorney

A healthcare power of attorney (HCPOA) is a written document through which an individual (the principal) gives another person (the agent) the authority to make healthcare decisions on the principal's behalf [103]. Unlike financial POAs, which generally become active when they are signed, a typical HCPOA only becomes active when a principal becomes incapacitated and is unable to make their own healthcare decisions. This limitation stems from the fundamental role of patient autonomy in medical decision-making and the deference that is given to patients' expressed wishes [104]. Furthermore, because the HCPOA applies in any circumstance of patient incapacity, regardless of severity, it encompasses a broader set of scenarios than a living will, which is exclusively intended for end of life. Like a POA, an agent's powers are defined in the document, and can typically include powers like making treatment decisions, hiring or firing providers, and transitioning the patient onto hospice. Some states prefer a single-form HCPOA and living will, where the two documents are combined and work together [105]. In these circumstances the HCPOA portion identifies the agent and the broad decision-making powers while the living will portion outlines the patient's end-of-life wishes. For cancer patients, a well-written HCPOA (along with a corresponding living will) is an essential component of effective ACP. They allow patients to ensure that their wishes regarding treatment will be honored even if they lose capacity. They also serve as a focal point for conversations regarding the principal's underlying values and beliefs as they pertain to treatment decisions.

### Living Will

A living will is a document that outlines a patient's wishes with respect to end-of-life treatment [103]. The document can include preferences regarding specific treatment options, such as chemotherapy, radiation therapy, cardiopulmonary resuscitation, ventilator support, and provision of nutrition and hydration. Because it is often intended to work with a broader HCPOA, the document is not required to designate a proxy decision maker. However, these documents can operate on their own and, in those circumstances, should identify a proxy to carry out the patient's expressed wishes.

Will of Estate

A will of estate (generally referred to as just a "will" or "final will") is likely the most commonly known ACP tool. A will is intended to reflect a patient's wishes with respect to their person, property, and assets upon their death. Although wills can be arranged to accomplish a number of goals in a variety of fashions and are governed almost exclusively by state law, they typically have some common basic elements. Most wills contain detailed instructions about the distribution and divestment of the individual's property and assets and often include burial instructions. They also identify, in detail, who is to receive the patient's property ("beneficiaries") and who is to assist in carrying out the instructions of the will ("executor/executrix").

Standby Guardianship

A standby guardianship is a document that allows cancer patients with minor children to appoint a caretaker for their children that would step in if the patient were to become incapacitated or pass away [106]. Some research suggests that parents with advanced cancer who have dependent children are more likely to be in denial of the terminal nature of their illness and more likely to choose treatment focused on life extension and not adequately prepare for their death [107]. Other studies have demonstrated that parents with metastatic cancer experience high rates of anxiety, panic, and depressive symptoms and that parenting concerns are correlated with these symptoms [107]. A standby guardianship can help ameliorate some of these issues. When executing these documents, it is important to check state law and determine if both parents, regardless of their connection to the child, must sign the document in order for it to be effective. States also differ on how to withdraw a standby guardianship, with some allowing revocation just in writing, while others requiring a court filing.

## *ACP Advocacy Tips*

There are a number of practical tips associated with advocacy around planning documents. First, MLP advocates should review any planning documents obtained online or through other sources with relevant state laws. For example, the Five Wishes document, which is used widely throughout the United States, is only legal as an advance directive in 42 states [108]. Second, advance care planning documents are only as good as the individuals and institutions who know of their existence. If a cancer patient has an executed planning document, they should provide copies to all of their providers and agents and have a discussion about the document's contents. Without knowledge of a document's existence, a provider or an institution cannot be obligated to follow its instructions. Finally, effective January

1, 2017, the Centers for Medicare & Medicaid Services issued new Current Procedural Terminology codes that allow physicians to bill for advance planning conversations [109]. These codes should incentivize cancer providers to have ACP meetings with their patients. However, many cancer centers may not have staff with the expertise to discuss the breadth of legal issues that the documents entail. Integration of lawyers through an MLP can help fill this gap.

**Case Vignettes**

What follow are two case examples that highlight the impact that legal determinants of health can have on low-income cancer patients and how interdisciplinary MLP intervention can work to address those needs.

**Carla**

Carla is a 38-year-old single mother who lives with her two sons, ages six and eight, in a two-bedroom apartment that she rents for $1800 per month. She earns $40,000–$50,000 per year working as a part-time paralegal for a single attorney and as a freelance web designer. She received her bachelor's degree 3 years ago. Based on her income and family size, she earns 200–250% of the Federal Poverty Level, which places her well above most government benefit programs. However, her children are eligible for insurance coverage under CHIP and she is covered through a plan on the individual marketplace for which she receives premium subsidies.

At some point Carla noticed a lump on her chest. A biopsy revealed that Carla had stage IIIA triple-negative breast cancer. After discussing her treatment options with her oncologists, she chose to pursue a lumpectomy followed by 4–6 weeks of radiation treatment and several months of chemotherapy.

Her treatment forced Carla to take an extended period of time off of work. The attorney for whom she worked was just beginning a long trial and had to hire a replacement. Carla could continue to work on websites from home, but her mental and physical ability to do that was diminishing. Since Carla had little savings, the loss in income severely jeopardized her ability to pay for her expenses, including her insurance premiums and her rent. She subsequently lost her health coverage and started receiving threatening letters from her landlord.

Shortly after she was diagnosed, Carla was referred by a social worker to Danielle, who is a legal aid attorney that provides free legal services through an MLP at the cancer center. When Carla lost her health coverage, Danielle was able to help her apply for Medicaid coverage under her state's BCCPT program. Danielle was also able to work with Carla's oncologist to prepare a tailored application for disability benefits. Danielle also participated in the family meeting arranged by Carla's care team. One of the main results of that meeting was a set of advance care planning documents, including a HCPOA and a standby guardianship that appointed Carla's sister the guardian of

Carla's children. Danielle also contacted Carla's landlord. Danielle was able to leverage the landlord's harassment of Carla into a grace period that allowed Carla to stay in the unit rent free for several months until she found a new apartment. As a result, Carla and her boys were able to move into a more affordable apartment. Following the first round of treatment, Carla's cancer entered remission.

Unfortunately, 6 months after she entered remission, Carla's cancer metastasized. In that time she was also told that her initial application for disability had been denied because the diagnosis did not sufficiently show that Carla would be unable to work for more than a year. Carla once again met with her care team and a new course of treatment was decided on. She submitted an appeal for the disability benefits, which Danielle was able to quickly expedite as a CAL case using medical records proving Carla's diagnosis was stage IV cancer. The benefits started on the first day of the following month. Although Carla's prognosis remained uncertain, with her MLP team's assistance, she was able to start on a new treatment plan, stabilize her income insurance and income, and move to a new apartment. She also knows that regardless of what happens, her children will be taken care of and that her treatment wishes will be adhered to.

**Rami**

Rami is 28 years old and fled Nepal to the United States after the 2015 earthquake destroyed his village. His mother had a permanent resident status and was able to legally travel, but Rami had no legal documentation. For the past month, Rami has had flu-like symptoms and discovered bruises over his body. Since he was undocumented, he was afraid that if he saw a doctor he could be deported. Eventually, he went to the ER of a NY safety net hospital, where he was reassured that his privacy was protected under HIPAA. He was diagnosed with Ph + acute lymphoblastic leukemia and began standard combination chemotherapy and tyrosine kinase inhibitors (TKI) which was covered by NY Emergency Medicaid, but because of his immigration status he was not eligible for allogeneic hematopoietic stem cell transplantation (HSCT). Without the transplant, it was unlikely that he would survive the year. With his consent, his physician referred him to the MLP attorney.

The MLP attorney met Rami in the hospital and realized that Rami qualified for a Nepal Temporary Protected Status (TPS), which granted him temporary protection against deportation. As a result of the pending TPS application, Rami was eligible for NY State Medicaid as a PRUCOL immigrant. Since he was inpatient and could not go to the Medicaid office, the attorney helped him complete a financial power of attorney so his mother could apply for Medicaid on his behalf. Rami was transferred to the adjacent academic hospital for the transplant and enrolled in a clinical trial. Fortunately, a matching donor was found and Rami could undergo the procedure.

Several weeks later, his physician reached out to the attorney in a panic. Rami received a notice that he was losing his Medicaid coverage due to lack of immigration status. The attorney requested an expedited fair hearing with aid to continue to contest the termination of coverage. Since the request was made before the coverage stopped, Rami had no disruption in care while the hearing was pending. At the fair hearing, the attorney saw that proof of TPS was not in his file even though the caseworker note showed that it was submitted. She pointed out the agency error and resubmitted the proof of immigration status directly to the judge. The error was corrected and Rami received a fair hearing decision confirming that he was in fact eligible for coverage.

After several difficult months, Rami continued to improve. The cancer was in remission, and he was granted TPS with work authorization. He wanted to start working but worried he could lose health coverage if he was over income. Additionally, his mother wanted him to move with her to New Jersey where a person with TPS is not eligible for Medicaid. The attorney explored Rami's options with him: If he stayed in New York then he could enroll in the Medicaid Buy-In Program for the Working Disabled. So long as he was working, this would allow him to maintain Medicaid with a low premium. If he moved to New Jersey he would lose Medicaid coverage but could purchase a plan on the individual marketplace.

Regardless of Rami's decision, his health and well-being are directly tied to the interdisciplinary efforts of the MLP team. Without their coordination at critical moments, Rami's access to coverage would have been in jeopardy and his life would have been at risk.

## Conclusion

As cancer treatment continues to shift towards an ambulatory setting, oncology care will be required to contend with the broader social and environmental circumstances impacting patients' lives. The services that MLP attorneys provide can aid not only with acute, emergency needs, but also with chronic and systemic issues. The MLP model is therefore uniquely situated to help augment the scope of patient care in order to address many of the short-term and long-term social determinants of patient health.

## References

1. Tyler ET. Aligning public health, health care, law and policy: medical-legal partnership as a multilevel response to the social determinants of health. J Health Biomed Law. 2012;VIII:211–347.
2. Krishnamurth B, Hagins S, Lawton E, et al. What we know and need to know about medical-legal partnership. S C Law Rev. 2016;67:377.
3. Sandel M, Hansen M, Kahn R, et al. Medical-legal partnerships: transforming primary care by address the legal needs of vulnerable populations. Health Aff. 2010;29:1697–705.
4. National center for medical legal partnerships [Internet]. http://medical-legalpartnership.org/. [Accessed 8 May 2017].

5. Partnerships across the U.S. [Internet]. National Center for Medical Legal Partnerships. http://medical-legalpartnership.org/partnerships/. [Accessed 8 May 2017].
6. NAPBC standards manual - patient navigation [Internet]. American College of Surgeons. https://www.facs.org/~/media/files/quality%20programs/napbc/2014%20napbc%20standards%20manual.ashx. [Accessed 8 May 2017].
7. Jean-Pierre P, Hendren S, Fiscella K, et al. Understanding the processes of patient navigation to reduce disparities in cancer care: perspectives of trained navigators from the field. J Cancer Educ. 2011;26(1):111–20.
8. Retkin R, Antoniadis D, Pepitone DF, et al. Legal services: a necessary component of patient navigation. Semin Oncol Nurs. 2013;29:149–55.
9. What is a legal hotline [Internet]. Center for elder rights advocacy. https://legalhotlines.org/. [Accessed 8 May 2017].
10. Social determinants of health [Internet]. World Health Organization. http://www.who.int/social_determinants/en/. [Accessed 8 May 2017].
11. Burris S. Law in a social determinants strategy: a public health law research perspective. Public Health Rep. 2011;126:22.
12. How civil legal aid helps health care address social determinants of health [Internet]. National Center for Medical Legal Partnerships. http://medical-legalpartnership.org/mlp-response/how-civil-legal-aid-helps-health-care-address-sdoh/. [Accessed 5 May 2017].
13. Marple K. Framing legal care as health care. Washington, DC: The National Center for Medical-Legal Partnership; 2015.
14. Dejong NA, Wood C, Morreale MC, et al. Identifying social determinants of health and legal needs for children with special health care needs. Clin Pediatr. 2016;55(2):272–7.
15. Zevon M, Schwabish S, Donnelly J, et al. Medically related legal needs and quality of life in cancer care. Cancer. 2007;109(12):2600–6.
16. Medical/professional relations [Internet]. Social Security Administration. https://www.ssa.gov/disability/professionals/answers-pub042.htm. [Accessed 5 Jun 2017].
17. Disability planner: what we mean by disability [Internet]. Social Security Administration. https://www.ssa.gov/planners/disability/dqualify4.html. [Accessed 5 Jun 2017].
18. Annual statistical report on the social security disability insurance program [Internet]. Social Security Administration. https://www.ssa.gov/policy/docs/statcomps/di_asr/2011/sect04.html. [Accessed 10 Jun 2017].
19. Evaluation of disability in general 20 C.F.R § 404.1520; 2017.
20. DI 10520.001 impairment-related work EXPENSES [Internet]. Social Security Administration. https://secure.ssa.gov/poms.nsf/lnx/0410520001. [Accessed 10 Jun 2017].
21. Listing of impairments – adult listings [Internet]. Social Security Administration. https://www.ssa.gov/disability/professionals/bluebook/AdultListings.htm. [Accessed 10 Apr 2017].
22. HALLEX - critical cases [Internet]. Social Security Administration. https://www.ssa.gov/OP_Home/hallex/I-02/I-2-1-40.html. [Accessed 10 Jun 2017].
23. Program operations manual system (POMS) DI 23020.045 terminal illness (TERI) cases [Internet]. Social Security Administration. https://secure.ssa.gov/poms.nsf/lnx/0423020045. [Accessed 10 Jun 2017].
24. Compassionate allowance conditions [Internet]. Social Security. https://www.ssa.gov/compassionateallowances/conditions.htm. [Accessed 10 Jun 2017].
25. Critical case criteria and exclusions [Internet]. Social Security Administration. https://secure.ssa.gov/poms.nsf/lnx/0302801001. [Accessed 10 Jun 2017].
26. Can i return to work while getting social security benefits [Internet]. Social Security Administration. https://faq.ssa.gov/link/portal/34011/34019/Article/3725/Can-I-return-to-work-while-getting-Social-Security-disability-benefits. [Accessed 10 Jun 2017].
27. The appeals process [Internet]. Social Security Administration. https://www.ssa.gov/pubs/EN-05-10041.pdf. [Accessed 10 Jun 2017].
28. December 2016 medicaid and CHIP enrollment data [Internet]. Centers for Medicare & Medicaid Services. https://www.medicaid.gov/medicaid/program-information/medicaid-and-chip-enrollment-data/report-highlights/index.html. [Accessed 10 Apr 2017].

29. Patient Protection and Affordable Care Act, Pub. L. No. 111-148, 124 Stat. 119; 2010.
30. Polite BN, Griggs JJ, Moy B, et al. American Society of Clinical Oncology policy statement on medicaid reform. J Clin Oncol. 2014;32(36):4162–7.
31. Financing & Reimbursement [Internet]. Centers for Medicaid & Medicare Services. https://www.medicaid.gov/medicaid/financing-and-reimbursement/. [Accessed 10 Apr 2017].
32. State Plans for Medical Assistance 42 U.S.C. § 1396a (a)(10)(A)(i); 2017.
33. State Plans for Medical Assistance 42 U.S.C. § 1396a (a)(10)(A)(ii)(XVIII); 2017.
34. Breast and Cervical Cancer Prevention and Treatment Act, Pub. L. No. 106-354, 113 Stat. 126; 2000.
35. National Breast and Cervical Cancer Early Detection Program [Internet]. Centers for Disease Control and Prevention. https://www.cdc.gov/cancer/nbccedp/. [Accessed 6 May 2017].
36. Lantz PM, Soliman S. An evaluation of a Medicaid expansion for cancer care: the Breast and Cervical Cancer Prevention and Treatment Act of 2000. Womens Health Issues. 2009;19:221–31.
37. Medicaid employment initiatives [Internet]. Centers for Medicare & Medicaid Services. https://www.medicaid.gov/medicaid/ltss/employmment/index.html. [Accessed 6 May 2017].
38. Medicaid eligibility [Internet]. Centers for Medicare & Medicaid Services. https://www.medicaid.gov/medicaid/eligibility/. [Accessed 27 Apr 2017].
39. Medicaid and CHIP eligibility levels [Internet]. Centers for Medicare & Medicaid Services. https://www.medicaid.gov/medicaid/program-information/medicaid-and-chip-eligibility-levels/index.html. [Accessed 6 May 2017].
40. Modified adjusted gross income [Internet]. U.S. Centers for Medicare & Medicaid Services. https://www.healthcare.gov/glossary/modified-adjusted-gross-income-magi/. [Accessed 5 Apr 2017].
41. State Plans for Medical Assistance 42 U.S.C. § 1396a(a)(3); 2017.
42. Greene v. McElroy, 360 U.S. 474, 496-97; 1959.
43. Goldberg v. Kelly, 397 U.S. 254, 296-71; 1970.
44. Social Security Act Amendments of 1965, Pub. L. No. 89-97, 79 Stat. 286; 1965.
45. Social Security Act Amendments of 1972, Pub. L. No. 92-603, 86 Stat. 1329; 1972.
46. Total number of medicare beneficiaries [Internet]. Kaiser Family Foundation. http://kff.org/medicare/state-indicator/total-medicare-beneficiaries/?currentTimeframe=0&sortModel=%7B%22colId%22:%22Location%22,%22sort%22:%22asc%22%7D. [Accessed 3 Apr 2017].
47. Narang AK, Hersch L. Out-of-pocket spending and financial burden among medicare beneficiaries with cancer. JAMA Oncol. 2017;3(6):757–65.
48. What part A covers [Internet]. U.S. Centers for Medicare & Medicaid Services. https://www.medicare.gov/what-medicare-covers/part-a/what-part-a-covers.html. [Accessed 3 Apr 2017].
49. Medicare 2017 costs at a glance [Internet]. U.S. Centers for Medicare & Medicaid Services. https://www.medicare.gov/your-medicare-costs/costs-at-a-glance/costs-at-glance.html. [Accessed 3 Apr 2017].
50. What part B covers [Internet]. U.S. Centers for Medicare & Medicaid Services. https://www.medicare.gov/what-medicare-covers/part-b/what-medicare-part-b-covers.html. [Accessed 3 Apr 2017].
51. Special things people with cancer need to think about [Internet]. American Cancer Society. https://www.cancer.org/treatment/finding-and-paying-for-treatment/understanding-health-insurance/health-insurance-options/medicare/medicare-part-d/things-people-with-cancer-need-to-think-about.html. [Accessed 5 Apr 2017].
52. Part B costs [Internet]. U.S. Centers for Medicare & Medicaid Services. https://www.medicare.gov/your-medicare-costs/part-b-costs/part-b-costs.html. [Accessed 5 Apr 2017].
53. How do medicare advantage plans work? U.S. Centers for Medicare & Medicaid Services. https://www.medicare.gov/sign-up-change-plans/medicare-health-plans/medicare-advantage-plans/how-medicare-advantage-plans-work.html. [Accessed 5 Apr 2017].
54. Costs for medicare drug coverage. U.S. Centers for Medicare & Medicaid Services. https://www.medicare.gov/part-d/costs/part-d-costs.html. [Accessed 5 Apr 2017].

55. Closing the coverage gap – medicare prescription drugs are becoming more affordable [Internet]. Centers for Medicare & Medicaid Services. https://www.medicare.gov/Pubs/pdf/11493.pdf. [Accessed 13 Apr 2017].
56. What's medicare supplement insurance (Medigap). U.S. Centers for Medicare & Medicaid Services. https://www.medicare.gov/supplement-other-insurance/medigap/whats-medigap.html. [Accessed 12 Apr 2017].
57. Extra help with medicare prescription drug plan costs [Internet]. Social Security Administration. https://www.ssa.gov/medicare/prescriptionhelp/. [Accessed 13 Apr 2017].
58. Prejudice to enrollment rights because of Federal Government misrepresentation, inaction, or error, 42 C.F. R. § 407.32; 2017.
59. Patient Protection and Affordable Care Act of 2012, Pub L No 11-148, 124 Stat 119; 2010.
60. Mariotto AB, Yabroff KR, Shao Y, et al. Projections of the cost of cancer care in the United States: 2010-2020. J Natl Cancer Inst. 2011;103(2):117–28.
61. Guy GP Jr, Ekwueme DU, Yabroff KR, et al. Economic burden of cancer survivorship among adults in the United States. J Clin Oncol. 2013;31(30):3749–57.
62. Ramsey S, Blough D, Kirchhoff A, et al. Washington State cancer patients found to be at greater risk for bankruptcy than people without a cancer diagnosis. Health Aff. 2013;32(6):1143–52.
63. Banega M, Guy G Jr, de Moor JS, et al. For working-age cancer survivors, medical debt and bankruptcy create financial hardships. Health Aff. 2016;36(6):54–61.
64. Fair Debt Collection Practices Act of 1977, Pub L No 95-109, 91 Stat 874; 1977.
65. Definitions 15 U.S.C. § 1692a; 2017.
66. Harassment or Abuse 15 U.S.C. § 1692d; 2017.
67. Marmot M. Health in an unequal world: social circumstances, biology, and disease. Lancet. 2006;368:2081–94.
68. Beck A, Klein MD, Schaffzin JK, et al. Identifying and treating a substandard housing cluster using a medical-legal partnership. Pediatrics. 2012;130(5):831–8.
69. Ko NY, Battaglia TA, Gupta-Lawrence R, et al. Burden of sociolegal concerns among vulnerable patients seeking cancer care services at an urban safety-net hospital: a cross-section survey. BMC Health Serv Res. 2016;16:196.
70. Housing choice voucher program guidebook [Internet]. U.S. Department of Housing and Urban Development. https://portal.hud.gov/hudportal/HUD?src=/program_offices/public_indian_housing/programs/hcv/forms/guidebook. [Accessed 26 Jun 2017].
71. Tun H. Project: special project on landlord-tenant law in the District of Columbia court of appeals: implied warranty of habitability. How L J. 1986;29:103–15.
72. NYC will be first in country to provide right to counsel in housing court [Internet]. National Coalition for Civil Right to Counsel. http://civilrighttocounsel.org/major_developments/894. [Accessed 26 Jun 2017].
73. Discrimination in the Sale or Rental of Housing and other Prohibited Practices 42 U.S.C. § 3604; 2017.
74. Reasonable accommodations under the fair housing act [Internet]. U.S. Department of Housing and Urban Development. https://portal.hud.gov/hudportal/HUD?src=/program_offices/fair_housing_equal_opp/ReasonableAccommodations15. [Accessed 5 Apr 2017].
75. Discrimination in the Sale or Rental of Housing and other Prohibited Practices 42 U.S.C. § 3604(f)(3); 2017.
76. Americans with Disabilities Act of 1990, Pub L No 101-336, 104 Stat 327; 1990.
77. Questions & answers about cancer in the workplace and the americans with disabilities act [Internet]. Equal Employment Opportunity Commission. https://www.eeoc.gov/laws/types/cancer.cfm. [Accessed 5 Apr 2017].
78. Definitions 42 U.S.C. § 12111; 2017.
79. Definition of Disability 42 U.S.C. § 12102; 2017.
80. Industry Affecting Commerce 29 C.F.R. § 401.3; 2017.
81. Family Medical Leave Act of 1993, Pub L No 103-3, 107 Stat. 6; 1993.
82. Leave Requirement 29 U.S.C. § 2612(a)((1)(D); 2017.
83. Definitions 29 U.S.C. § 2611(11); 2017.

84. Continuing Treatment 29 C.F.R. § 825.115(e)(2); 2017.
85. Leave Requirement 29 U.S.C. § 2612(a); 2017.
86. Definitions 29 C.F.R. § 825.102; 2017.
87. Leave Requirement 29 U.S.C. § 2612(e)(1); 2017.
88. Retkin R, Rodabaugh K, Mochizuki T. Cancer patients, survivors and their families, poverty, health and law. In: Tyler ET, Lawton E, Conroy K, et al., editors. Poverty, health and law, readings and cases for medical-legal partnership. Durham: Carolina Academic Press; 2013. p. 395–429.
89. Plyer v. Doe, 457 U.S. 202; 1982.
90. Removal Proceedings 8 U.S.C. § 1229a; 2017.
91. Siskin, A. Noncitizen eligibility for public assistance: policy overview [Internet]. Congressional Research Service. https://fas.org/sgp/crs/misc/RL33809.pdf. [Accessed 26 Jun 2017].
92. Personal Responsibility and Work Opportunity Reconciliation Act of 1996, Pub L No 104-193, 110 Stat 2105; 1996.
93. Jost T. Health insurance exchanges and the affordable care act: eight difficult issues [Internet]. The Commonwealth Fund. http://www.commonwealthfund.org/publications/fund-reports/2010/sep/health-insurance-exchanges-and-the-affordable-care-act. [Accessed 26 Jun 2017].
94. Gusmano M. Undocumented immigrants and health care access in the United States [Internet]. The Hastings Center. http://undocumentedpatients.org/issuebrief/health-policy-and-access-to-care/. [Accessed 26 Jun 2017].
95. Examination and treatment for emergency medical conditions and women in labor 42 U.S.C § 1395dd; 2017.
96. Diaz-Mentes TP, Johnson ML, Giuntoli RL 2nd, et al. Importance and timing of end-of-life care discussions among gynecologic oncology patients. Am J Hosp Palliat Care. 2013;30(1):59–67.
97. Clark M, Ott M, Rogers M, et al. Advance care planning as a shared endeavor: completion of ACP documents in a multidisciplinary cancer program. Psych Oncol. 2013;26:67.
98. Detering KM, Hancock AD, Reade MC, et al. The impact of advance care planning on end of life care in elderly patients: randomized controlled trial. BMJ. 2010;340:c1345.
99. Silveira MJ, Kim SY, Langa KM. Advance directives and outcomes of surrogate decision making before death. N Engl J Med. 2010;362(13):1211–8.
100. Noah B. In denial: the role of law in preparing for death. Elder L J. 2013;21:1–11.
101. Rodabaugh KJ, Hammond M, Myszka D, et al. A medical-legal partnership as a component of a palliative care model. J Palliat Med. 2010;13(1):15–8.
102. Jeffrey M. Power of attorney – key issues for elder care planning. PA Bar Q. 2003;74:160.
103. Tucker K. Elder law: counseling clients who are terminally ill. William Mitchell L Rev. 2010;37(1):117–31.
104. Dolgin J. Dying discourse: contextualizing advance care planning. Quinnipiac L Rev. 2016;34(2):235–98.
105. As an example, Pennsylvania law provides for a dual form HCPOA and Living Will. 20 Pa.C.S.A § 5451–5465.
106. Standby guardianships [Internet]. Child Welfare Information Gateway – Department of Health & Human Services. https://www.childwelfare.gov/topics/systemwide/laws-policies/statutes/guardianship/. [Accessed 11 Jun 2017].
107. Park EM, Check DK, Song M, et al. Parenting while living with advanced cancer: a qualitative study. Palliat Med. 2017;31(3):231–8.
108. Five wishes [Internet]. Aging With Dignity. https://www.agingwithdignity.org/five-wishes/about-five-wishes. [Accessed 16 Apr 2017].
109. Advance care planning [Internet]. Centers for Medicare & Medicaid Services. https://www.cms.gov/Outreach-and-Education/Medicare-Learning-Network-MLN/MLNProducts/Downloads/AdvanceCarePlanning.pdf. [Accessed 13 Jun 2017].

# Chapter 12
# Palliative Care for Cancer and Treatment-Related Changes for Inpatients

**Geoffrey P. Dunn, Jennifer Pruskowski, and Lisa K. Simonian**

## Introduction

The past decade has witnessed marked proliferation of palliative care programs for hospitalized cancer patients ranging in size from one or two committed practitioners to sizeable departments including physician fellowship training programs in the now-certifiable subspecialty of hospice and palliative medicine. However, variations in access to palliative care based on region, profit status, and hospital size persist [1].

The American Society for Clinical Oncology (ASCO) issued a provisional clinical opinion [2] that supports the consideration of the combination of standard oncology care and palliative care early in the course of treatment for any patient with metastatic cancer and/or high symptom burden. Furthermore, it supports strategies to optimize concurrent palliative care and standard oncology care, with evaluation of its impact on important patient and caregiver outcomes (e.g., QOL, survival, healthcare service utilization, and costs) and on society. In 2012 the Commission on Cancer included access to palliative care services among its Cancer Program Standards [3]. In the Standard's most recent iteration it states: "The availability of palliative care services is an essential component of cancer care, beginning at the time of diagnosis and being 'continuously available' throughout treatment, surveillance, and, when applicable, during bereavement" [4]. Although the potential benefit of these programs to cancer patients and their families has been increasingly

G. P. Dunn, MD, FACS (✉)
Department of Surgery, Palliative Care Consultation Service, UPMC Hamot, Erie, PA, USA

J. Pruskowski
Department of Pharmacy and Therapeutics, University of Pittsburgh Medical Center, Palliative Supportive Institute (PSI), Pittsburgh, PA, USA
e-mail: pruskowskija@upmc.edu

L. K. Simonian
Palliative Care Consultation Service, UPMC Hamot, Erie, PA, USA



P. Hopewood, M. J. Milroy (eds.), *Quality Cancer Care*,
https://doi.org/10.1007/978-3-319-78649-0_12

proven and recognized, in-hospital palliative care consultation rates for cancer patients remain low [5].

The barriers to access include lack of trained personnel; program costs; association of palliative care with hospice in the minds of patients, their families, and practitioners; and lack of knowledge about the scope and potential of palliative care services. Several in-hospital specialties, critical care and surgery, for example, which are frequently involved in cancer management, have only recently begun to recognize and assimilate the principles of palliative care.

## Palliative Care: What Is It?

The conceptual framework for palliative care evolved from the hospice concept of care introduced by the late Dr. Cicely Saunders in the 1960s. The hospice concept has subsequently been modified and extended to apply to individuals with more favorable prognoses and it has always been applied to patients with cancer *and* non-cancer diagnoses, a fact that still often eludes both professionals and the public. Palliative care has been defined as "… an approach that improves the quality of life of patients and their families facing the problems associated with life-threatening illness, through the prevention and relief of suffering by means of early identification and impeccable assessment and treatment of pain and other problems, physical, psychosocial and spiritual" [6]. It can be further characterized as interdisciplinary care that is offered simultaneously with all other appropriate medical treatments including those anticipating potential curative cancer treatment. The choice of therapy is based on the ability of the treatment to meet the agreed-upon goals of care, including the goal of remission or cure, not its impact on the underlying disease process. The concept of palliative care for surgical patients has been endorsed by the American College of Surgeons. Because of the association of death with palliative care in the minds of the public and practitioners, some have proposed the use of the term "supportive care" to enhance the number and timeliness of referrals [7].

## Indications and Referral for Palliative Care

The broadest indication for palliative care is the seriously ill patient and the patient's family's desire for relief of distress in any of its forms as well as the wish to improve the quality and promise of life regardless of diagnosis or prognosis. Specific indications for palliative care referral (Table 12.1) include pain and non-pain symptom management, psychosocial support for patients and their self-identified families, clarification of goals of care, conflict resolution when occurring within patient-family unit or staff or between staff and patient family-unit, and evaluation for hospice referral. Validated screening tools and "triggers" for palliative care referral are available although their use and utility depend much upon the experience and resources of the hospital.

**Table 12.1** Indications for referral for palliative care consultation

| | |
|---|---|
| **Qualitative** | |
| | Patient has an illness typified by progressive deterioration and worsening symptoms, often ending fatally. |
| | Patient has limiting/threatening conditions with declining functional status, or mental or cognitive function. |
| | Suboptimal control of pain or other distressing symptoms. |
| | Patient/family would benefit from clarification of goals and plan of care, or resolution of ethical dilemmas. |
| | Patient/surrogate declines further invasive or curative procedures, preferring comfort-oriented symptom management only. |
| | Patients on medical/surgical or critical care units who are expected to die imminently or shortly following hospital discharge. |
| | Bereavement support of hospital workers, particularly after the death of a colleague under care. |
| **Quantitative** | |
| | Advanced-stage cancer |
| | ECOG performance status of 3 |
| | Karnofsky status of 50% or less |
| | ICU stay of longer than 10 days |
| | Cancer recurrence or documented progression |

For ICU consultations, the usual goal of the palliative care consultant is to perform an independent evaluation to assist in the creation of a consistent, consensus-based medical narrative. One of the most common and bitter complaints of patients and families in hospitals, particularly in the ICU, is “mixed messages” from physicians and nurses.

Palliative care teams can be helpful negotiating the differences between ICU and oncology cultures. Older cancer patients are more likely to have life-limiting comorbidities (COPD, CHF) for which palliative care consultation might be indicated in addition to a cancer diagnosis. Oncologists often have long-term outpatient relationships with patients creating strong emotional connections though they may not fully appreciate the adverse long-term consequences of critical illness and the extremely high burden of acute critical illness. Intensivists have more brief relationships with patients and families and encounter them in a time of crisis. This may make it more difficult for them to divine patient/family values and the meaning of their past cancer experience [8].

## Palliative Care Screening

An expert consensus panel convened by the Center for the Advancement of Palliative Care (CAPC) proposed criteria that should be used for hospitals to conduct prospective case finding, via a checklist, for patients with unmet palliative care needs [9].

It proposed two checklists—a screening at the time of admission to identify for obvious candidates for basic palliative care assessment (chronic progressive illness, debility) and a daily rounds checklist to identify patients with ongoing uncontrolled symptoms or lack of clarity about goals of treatment for whom a basic palliative care assessment is needed.

Each checklist comprises primary global criteria for high likelihood of unmet palliative care needs, e.g., the "surprise question," *Would you not be surprised if the patient died within 12 months or before adulthood,"* and secondary more specific criteria that include potential interventions with palliative implications such as placement of a feeding tube, initiation of dialysis, or referral to hospice. The primary palliative care assessment triggered by these screenings includes pain/non-pain assessment, social and spiritual distress, comprehension of illness with its prognosis and treatment choices, patient's preferences, and disposition considerations (ongoing cancer treatment, hospice, etc.).

## Making a Referral for Palliative Care Services

The manner of referral is critical for engaging palliative support for a patient. If referral is clumsily handled or if it is perceived as abandonment by the patient or the patient's family, the result, no matter how well intentioned and appropriate the referral, will be counterproductive with respect to fostering trust, clarification of goals, and expeditious management of symptoms. Palliative care services have been available long enough in enough hospitals with an ever-growing number of families who have had direct experience with palliative care that a clinician's decision to refer for services is now much more likely to precipitate anxiety for providers or the patient/family. The physician may avoid or delay consultation because of fear of adverse emotional reactions or incorrect ideas about palliative care, i.e., "They just want to give morphine and put her to sleep," "All they do is talk about death," or "He is not ready for hospice." Instead of abandoning the patient by saying, *"There is nothing more we can do."* Arnold and Weissman [10] suggest proactively stating: "*To best meet some of the goals we've been discussing* (fill in with the goals mentioned by the family/patient) *I'd like to have some consultants from the Palliative Care Team visit with you.* This may be followed with, "*They are experts in treating the symptoms you are experiencing* (fill in symptom*). They are also good at helping your family deal with all the changes brought on by your illness; they can answer your questions about* (fill in previously discussed patient questions)." The patient should be reassured that the palliative care team works *with* other providers active in his or her care and not in their stead. In-hospital palliative care referrals are initiated by the attending physician's order or by other providers involved in the patient's care. Recently, the potential benefit of palliative care team engagement in critical care [11] and emergency room settings [12, 13] has been recognized not only because of the high levels of multi-dimension distress for patients and families there but also because these venues offer the greatest opportunity for proactive prevention of even greater distress.

## Patient Assessment for Palliative Care

Identification of patients likely to benefit from palliative care is followed by palliative care assessments, which, in aggregate, amount to a "whole-person" assessment, a reframing of the traditional biophysical medical interview that has been dominant since the late nineteenth century. Patient assessment for palliative treatment indexes the physical, psychological, social, and spiritual dimensions of the person's experience of illness rather than interrogates for signs and symptoms related to a list of organ systems. An important feature of palliative care screening is the opportunity for the patient to designate the degree of relevance of identified problems. The ideal assessment obtains the patient's self-report of symptoms and problems, while building a therapeutic alliance, and then conveys this information to the interdisciplinary team (IDT) for its deliberations and recommendations. Validated, disease-specific, and venue-specific screening tools exist for each of these entities in addition to more specific, in-depth instruments (see Table 12.2). See Case Example 12.1 for a composite example of an in-patient palliative care initial consultation report. The consultation emphasizes achieving prompt relief from the most pressing self-identified problems before addressing issues such as cancer treatment, code status, and

**Table 12.2** Selected palliative care assessment tools for cancer patients

| Tool | Measures | Scoring | Report | Comments |
|---|---|---|---|---|
| POS | Ten questions addressing physical, psychological, and spiritual domains | Numeric grading | Patient and staff versions available | Allows listing of "main problems" occurring during the previous 3 days |
| ESAS | Nine questions addressing nine symptoms: pain, fatigue, drowsiness, nausea, lack of appetite, depression, anxiety, SOB, well-being, and option to add symptom | Visual analogue scale of severity. Higher score = greater severity | Patient; caregiver if patient unable | The ESAS graph also contains space to add the patient's mini-mental status exam score. The "normal" box refers to the normal range for the patient, based on age and education level<br>Space for the Palliative Performance Scale (PPS) is included. Available in multiple languages and faces |
| PPSv2 | 11 categories measuring ambulation, activity level, evidence of disease, self-care, PO intake, and level of consciousness | Highest category (100%): Full function, no evidence of disease, full self-care, normal intake, full consciousness<br>Lowest category (0%): death | Medical staff assessment | Allows common language about performance status that is more relevant in palliative care than the Karnofsky performance scale on which it is based |

existential distress. Symptom management, practical home needs, possible spiritual distress, and family psychosocial support identified during this consultation would be discussed at the next IDT for its input and subsequent support.

**Case**

**Case Example 12.1** Supp and Pall Care Consult

Patient: **XXX**

Age: **54** Sex: **Female** DOB: **4/15/1953**

Author: Simonian CRNP, Lisa K.

**Basic Information**

**Visit information:** Patient seen on 5/12/2016

**Consultation information:**

**Requesting Physician**: Wong MD, Edward.

**Consultation Reason**: Goals of Care.

**Service Requesting Consult**: General Medicine/Hospitalist.

**Subjective**

We are asked to see this 54-year-old married female who presented in the ER on 5/8/2017 with intractable abdominal pain associated with nausea and vomiting and a 20-pound unintentional weight loss over the past few weeks. CT abdomen demonstrated a 7.3 × 5.2 cm irregular mass in the tail of the pancreas. Multiple hypodense lesions were noted in both lobes of the liver. No biliary ductal dilatation or ascites noted. A liver lesion was biopsied and showed poorly differentiated carcinoma consistent with pancreatic primary. She was seen by the medical oncology service that recommended a paclitaxel and gemcitabine-based treatment regimen. She is scheduled to commence treatment as an outpatient following discharge. Patient was scheduled for discharge yesterday but this was cancelled because of ongoing uncontrolled pain and nausea. She is currently receiving IV Dilaudid.

The patient is seen at bedside. Her husband, two sons, and a daughter are all present. The patient's family still feels that she is "pretty miserable." They believe "her oxygen sats are not where they should be." Initially she had some pain relief with hydrocodone and acetaminophen though her pain is becoming worse. She had previously expressed concerns that using pain medicine will make her "become addicted." However, the patient states that she has good relief with Dilaudid, "it takes away most of it. I feel like I can do things if my oxygen level is o.k. but then there is this nausea and gagging." The patient has had two bowel movements yesterday with the use of MiraLax.

Prior to this hospitalization, the patient was fairly independent at home with ADLs. She has noted that she can complete tasks but then "is completely exhausted."

The family who thought that her difficulties were related to her COPD provided her with a shower chair and walker. The husband states that grab rails in the shower would be helpful. She still was able to get in and out of bed.

The patient has been married 33 years to her high school sweetheart. They have two sons and a daughter all of whom live nearby as well as ten grandchildren. Prior to her illness, the patient worked in retail. She also loved to walk with her neighbors, which she can no longer do. Nor can she bowl, garden, and mow the grass. "I love yard work." The patient has a pet cat named Witch Hazel. The patient describes herself as a "lapsed" Roman Catholic who has not been to church in some time.

**Past Medical History**
COPD
Hypertension
Hypothyroidism
Active smoker

**Surgical History**
Tonsillectomy
Tubal ligation

**Social History**
(See above)
No alcohol or substance abuse
No prior military service
Health insurance through husband's employer

**Medications**
Albuterol inhaler
Synthroid 0.1 mg daily
Atenolol 50 mg daily

**Allergies**
None

**Review of Systems**

**Modified Edmonton Symptom Assessment Scale**

**All Obtainable**

Pain: 3-severe.
Anorexia: 3-severe.
Tiredness (fatigue): 2-Moderate.
Drowsiness: 1-Mild.
Initial Depression Screen: Past 2 weeks, down/depressed/hopeless? No.
Initial Anxiety Screen: Prev. 4 weeks, worried, tense, anxious? Yes.
Nausea: 3-Severe.
Shortness of breath: 3-Severe.
Constipation: Yes.
Delirium: Negative.

**PPS (Palliative Performance Scale):**
PPS 50.
**General State of Health:** Fair.

**Objective**
**Vital Signs** *Most Recent (Vitals in past 36 h; Dosing Wt and BMI this visit).*
**Temp C** 36.6 (36.5–37.4) **SBP** 127(118–131) **DBP** 79(72–79) **Pulse 91** (87–105) **RR** 16 (16–16).

**$SaO_2$** 92 (87–96) **$FiO_2$-$O_2$ (L/m)** 3 L/m (3 L/m-3 L/m) **Dosing Wt** 91.4 kg **BMI** 29.8.

**Gen:** Alert middle-aged female in moderate distress.

**HEENT:** Normocephalic. Mucous membranes moist. No JVD.

**Chest:** Clear bilaterally to auscultation and percussion. Equal inspiratory expansion.

**CV:** RRR. No murmur or rub.

**Abd:** Bowel sounds present. Soft, tender to palpation across epigastrium. No organomegaly.

**Skin:** No rash, purpura, jaundice.

**Ext:** No deformity. Normal range of motion. Trace pedal edema.

**Neuro:** Alert, oriented. CII-X11 grossly intact. Sensorimotor intact.

**Psych:** Cooperative, anxious. Judgment appropriate.

**Results Review.**

**Labs** (Past 24 h)

Hct = 24

WBC = 9000

Plt = 310,000

Na = 138

Cl-108

K = 3.8

HCo3 = 23

BUN = 22

CRT = 1.5

Ca + 2 = 8.5

Phos = 3.0

**Other labs/diagnostics**

**CTABDPELX**

Indication: Abdominal pain.

CT abdomen and pelvis without contrast. No prior study available.

CT abdomen: The visualized portions of the lungs and mediastinum demonstrate a small left pleural effusion. There is right lower lobe and right middle lobe atelectasis. There is a 7.3 × 5.2 cm irregular mass in the tail of the pancreas. Multiple hypodense lesions are noted in both lobes of the liver. Several enlarged celiac nodes are seen. No biliary ductal dilatation or ascites noted. Spleen, kidneys, and adrenal glands are unremarkable. There is no small- or large-bowel distention. There is moderate calcification of the aorta without aneurysmal change. There is no periaortic adenopathy. Edema of subcutaneous tissues is noted.

CT pelvis: Uterus and adnexa are noted and unremarkable. Bladder is non-distended and unremarkable.

Impression: 7.3 × 5.2 cm irregular mass in tail of the pancreas with multiple liver lesions and enlarged celiac nodes consistent with metastatic disease. No other remarkable findings.

Dictated by: Carl B Learner.

Signed by: Carl B Learner.

Signed on: 05/08/2017.

**Impression and recommendations**

**Diagnosis**

Encounter for Palliative Care ICD10-CM Z51.5.
Abdominal pain, acute, right upper quadrant (ICD10-CM R10.10)
Pancreatic cancer (ICD10-CM C25.9, Working, Diagnosis)

1. *Pain*: She had poor relief with low-dose oxycodone and is skeptical about the efficacy of PO pain medication. We recommend starting with oxycodone 10 mg Q4 hours with oxycodone 5 mg Q2 hours for breakthrough pain and Dilaudid 0.5 mg Q3 hours for severe pain. We will titrate from there with the goal of using an extended-release oxycodone + immediate-release oxycodone regimen for discharge. We could consider a celiac plexus block should her pain progress or should opioid side effects become problematic. Patient's concerns about addiction might be lessened by an explanation about the difference between physical dependence on opioids and addiction in addition to safeguards for the use of opioids for persons at risk for addiction. Currently she is a low risk (<4) for opioid addiction by ORT screening.
2. *Nausea*: Patient states that nausea has been well controlled with Compazine that has recently been ordered around the clock. Metoclopramide would be a good alternative because of its impact on the anticipated gastric dysmotility caused by her tumor.
3. *Weight loss*: Will ask a nutritionist to assess patient's nutritional status and needs. Patient's son had inquired about "IVs" and a "feeding tube" to address her nutritional decline. When the patient's main distracting symptom (pain) is better controlled, family and patient will need further counseling about risks and benefits of artificial nutrition and hydration in addition to the range of available options for appetite stimulation.
4. *Respiratory issues*: Family member had stated, "her oxygen sats are not where they should be." Will clarify for patient and family about the different implications of hypoxemia, shortness of breath, and rapid breathing.
5. *Advance care planning*: Patient has no advance directives. Patient and family overwhelmed by active symptoms. When these are better controlled, will broach their knowledge and insight about her disease process as a first step towards assessing their goals and the implications for cancer treatment, code status, and posthospital disposition.

Discussed with Dr. Wong

**Credentials: Professional Services**

**Credentials Title and Author**

CRNP

Title: CRNP

Supervising MD: Dunn MD, Geoffrey P

Attending Note and Attestation

**Review/Management**

**Spirituality**
Inquired about Religious/Spiritual Views: Yes: Roman Catholic—not active.
**Advance Care Planning:**
Inquired about durable POA/Surrogate: Not Done: Patient is decisional.
Is there an advance care plan in the chart? None.
**Was prognosis discussed?** Not requested.
**Long/Short-Term Goals discussed?** See notes.
**Patient Education & Discharge Planning:**

Is patient going to desired setting of care? Discharge planning not discussed.

**Treatment Recommendations:**

Laxative recommended if pt on opioids: Yes.
Chaplain Referral: Patient-family declines.
Depression Treatment/Referral Made: Clinically not indicated.
Spoke about Goals of Care: Both patient and family.
POLST completed if limited code? Patient is not limited code.

## The Palliative Care Team

The palliative care team uses an interdisciplinary, not multidisciplinary, approach in its deliberations. An interdisciplinary team is structured to encourage collaboration in sharing information for the purpose of setting goals. Leadership shifts depending on the specific issue being addressed while responsibility is shared. Team meetings typically occur on a daily basis.

The core members of a palliative care team include physician, an advanced-practice nurse, social worker, and chaplain. Certification of hospice and palliative care expertise exists for each of these entities (Table 12.3). The rationale for the core team composition can be traced back to Dame Cicely Saunders's concept of "total pain" in which she described [14] the experience of total pain as the totality of distress stemming from four dimensions of human experience: physical, psychological, socioeconomic, and spiritual. Other team members may include phar-

**Table 12.3** Certification in palliative care

| |
|---|
| • *Physicians*: In September 2006, ABMS approved the creation of hospice and palliative medicine (HPM) as a subspecialty of ten participating boards. Currently, approximately 2500–3000 physicians are certified. |
| • *Nurses*: Nursing certification examinations for advance-practice nurses, registered nurses, licensed practical nurses, and certified nursing assistants are offered by the National Board for Certification of Hospice and Palliative Care Nurses. 16,000 nurses are certified. |
| • *Social workers*: Certified Hospice and Palliative Social Worker (CHP-SW) and Advanced Certified Hospice and Palliative Social Worker (ACHP-SW) credentialing developed by collaboration of NHPCO and NASW. |

macists, case managers, psychologists, dieticians, nurses and nurse assistants, physician assistants, massage/art/music therapists, and volunteers. Depending on hospital size and resources, team members may participate with the palliative care service on a full-time or part-time basis. There is significant variation nationally in staffing models, reporting structures, and staffing ratios. Active participation by a pharmacist in the interdisciplinary team's activities is particularly valuable given the importance of pharmacologic approaches to symptom management and the predictable adverse quality of life impact (e.g., delirium, burdensome costs, withdrawal syndromes) encountered with polypharmacy occurring in a vulnerable population. See Table 12.4 for charts of commonly used medications and their indications in the palliative care setting.

**Table 12.4** Medications commonly used for pain and other symptoms

| Pain | | | | |
|---|---|---|---|---|
| | Class or drug | Starting dose/route | Maximum daily dose (MDD) and duration | Comments |
| Inflammatory pain | APAP | 650 mg PO/PR q4h<br>1000 mg IV q6h | • MDD: 3–4000 mg; 2000 mg/day for alcoholics and elderly | • Lacks anti-inflammatory effects of NSAIDs<br>• Avoid in severe hepatic disease |
| | NSAIDs | **Ibuprofen** 400 mg PO q8h | • MDD: 3200 mg | • Avoid use in severe hepatic and renal impairment |
| | | **Naproxen** 250 mg PO q6h | • MDD: 1250 mg | • CrCl <30 mL/min: use is not recommended<br>• Use lowest possible dose in advanced liver disease |
| | | **Ketorolac** 15–30 mg IM/IV q6h | • MDD: 120 mg<br>• Duration: 3–5 days | • Elderly, renally impaired, and/or weight < 50 kg/dose = 10–15 mg IM/IV<br>• Use caution in hepatic impairment |
| Neuropathic pain | Antiepileptics | **Gabapentin** 300 mg PO HS | • MDD: 3600 mg<br>• No benefit seen >1800 mg/day | • Must reduce in renal insufficiency<br>• Requires post-dialysis supplementation dose |
| | SNRIs | **Venlafaxine** 37.5 mg XR PO once daily | • MDD: 300 mg/day<br>• No benefit seen >150 mg/day | • Must reduce in renal insufficiency<br>• Avoid in severe renal and hepatic insufficiency |

(continued)

**Table 12.4** (continued)

Pain

| | Class or drug | Starting dose/route | Maximum daily dose (MDD) and duration | Comments |
|---|---|---|---|---|
| Nociceptive pain | Opioids | **Morphine**<br>7.5–15 mg PO IR q4-6 h PRN | • N/A<br>• Opioid-naïve patients should only be prescribed IR medications PRN<br>• Can consider transitioning to long-acting agent if appropriate | • Avoid in renal dysfunction (CrCl <30 mL/min); however safe in patients receiving hemodialysis<br>• Avoid in patients with true morphine allergy<br>• Treat OIC empirically with bowel regimen<br>• Monitor for signs of opioid misuse, abuse, diversion |
| | | **Oxycodone**<br>2.5–5 mg IR PO q4-6 h PRN | | • Treat OIC empirically with bowel regimen<br>• Monitor for signs of opioid misuse, abuse, diversion |

Key: *IV* intravenous, *PO* by mouth, *APAP* acetaminophen, *NSAIDs* nonsteroidal anti-inflammatory drugs, *IR* immediate release, *PRN* as needed, *CrCl* creatinine clearance, *OIC* opioid-induced constipation

Dyspnea

| Class | Starting dose/route | Maximum daily dose (MDD) and duration | Comments |
|---|---|---|---|
| Opioids | Morphine<br>• 7.5–15 mg PO IR q4-6 h PRN<br>• 0.5–1 mg IV q4-6 h PRN | • N/A<br>• Opioid-naïve patients should only be prescribed IR medications PRN<br>• Can consider transitioning to long-acting agent (or continuous infusion) if appropriate | • Avoid in renal dysfunction (CrCl <30 mL/min); however safe in patients receiving hemodialysis<br>• Avoid in patients with true morphine allergy<br>• Treat OIC empirically with bowel regimen<br>• Monitor for signs of opioid misuse, abuse, diversion |
| | **Oxycodone**<br>2.5–5 mg IR PO q4-6 h PRN | | • Treat OIC empirically with bowel regimen<br>• Monitor for signs of opioid misuse, abuse, diversion |
| | **Hydromorphone**<br>0.5 mg IV q4-6 h PRN | | • Treat OIC empirically with bowel regimen<br>• Monitor for signs of opioid misuse, abuse, diversion |

**Table 12.4** (continued)

| Dyspnea | | | |
|---|---|---|---|
| Class | Starting dose/ route | Maximum daily dose (MDD) and duration | Comments |
| Benzodi-azepines* | **Lorazepam**<br>0.5–1 mg PO q4-6 h PRN | • Usually no more than 4 mg/dose<br>• Benzodiazepine-naïve patients should only be prescribed IR medications PRN | • Monitor for sedation |

Key: *Benzodiazepines have only been shown to be effective for the anxiety component of dyspnea. Will not improve subjective feeling of dyspnea alone; *IV* intravenous, *PO* by mouth, *IR* immediate release, *PRN* as needed, *CrCl* creatinine clearance, *OIC* opioid-induced constipation

| Nausea and vomiting | | | | |
|---|---|---|---|---|
| Drug | Common clinical indication | Starting dose/ route | Maximum daily dose | Comments |
| Metoclopramide* | • N/V of unknown etiology<br>• Impaired GI motility<br>• Opioid-induced /v | 5–20 mg PO/ SC/IV AC and HS | 60 mg | Risk of EPS with prolonged use (>12 weeks) |
| Haloperidol | • Opioid-induced n/v | 0.5–4 mg PO/ SC/IV q6h | 5 mg | IV has higher risk of EPS and QTc prolongation than PO |
| Prochlorperazine | • Opioid-induced n/v | 5–10 mg PO/ IV q6 h or 25 mg PR q6h | 40 mg | Risk of EPS<br>Common ADR: sedation |
| Ondansetron | • Chemotherapy- or radiation-induced n/v | 4–8 mg PO/ IV q4-8 h | 32 mg | Common ADRs: headache, fatigue, and constipation |
| Scopolamine | • Motion-induced n/v | 1.5 mg patch q72h | 1 patch q72h | Common ADRs: dry mouth, blurred vision, ileus, urinary retention. Considered a higher cost agent |
| Dexamethasone | • N/V related to increased ICP | 4–8 mg PO/ IV qAM or BID | 8–16 mg | Common ADRs: agitation, insomnia, and hyperglycemia |

Key: *Metoclopramide is considered first line for empiric therapy; *N/V* nausea/vomiting, *GI* gastrointestinal, *PO* by mouth, *SC* subcutaneous, *IV* intravenous, *PR* rectal, *AM* morning, *BID* twice a day, *ADR* adverse drug reactions, *EPS* extrapyramidal syndrome

**Table 12.4** (continued)

Anxiety/depression

| Category | Medication | Starting dose | Target daily dose | Adverse drug reactions | | |
|---|---|---|---|---|---|---|
| | | | | Anticholinergic | Insomnia | GI distress |
| SSRIs | Citalopram | 10–20 mg daily | 10–40 mg | + | + | ++ |
| | Escitalopram | 5–10 mg daily | 10–20 mg | + | +++ | ++ |
| | Sertraline | 25–50 mg daily | 50–200 mg | – | + | +++ |
| SNRIs | Venlafaxine (IR and XR)* | 75 mg/day (either qAM (XR) or divided TID (IR) | 150–375 mg | + | ++++ | ++ |
| | Duloxetineʊ | 20 mg BID | 30–60 mg | + | ++ | ++ |
| Stimulant | Methylphenidate ɷ | 2.5–5 mg BID (at 08:00/12:00) | 5–40 mg | – | ++++ | + |

Key: * Dual-serotonin/norepinephrine action at doses of 150–225 mg which is effective in neuropathic pain and is mildly activating. On switching from the venlafaxine XR to venlafaxine, the shorter half-life of venlafaxine requires frequent dosing to reach the same dose of venlafaxine XR. Use with caution in patients with hypertension, ʊ Do not use in patients with liver dysfunction, ɷ Energizing, may increase appetite

Agitation/delirium

| Medication | Starting dose | Maximum daily dose | Adverse drug reactions | | | |
|---|---|---|---|---|---|---|
| | | | EPS | Anticholinergic | Sedation | QTc prolongation |
| Haloperidol ^ | 0.5–1 mg BID to q8h | 20 mg | PO: ++ IV: +++ | + | 0/– | PO: + IV: ++ |
| Risperidone ^ * | 0.25–1 mg BID, up to q6h | 6 mg | ++ | + | ++ | ++ |
| Olanzapine * | 2.5–10 mg daily | 20 mg | + | ++ | +++ | + |
| Quetiapine | 12.5–50 mg BID | 800 mg | + | ++ | +++ | ++ |
| Aripiprazole ^ * | 5–15 mg qAM | 30 mg | ++ | + | ++ | 0/– |

Key: The FDA has determined that the use of antipsychotic medications in the treatment of behavioral disorders in elderly patients with dementia is associated with increased mortality. This risk appears to be highest during the first 2 weeks of use; ^ available in oral solution, * available in oral disintegrating formulation, *PO* by mouth, *AM* morning, *BID* twice a day, *EPS* extrapyramidal syndrome

**Table 12.4** (continued)

| Secretions | | | |
|---|---|---|---|
| Medication (route) | Starting dose | Onset of action | Maximum daily dose |
| Glycopyrrolate (PO)* | 1 mg q4-6 h PRN | 30 min | 8 mg |
| Glycopyrrolate (SC/IV) * | 0.2 mg q4-6 h PRN | 1 min | 8 mg |
| Atropine (IV) | 0.1 mg q4-6 h PRN | 1 min | 2 mg |
| Atropine (SL drops ◯) | 1 gtt (1%) q4-6 h PRN | 30 min | 48 drops |
| Scopolamine (transdermal patch) | 1 mg patch q72h | 12 h | 1 patch q72 h |
| Hyoscyamine (tabs, and SL tabs) | 0.125 mg TID-QID PRN | 30 min | 1.5 mg |

Key: * Glycopyrrolate will not cross the blood-brain barrier, reducing the risk of CNS toxicity (sedation, delirium). ◯ Use atropine ophthalmic drops, *PO* by mouth, *SC* subcutaneous, *IV* intravenous, *PRN* as needed, *SL* sublingual

## "Ethical" Issues Relevant to Palliative Care

In many hospitals palliative care services saw their origin in ethics committees because until relatively recently a consistent moral, ethical, and legal framework for the application of palliative approaches such as withholding or withdrawal of life support did not exist. Even when such a framework was available by the end of the 1990s, most practitioners were not knowledgeable or comfortable with it. Many of the "ethical" dilemmas with patients with advanced or critical illness brought to ethics committees were not true legal or ethical breaches but education deficits about the nature of individual autonomy and appropriate symptom control. The more common of these recurrent issues include extent of disclosure of unfavorable news to patients; withholding or withdrawal of life support, especially artificial hydration and nutrition; and ongoing medical treatment without any predictable benefit (futility) (Table 12.5).

## Reimbursement

In-hospital palliative care services are not billed to the patient/family though there is a physician reimbursement mechanism in place that offsets some of the costs for the hospital. The hospital's cost avoidance can increase through palliative care services because of their impact on prompt resolution of patient symptoms, avoidance of costly and burdensome interventions not likely to improve function or survival, and improved discharge planning for patients. Physician coding and reimbursement for palliative care services are the same as with any other medical specialties—each patient encounter is coded for a procedure code and a diagnosis. Diagnosis codes are selected from the International Classification of Diseases (ICD). The procedure

**Table 12.5** Ethical issues relevant to palliative care

| Issue | Commentary |
|---|---|
| Disclosure of bad news | Broad legal and ethical consensus supporting disclosure of bad news *when permitted* by patient or surrogate. No evidence that disclosure of bad news "takes away hope" if conveyed gently and in the spirit of non-abandonment. Empathic truth telling fosters trust that is the basis of hope. |
| Perioperative do-not-resuscitate (DNR) orders | The American College of Surgeons, the Association of Operating Room Nurses, and the American Society of Anesthesiologists position papers condemn policies requiring automatic cancellation of existing DNR orders for patients undergoing anesthesia based on the principle of patient autonomy. All recommend preoperative discussion ("required reconsideration") during which patient or surrogate confirms patient's treatment goals and limits of care including revision or implementation of a DNR order; risks of patient's care plan; and recommendations by anesthesiologist and surgeon. During this discussion the anesthesiologist and patient can set the parameters for resuscitation for the procedure itself and in the recovery room. |
| Withhold/withdraw of life support | The withholding and withdrawal of medical treatments are considered legally and ethically equivalent and are based on the right to bodily integrity. It is more difficult to withdraw a life-supporting treatment once it has been started than to not initiate it at all. A surrogate's persistent reluctance to consider termination of life support is usually related to their fear that they will be "killing the patient" or their fear that withdrawing life support will cause suffering. Legally and ethically, termination of undesired medical treatment of the properly informed patient/surrogate is not considered homicide or suicide. |
| Aggressive symptom management | • Aggressive symptom management of unbearable symptoms is a moral imperative if effective treatment is available, even at the risk of hastening or causing death, as long as causing death is not the intention of treatment. The risk of hastening death is present with any surgical treatment for serious illness, including attempts to cure.<br>• In situations where rapid escalation of dosing is necessary to relieve intractable severe symptoms (pain, dyspnea, agitated delirium) in the imminently dying patient, the rule of double effect, broadly accepted by ethicists, is invoked.<br>RDE is comprised of these elements:<br>• The act must be good or morally neutral<br>• Bad effects are foreseen but not intended<br>• A good end cannot justify a bad means<br>• The risk/benefit ratio must be reasonable |
| Terminal sedation | Rarely indicated in palliative care. Reserved for severe, intractable symptoms when death is imminent. The goal of palliative sedation is to use the minimum amount of sedation necessary to relieve severe physical symptoms to the point of unconsciousness, if necessary, not deliberate induction of coma or hastening of death. Consultation with ethics committee, neuropsychiatric consultant (to determine competency), and palliative care specialist is recommended. |

code reflects the degree of difficulty, setting, and effort (time) while the diagnosis codes include not only disease codes (e.g., pancreatic cancer) but also symptom codes (e.g., dyspnea).

## Palliative Care: Outcomes, Metrics, and Quality

Not surprisingly, given its patient/family focus and timeliness in addressing acutely distressing issues, in-hospital and outpatient palliative care programs have enjoyed favorable public perception and other desirable outcomes, especially if consultation is early [15]. Other reviews have documented much better outcomes for hospital-based palliative care teams than "standard care" for management of pain, non-pain symptoms, patient and family satisfaction, hospital costs, and hospital length of stay [16–19].

In 2006 the National Quality Forum (NQF) issued its report, *A National Framework and Preferred Practices for Palliative and Hospice Care* [20]. The report details a framework for palliative and hospice care intended to serve as a foundation upon which a quality measurement and reporting system should be built. The report listed 38 preferred practices designed to improve palliative and hospice care. Both the framework and the preferred practices were endorsed by NQF in 2006. Subsequently NQF has endorsed roughly 20 palliative care quality measures including 5 that were stewarded by the American Society of Clinical Oncology (ASCO). ASCO-sponsored measures relevant to hospitalized patients include the proportion of patients admitted to hospice for less than 3 days (NQF#0216), proportion of patients admitted to ICU in the last 30 days of life (NQF#0213), and proportion receiving chemotherapy in the last 14 days of life (NQF#0210) [21]. As the number of hospital-based palliative care programs continues to grow across the country, measurement tools such as these will be necessary to ensure consistent appropriate and compassionate care.

## Conclusion: Living Beyond the Diagnosis

Accumulating public and professional experience with a growing evidence base has established palliative care support as an integral part of cancer care, ideally from the time of diagnosis in most instances. As palliative care continues to mainstream itself, the dated and dichotomous view of "cure versus palliation" should fade as curable patients are comforted and incurable patients live better and longer. Although the in-hospital admission for the cancer patient hazards dignity, comfort, and quality of life, it now provides the opportunity through palliative care support to transform the cancer journey from one shadowed by despair to a purposeful one of affirmation.

## References


1. CAPC (Center to Advance Palliative Care) Analysis of U.S. Hospital Palliative Care Programs, 2010 Snapshot. 2010. http://www.capc.org/news-and-events/rleases/analysis-of-us-hospital-palliative-care-programs-2010-snapshot.pdf/file_. Accessed 5 Jun 2017.
2. Smith TJ, Temin S, Alesi ER, Abernethy AP, et al. American Society of Clinical Oncology provisional clinical opinion: the integration of palliative care into standard oncology care. J Clin Oncol. 2012;30(8):880–7.
3. Commission on Cancer. Cancer program standards 2012: ensuring patient-centered care. Chicago: American College of Surgeons; 2012. p. 70–1.
4. Commission on Cancer. Cancer program standards, 2016 ed., Ensuring Patient-Centered Care. Chicago: American College of Surgeons; 2016. p. 53.
5. Roeland EJ, Triplett DP, Matsuno RK, Boero IJ, Hwang L, Yeung HN, et al. Patterns of palliative care consultation among elderly patients with cancer. J Natl Compr Cancer Netw. 2016;14(4):439–45.
6. www.who.int/cancer/palliative/definition/en/. Accessed 9 Mar 2017.
7. Dalal S, Bruera S, Hui D, Yennu S, Dev R, Williams J, et al. Use of palliative care services in a tertiary cancer center. Oncologist. 2016;21(1):110–8.
8. Bhatnagar M, Arnold R. Fast facts and concepts #310. The oncology-ICU-palliative care interface. Palliative Care Network of Wisconsin. https://www.mypcnow.org/fast-facts. Accessed 4 Jun 2017.
9. Weissman DE, Meier DE. Identifying patients in need of a palliative care assessment in the hospital setting. A consensus report from the center to advance palliative care. J Palliat Med. 2011;14(1):1–6.
10. Arnold R, Weissman DE. Fast facts and concepts #42. Broaching the topic of palliative care consultation with patients and families. Palliative Care Network of Wisconsin. https://www.mypcnow.org/fast-facts. Accessed 4 Jun 2017.
11. Aslakson RA, Curtis JR, Nelson JE. The changing role of palliative care in the ICU. Crit Care Med. 2014;42(11):2418–28.
12. Lamba S, Nagurka R, Walther S, Murphy P. Emergency-department-initiated palliative care consults: a descriptive analysis. J Palliat Med. 2012;5(6):633–6.
13. Choosing Wisely Campaign- American College of Emergency Physicians. https://www.acep.org/Clinical—Practice-Management/ACEP-Announces-List-of-Tests-As-Part-of-Choosing-Wisely-Campaign. Accessed 4 June 2017.
14. Saunders C, Sykes N. The management of terminal malignant disease. 3rd ed. London: Edward Arnold; 1993.
15. Casarett D, Pickard A, Bailey FA, et al. Do palliative consultations improve patient outcomes? J Am Geriatr Soc. 2008;56:593–9.
16. Jordhøy MS, Fayers P, Saltnes T, Ahlner-Elmqvist M, Jannert M, Kaaasa S. A palliative-care intervention and death at home: a cluster randomized trial. Lancet. 2000;356(9233):888–93.
17. Finlay IG, Higginson IJ, Goodwin DM, et al. Palliative care in hospital, hospice, at home: results from a systematic review. Ann Oncol. 2002;13:257–64.
18. Finlay IG, Higginson IJ, Goodwin DM, et al. Do hospital-based palliative teams improve care for patients or families at the end of life? J Pain Symptom Manag. 2002;23:96–106.
19. Morrison RS, Penrod JD, Cassel JB, Caust-Ellenbogen M, Litke A, Spragens L, Meier DE, Palliative Care Leadership Centers' Outcomes Group. Cost savings associated with US hospital palliative care consultation programs. Arch Intern Med. 2008;168(16):1783–90.
20. A national framework and preferred practices for palliative and hospice care quality, a consensus report. Dec. 2006. http://www.qualityforum.org/. Accessed 4 Jun 2017.
21. National quality forum endorses cancer measures article and search pages. http://www.qualityforum.org. Accessed 4 Jun 2017.

# Chapter 13
# Ambulatory Palliative Care

**John D. Halporn, Simone P. Rinaldi, and Vicki A. Jackson**

## Introduction

Palliative care, and the medical subspecialty of palliative medicine, is a specialized medical care for people living with serious illness. It focuses on providing relief from the symptoms and stress of a serious illness. The goal is to improve quality of life for both the patient and the family. Palliative care is provided by a team of palliative care doctors, nurses, social workers, and others who work together with a patient's other doctors to provide an extra layer of support. It is appropriate at any age and at any stage in a serious illness and can be provided along with curative treatment. This definition, from the Center to Advance Palliative Care [1], is helpful to define the goals, providers, and scope of palliative care—it is impressively broad! It is important to clarify that hospice is specialized form of palliative care for patients with a limited life expectancy (usually 6 months or less) provided by a multidisciplinary team-based agency or organization; hospice always includes the provision of palliative care, but palliative applies to a broader range of illnesses, disease trajectories, and prognoses not included in hospice. Palliative care is

J. D. Halporn (✉)
DFCI – POPC, Adult Palliative Care Clinic, Dana-Farber Cancer Institute,
Harvard Medical School, Boston, MA, USA

Harvard Medical School Center for Palliative Care, Harvard Medical School,
Boston, MA, USA
e-mail: john_halporn@dfci.harvard.edu

S. P. Rinaldi · V. A. Jackson
Division of Palliative Care and Geriatrics, Department of Medicine, Massachusetts General
Hospital, Boston, MA, USA

Harvard Medical School Center for Palliative Care, Harvard Medical School,
Boston, MA, USA
e-mail: sprinaldi@partners.org; vjackson@mgh.harvard.edu

 
P. Hopewood, M. J. Milroy (eds.), *Quality Cancer Care*,
https://doi.org/10.1007/978-3-319-78649-0_13

recognized as an increasingly important component of medical care for cancer that can improve quality of life, extend survival in some cases, and help to tailor patients' medical care to their individual beliefs and values, termed goal-concordant care.

Palliative care is commonly understood to be delivered at a specialty level by fellowship-trained, board-certified practitioners in a hospital or hospice setting; however, the clear majority of this work is "primary palliative care" delivered by surgeons, primary care physicians, hospitalists, and specialists as an integral part of their existing practice. Basic management of pain, depression, anxiety, and other symptoms as well as discussing prognosis, goals of care, suffering, and code status are primary palliative care tasks common to all physicians [2]. Specialty-level palliative care includes management of complex and refractory symptoms, existential distress, complicating psychiatric illness or substance abuse, and conflicts regarding goals of care.

The initial imperative in promoting quality of life is expert symptom management, particularly in cancer, when symptoms can be rapid and severe and herald a significant worsening of disease. Uncontrolled symptoms represent immediate and compelling suffering caused by both disease and treatment; little progress can be made without addressing them directly, beginning at the first encounter. In cancer patients, active symptoms drive anxiety about progressing or recurrent disease, impede understanding and coping, and diminish quality of life. Once symptoms are improved or relieved—sometimes requiring multiple interventions over several encounters—the more cerebral and existential palliative care issues of survival, prognosis, and personhood can be addressed.

This chapter begins with a review of common ambulatory palliative care symptom management followed by sections on the aims and potential of ambulatory palliative care and the sophisticated communication skills needed to achieve these aims. Several sources [3–5] on palliative care symptom management are included in the reference section for further study. There are aspects of palliative care that are specific to surgeons, such as communication about high-risk procedures, placing procedure outcomes in the context of patient clinical condition and future goals, and interventions in exclusively surgical populations; several of these are highlighted in the communication section below.

## Symptom Management

### *Pain*

Pain is the physical sensation of actual or imagined tissue injury—("imagined" referring to neuropathic mechanisms where pain is present without a precipitating injury). For patients with cancer, pain is a common experience of disease, and it is nearly universal in recurrent or advanced disease. Patients in moderate or severe pain are unable to appreciate quality of life, they are distracted and diminished by the symptom, and often their discouragement leads to wishes for an early death for relief. As patients contemplate worsening disease and the dying process, pain is often a strong central fear. Perceptions and meaning of pain and cultural and social ideas about pain treatment influence the experience for patients, providers, and families alike. When pain is accurately diagnosed and expertly treated, quality of life can be improved and the patient can be sustainably cared for, particularly by family members at home. Barriers to effective pain relief are many, from logistic, financial, and regulatory challenges as well as social, emotional, and religious beliefs complicating diagnosis and treatment. Women, minorities, poor, aged, and nursing home groups are at increased risk of ineffective pain relief treatment, and maladaptive behaviors and attitudes commonly lead to undertreatment and conflict.

## Pain: Assessment

Assessment of pain includes a careful history, review of systems, physical examination, and collection of radiographic and laboratory data. Complete characterization of pain requires elucidation of the mechanism (somatic, visceral, or neuropathic), severity, location, referral pattern, timing, and aggravating and relieving features. Attributing symptoms to recognized pain syndromes, such as burning mouth syndrome, bone pain from lytic metastases, or chemotherapy-induced peripheral neuropathy, allow for specific and effective treatment strategies. The cancer patient with new or unexplained pain should always raise the question of disease spread or complications or even a new diagnosis. Treating pain empirically, without understanding cause and contributing factors, is regrettably common and contributes to delay in diagnosis, ineffective treatment, and overuse of pain medications.

Ambulatory palliative care requires expertise with common analgesics in oral, sublingual, and topical forms as well as skills in patient education and risk management. For cancer pain, treatment is rarely a single prescription for an as-needed analgesic, and requires a practice with regular follow-up visits with monitoring and compliance functions in place to assure safe and effective use.

## Pain: Opioid Risk Management and Patient Education

As opioids are considered first-line therapy for the management of moderate-to-severe cancer pain, it is essential that providers be familiar with the known risks of opioids and that they implement a "universal precaution strategy" to manage patients safely and effectively [6]. Opioid therapy begins with risk assessment/stratification and subsequent implementation of management strategies proportionate to patient's individual risk. Validated screening tools, like the Opioid Risk Tool [7] (ORT) or the Revised Screener and Opioid Assessment for Patients in Pain [8] (SOAPP-R), can help identify patients at risk for developing opioid addiction or aberrant drug-taking behaviors, and are easily incorporated into clinical practice. However, providers should not overestimate the ability of these tools to rule out risks from long-term opioid therapy [9, 10]. This is particularly true when screening tools are applied in the intake process, but risk is not reassessed continually by active surveillance over ensuing weeks or months of use. It is also necessary, and in many states mandatory, for the provider to review the patient's history in the state prescription drug monitoring database prior to prescribing opioids and other controlled substance medications.

Opioid therapy should also include patient education on the risks and benefits of opioid use; potential side effects; goals of treatment; behavioral expectations; safe storage and disposal of opioids; state driving law; and the clinic's opioid prescription process [9, 10]. The use of a medication management agreement can be helpful in establishing and documenting informed consent, treatment goals, expected behaviors, and consequences should aberrant opioid-related behaviors occur. There are challenges with the use of medication agreements in palliative care and cancer populations, and historically these agreements have only been implemented with those patients considered to be at higher risk. However, many insurers now require evidence of a medication management agreement in their coverage determination process for opioids. As the regulatory climate in the United States evolves, there is a march toward wider and compulsory use of these agreements—prescribers should understand the current standards required by their institutions, societies, and state medical boards.

Comprehensive and ongoing opioid education and monitoring are appropriate for all patients, including those at low risk for misuse. Other components of the "universal precaution strategy" include identification of primary prescribing team/provider and pharmacy; regular review of prescription monitoring program; and optimization of non-pharmacological, non-opioid, adjuvant, and/or interventional therapies for the potential opioid-sparing effect. At each visit, reassessment of opioid therapy should occur with documentation of efficacy, adverse effects, patient functionality, and any aberrant opioid-related behaviors. Documentation should also include rationale of whether to continue, modify, or discontinue opioid therapy.

Additional structure/interventions should be implemented for those patients at moderate to high risk. This includes patients with active substance-use disorder exhibiting aberrant drug-taking behavior; patients without substance-use disorder history but exhibiting aberrant behaviors; and lastly patients with a history of substance-use disorder in active recovery with no current aberrant drug behaviors. Providers must stop prescribing opioids when there is significant concern or high probability that diversion is occurring. However, for other aberrant opioid-related behaviors, providers can consider additional mitigation strategies, tailored to the individual patient, and titrated over time. These include: use of toxicology screens; shortened prescribing intervals; smaller quantities; more frequent provider visits; pill counts; limited use of short-acting opioids; selection of opioid drug and route to optimize compliance (e.g., fentanyl patch or methadone); use of lockboxes and home opioid dispensing by a trusted individual; prescription of naloxone rescue kits; and consultation with social work, chaplaincy, homecare agencies, psychiatry, and/or an addiction specialist. The team must reevaluate the risks and benefits of continuing to prescribe opioids if aberrant drug-taking behavior persists. If the ability to safely manage opioids in the outpatient setting has been exceeded, despite risk mitigation strategies, opioid therapy may be discontinued. Alternatively, the team can consider options for inpatient or extended-care-facility placement (based on patient's clinical status and prognosis) to optimize symptom management while ensuring safe opioid use.

## Pain: Initial Opioid Prescribing

Treating pain in cancer often requires opioids early on for severe symptoms, but the progression initially follows the WHO pain ladder with acetaminophen or nonsteroidal anti-inflammatory medication for mild and intermittent symptoms. With appropriate monitoring, these strategies can be effective for months or more in slow-moving diseases, particularly for somatic bony pain. Visceral, neuropathic, or steadily escalating symptoms require opioids for control. In cancer patients, combination agents with opiate and nonsteroidal anti-inflammatory agents or acetaminophen are not used due to frequent contraindications for the non-opioid component and likelihood of escalation beyond the allowable ceiling of this component. The commonly available short-acting agents—oxycodone, morphine, and hydromorphone—are routinely used, starting with an every-3-h as-needed regimen. The three opioids are equally effective for somatic and visceral pain but with differing potencies; the equivalent starting doses of each agent for oral or enteral administration are oxycodone 5 mg, morphine 7.5 mg, and hydromorphone 2 mg (1.875 mg to convert exactly). Each reaches peak effect within 30–60 min, and the effective duration is 3–4 h. Selection of a particular agent depends on previous tolerance experience and compatibility with other medical issues, detailed in Table 13.1.

Dose adjustment is determined by the degree and duration of pain relief from each dose. For example, 7.5 mg oral morphine may improve pain from 8/10 to 6/10, whereas 15 mg brings it from 8/10 to 4/10. It is helpful to establish a goal pain score with the patient; this gives a valuable opportunity to teach that eliminating pain is unlikely with opiates and that there is a balance between the burden of frequent dosing and side effects and the degree of relief achieved. Dose frequency is assessed by how long episodes of pain last or how long the relief from medication lasts. When patients take more of their as-needed doses (up to eight times per day for an every-3-h as-needed prescription) it indicates frequent or nearly constant pain. Five or more as-needed opioid doses per day signal the need to consider long-acting opioids.

**Table 13.1** Properties of common opioids

| | Form | Onset—minutes | Peak—minutes | Duration—hours |
|---|---|---|---|---|
| Morphine | Oral—IR[a] | 15–60 | 30–60 | 3–4 |
| | Oral—ER[a] | 2–4 h | | 8–12 |
| | IV | 1–5 | 3–4 | 3–4 |
| Oxycodone | Oral—IR | 10–15 | 30–60 | 3–4 |
| | Oral—ER | 2–4 h | | 8–12 |
| Hydromorphone | Oral IR | 15–30 | 30–60 | 3–4 |
| | IV | 1–2 | 5–20 | 3–4 |
| Fentanyl | Oral transmucosal | 5–15 | 20–30 | 1–2 |
| | Transdermal patch | <12 h | | 48–72 |
| | IV | <1 | 5–15 | 0.5–2 |

[a]*IR* immediate-release formulation, *ER* extended-release formulation

## Pain: Long Acting Opioids

With increased severity and duration of pain, patients are more comfortable with the addition of a long-acting agent for constant pain control and as-needed doses of short-acting opioids for incident or fluctuating pain. The commonly available long-acting agents are oral extended-release morphine (MS-Contin) and oxycodone (OxyContin) in 2- or 3-times-daily dosing, or the topical fentanyl patch that provides 48–72 h of coverage. Long-acting agents should provide 70% of total daily opioid intake, with the balance provided by short-acting agents on an as-needed basis. The short-acting or breakthrough dose should be 10–15% of the total daily opioid dose, administered every 3–4 h as needed. See Example 13.1 below.

**Example 13.1** Opioid Escalation

Outpatient taking morphine 15–30 mg every 3 h as needed for pain with a total of 11 daily tablets of 15 mg each.

Daily PO morphine = 11 × 15 mg = 165 mg morphine daily.

Long-acting morphine—The nearest available pill size gives an extended-release morphine dose of 60 mg two times daily for 120 mg daily total. This is close to the target of 70% of the daily total provided in extended-release form.

Short-acting morphine—Breakthrough dosing is 10–15% of 165 mg daily total, or 15 mg every 3 h as needed using the nearest available pill size of 15 mg.

Note that the usual 50–75% safety factor reduction is NOT required because there is no conversion between opioids. Although the 120 mg of long-acting morphine is less than the current 165 mg taken in the 11 short-acting doses initially, the patient has access to eight as-needed doses of 15 mg over the course of the day, giving a final dose range of 120 mg (no as-needed doses) to 240 mg (eight as-needed doses). At the follow-up encounter after this change, review of the pattern and number of short-acting doses should guide further adjustment of both agents.

## Pain: Conversion Between Opioids

On admission and discharge of hospitalized patients, providers often have to convert between IV and oral routes and among different opiate agents. For example, a patient admitted with sudden onset of severe pain and vomiting from progressive cholangiocarcinoma with biliary obstruction may require intravenous opioid for initial relief, followed by introduction of a long-acting oral agent once oral intake is reestablished, and then transition from an IV to oral short-acting as-needed agent before discharge. Conversion of opiate doses is accomplished by creating a proportion between equianalgesic amounts of the different opioids and using this to convert to the equivalent dose of the new drug; see Example 13.2 below. A 25–33% safety factor reduction in the destination dose of the new opioid is recommended to allow for patient variation in absorption, drug sensitivity, metabolism, and secretion (Table 13.2).

**Table 13.2** Equianalgesic doses of common opioids

| Opioid | Intravenous dosing | Oral dosing |
|---|---|---|
| Morphine | 10 mg | 30 mg |
| Oxycodone | | 20 mg |
| Hydromorphone | 1.5 mg | 7.5 mg |
| Fentanyl | 0.1 mg | |
| Fentanyl | 25 μg/hour patch = 50 mg of oral morphine in 24 h | |

## **Example 13.2** Equianalgesic Conversion

Opioid Conversion Calculation:

$$\frac{\text{Old Opioid equivalent dose from table 13.2}}{\text{New Opioid equivalent dose from table 13.2}} = \frac{\text{Old Opioid Dose/24 h}}{X} \quad X = \text{New Opioid Dose/24 h}$$

Opioid conversion—Hospitalized patient receiving 3 mg IV hydromorphone every 6 h and 20 mg of oral oxycodone three times daily with good pain control. Convert this to a long- and short-acting morphine regimen for discharge.

Daily IV hydromorphone = 4 doses/day × 3 mg/dose = 12 mg IV hydromorphone daily.

Daily PO oxycodone = 3 doses/day × 20 mg/dose = 60 mg PO oxycodone daily.

Convert to daily PO morphine doses.

Hydromorphone Conversion Calculation:

$$\frac{\text{30 mg Oral morphine}}{\text{1.5 mg IV hydromorphone}} = \frac{X}{\text{12 mg/day}} \quad X = \text{240 mg daily morphine from hydromorphone}$$

Oxycodone Conversion Calculation:

$$\frac{\text{30 mg Oral Morphine}}{\text{20 mg Oral Oxycodone}} = \frac{X}{\text{60 mg/day}} \quad X = \text{90 mg daily morphine from oxycodone}$$

Total equivalent daily PO Morphine Dose = 240 mg + 90 mg = 330 mg per day

Apply safety factor reduction – 75% of 330 mg = 248 mg daily PO morphine.

In practice, it is best to use 75% as the upper limit of the safety conversion factor, with lower doses selected mainly to accommodate available pill sizes as long as the safety factor is between 67 and 75%. For this example, we will round to 240 mg for simplicity.

Extended-release morphine—For the long-acting component we aim for 70% of the daily total 240 mg range giving a target of 168 mg and calculate using the nearest pill size yielding 60 mg three times daily or 180 mg daily total. (The slight extra dosing to accommodate the pill size remains well below the 240 mg total goal).

Breakthrough dose = 10–15% of the 240 mg daily total dose range = 30 mg PO every 3 h as needed with the available 30 mg pill size.

## Pain: Opioid Toxicity

The common adverse effects of opiates are nausea, somnolence, delirium, rash, itching, constipation, and ataxia. Except for constipation, these are all usually more pronounced during the first 3 days and the patient can be advised to try to endure until the symptoms fade or disappear. In some patients, however, the side effect will continue past the first several days or be severe enough that the patient will require a change in agent or occasionally an additional drug to control the side effect. The differences between the drugs in metabolism and clearance usually allow patients to tolerate an alternative to the initial agent.

Constipation occurs with all opiate drugs and requires regular use of osmotic and stimulant laxatives; a bowel regimen should be started on a standing basis with all new opioid prescriptions [11]. Polyethylene glycol is a very effective single-daily-dose treatment, and senna and lactulose may be necessary additions for more difficult cases. Soluble fiber, especially prune juice, is more helpful for opioid constipation than non-soluble fiber (psyllium) which when combined with opiates can lead to very dense stool that is difficult to pass. New agents are available for opioid-induced constipation that target the specific mesenteric plexus effects of opioids; these include methylnaltrexone and lubiprostone and can be helpful in severe cases. Recent meta-analysis suggests that docusate (Colace) is no more effective than placebo for constipation [12].

The principal danger with exposure to opioids, particularly new prescriptions or dose increases, is drug-mediated suppression of the respiratory drive. Opioids inhibit the respiratory stimulant effects of both hypercarbia and hypoxia, allowing the patient to tolerate these non-physiologic conditions. Opioid-naive patients and those with additional contributors to somnolence—metabolic derangement, neurologic injury, or medications such as benzodiazepines or alcohol—are most at risk. It is important for physicians to monitor the level of consciousness, respiratory rate, and oxygenation in the patient with acute pain treated with new or escalating doses of opiates. The highest risk of respiratory suppression occurs with intravenous opiates when doses are "stacked" at frequency intervals less than the drug's time to peak effect. Capnography is a more sensitive and earlier warning for respiratory depression and is beginning to be used in monitoring of high-risk opiate situations in hospitals.

At very high doses of opiates, neuro-excitatory side effects of myoclonus and hyperesthesia emerge due to increasing activation of lower affinity opiate receptors. These unusual symptoms are intolerable and require reduction in total opioid dosing or rotation to a different opioid, often methadone, or both. Palliative care or anesthesia-pain consultation is helpful in these cases.

## Pain: Buprenorphine and Methadone

Two special opioids are important for their utility in chronic pain management, neuropathic pain, and opioid abstinence settings. Methadone is unique due to its long half-life, availability in liquid form, and additional antagonist action at the NMDA receptor; this last quality provides additional benefit in cases of neuropathic pain or in cases of hyperesthesia caused by other opioids at extreme doses. The liquid form is useful for patients with a feeding tube who need a long-acting opioid. Two unique risks with methadone are due to the long and variable half-life of up to 60 h causing delayed emergence of somnolence and respiratory depression, and potentially significant prolongation of QT interval requiring EKG monitoring and awareness of other medications that will compound this effect. Methadone used for pain management is usually dosed in two- or three-times-daily regimens and can be prescribed by all licensed physicians with a notation of "for chronic pain" or "for cancer-related pain" noted on the prescription. Consultation or review with a pain or palliative care specialist is recommended given the unique challenges in methadone use.

Patients on once-daily methadone maintenance for opioid dependence at an addiction treatment center can be given additional short-acting opioids for acute pain while continuing their methadone maintenance dose. Treatment centers will usually allow this with advanced notice from the prescriber. To avoid overdose, it is critically important to confirm the current dose and last administration of methadone with their maintenance program before continuing it in the inpatient setting.

Buprenorphine (suboxone) has both opioid agonist and antagonist properties, and it is increasingly used to treat opioid dependence. Buprenorphine reduces opioid craving and offers mild analgesic effects by its agonist effects while blocking further euphoric (and analgesic effects) of additional opioids, either illicit or prescribed. Buprenorphine is prescribed as a three-times-daily tablet or sublingual film and a newly released depot IM injection. The patient on maximal dose buprenorphine for abstinence treatment with increasing cancer pain must be switched to a traditional opioid for pain relief; assistance of a pain, addiction, or anesthesia-pain provider is usually necessary.

## Pain: Adjuvant Pain Medications

Additional medications and modalities are useful treatments that can lessen the overall opioid dose or add additional potency for neuropathic symptoms. Acetaminophen, NSAIDS, and corticosteroids can be extremely effective in the short term for inflammatory and bone pain if the agents are compatible with the patient's illness and other medications. Several anti-epileptic and antidepressant agents are effective alone or in combination for neuropathic pain. These symptoms are common with taxane- or platinum-based chemotherapy and respond well to agents such as gabapentin, pregabalin, amitriptyline, venlafaxine, or duloxetine. Bisphosphonates can help with pain and prevention of pathologic vertebral compression fractures from lytic bone lesions.

## Pain: Procedural Pain Interventions

Anesthesia-pain specialists can perform regional nerve blocks for cancer pain by infiltrating around a nerve or nerve root with local anesthetic (marcaine), steroid, and sometimes a nerve ablative agent such as ethanol or phenol. The ablative agent can extend the effect of the block for up to 3 months although the average duration of relief is 1 month. Common nerve blocks are at the celiac or hypogastric plexus for abdominal and pelvic pain, intercostal and paravertebral blocks for chest wall and abdominal wall pain, and trigeminal block for facial nerve symptoms. Pain blocks are relatively easy to perform under ultrasound or fluoroscopic guidance, they have few to no side effects, and they can offer significant and prolonged relief and allow decrease in opioid dosing.

## *Nausea*

Nausea is a very common symptom in most serious illnesses with several independent mechanisms and associated targets for treatment. Nausea is a disabling and discouraging symptom common in cancer patients that causes significant suffering from discomfort, inability to eat, weight loss, inactivity, isolation, and depressive symptoms. It is caused by several independent mechanisms and in cancer is associated with CNS disease, humoral agents released by tumor, infiltration or obstruction of GI organs, and common chemotherapeutic agents.

### Nausea Mechanism

There are four routes of nervous system input that stimulate nausea, all leading to the medullary vomiting center with afferent output to the stomach and diaphragm via the vagus nerve. The fourth ventricle's area postrema is termed the chemoreceptor trigger zone (CTZ)—many exogenous (and some endogenous) substances are antagonists here leading to nausea. This brain region is also sensitive to compression from obstruction, edema, or tumor and mediates the nausea caused by increased intracranial pressure. Vagus afferent signals originate from mechano- and chemoreceptors in the liver, stomach, peritoneum, and intestinal walls. Triggers include many cancer-related processes including vascular edema, excessive osmotic load, physical distension, compression from tumor or ascites, and specific toxins. Visual and motion-related nausea is transmitted from disordered vestibular and ophthalmic input or caused by impaired processing of these signals, and higher cortical stimuli trigger nausea from heightened anxiety states.

### Nausea Treatment

Strategies for nausea and vomiting treatment should be tailored to the operative mechanism (often more than one), shown in Table 13.3. Several agents may be necessary to control severe symptoms. Gastric and small-bowel decompression and drainage may be required for persistent vomiting from obstruction, related to gastric outlet or small-bowel obstruction common in gynecologic and gastrointestinal cancers. Maximal medical treatment with steroids and antisecretory agents can sometime allow removal of a nasogastric tube, but often a more permanent percutaneous drainage or surgical entero-enteral bypass is required to control vomiting.

**Table 13.3** Nausea mechanisms and medication strategies

| Nausea mechanism | Causes | Treatment strategy | Medication and receptor activation |
|---|---|---|---|
| Chemoreceptor trigger zone | Chemotherapeutic drugs, toxins, cytokines | Block CTZ activation<br>Remove causative external drug or decrease internal production | 5HT3—Ondansetron<br>NK-1—Aprepitant<br>D2-metoclopramide, chlorpromazine, haloperidol<br>Multiple HT and D plus others—olanzapine |
| GI injury, toxins, and inflammation - Vagus | Gastroparesis, bowel wall edema, distention, tumor, mucosal inflammation | Reduce distention and inflammation | 5HT3 and D2 agents above<br>ACH—scopolamine<br>Dexamethasone for inflammation and malignant obstruction |
| Hepatic insufficiency and biliary obstruction - Vagus | Loss of functioning liver due to tumor or cirrhosis, biliary obstruction, hepatic congestion | Reduce liver inflammation or ongoing injury, improve biliary drainage, reduce venous pressure | Corticosteroids<br>D2-haloperidol, multiple HT and D plus others—olanzapine |
| Vestibular dysfunction, higher CNS lesions | Tumor invasion, drug or radiation toxicity | Reduce vestibular sensitivity, reduce swelling and inflammation | ACH—scopolamine<br>Histamine—meclizine<br>Dexamethasone |
| Higher cortical—anxiety, fear, conditioning | Anxiety, fear, emotional upset | Pharmacologic and behavioral strategies | Lorazepam<br>Olanzapine<br>Relaxation<br>Behavioral techniques |

## *Dyspnea*

Dyspnea is the distressing sensation of tightness in the chest, air hunger, and suffocation with attendant extreme anxiety and fear of dying. Cancer leads to dyspnea through cardiac, pulmonary, neurologic, and metabolic derangements and is a common symptom in late-stage disease accompanying pain, anemia, and cachexia. Recognizing the pathophysiology of dyspnea is the essential first step to guide treatment [13], and most of the physiologic causes can be improved with medications and procedures (listed in Table 13.4) resulting in reduced dyspnea. Careful medical evaluation is essential to allow these effective treatments.

Oxygen is an immediately available tool for relief of dyspnea related to hypoxia, and it can be administered continuously in home settings; it is not helpful when oxygenation is normal beyond the mild sensation of positive airway pressure it provides. More helpful for normal oxygenation is a fan directed at the face to reduce dyspnea; this strategy is helpful at any level of oxygenation. Opioids reduce dyspnea by dampening the brain's sensitivity to mechanoreceptors in the lungs and chest, and chemoreceptors in the carotid bodies and brain, allowing the brain's

**Table 13.4** Common dyspnea mechanisms and associated disease processes

| Mechanism | Pathophysiology | Clinical setting |
|---|---|---|
| Increased respiratory drive | Metabolic disturbance, respiratory insufficiency | Hypoxia, hypoxemia, acidemia, low cardiac output |
| | Increased cardiac filling pressures | CHF, aortic stenosis, pericardial effusion |
| | Loss of lung volume | Effusion, tumor, surgery, COPD |
| | Inadequate perfusion | Anemia, CHF, COPD |
| | Psychiatric symptom overlap | Anxiety, panic |
| Decreased ventilation | Neuromuscular compromise | Spinal cord injury, ALS |
| | Chest wall and diaphragm dysfunction | Tumor infiltration, pleural effusion |
| | Bronchial constriction/obstruction | Tumor infiltration, radiation effects, COPD |
| | Fibrosis | Radiation effects, chemotherapy, idiopathic pulmonary fibrosis |

respiratory center to tolerate both hypoxia and hypercarbia without increasing respiratory drive. Opiates also relax pulmonary vasculature, further reducing mechanoreceptor stimulation and increasing pulmonary perfusion. These multiple effects of opioids are essential in allowing the patient to tolerate acute and chronic respiratory insufficiency with comfort. Coupled with oxygen, patient's exertional capacity can often be increased enough to make a meaningful difference in their activity level. A low dose of opioid—morphine 0.5 mg IV, or 5 mg of oral morphine elixir every 3 h as needed—may be all that is required to improve dyspnea.

It is essential to prepare patients and families for the consequences of increasing use of opioids to tolerate dyspnea in patients with marginal respiratory function; decreasing respiration and ventilation will lead to respiratory failure, intubation, or death. Appropriate advanced directives should be in place. Benzodiazepines are a useful adjunct to reduce the extreme anxiety caused by dyspnea; these agents will compound sedation and slowed respiratory drive.

## *Anorexia*

Anorexia, a diminished appetite and aversion to food, is frequently attributed to nausea alone; however, once nausea is controlled, anorexia may remain and require additional interventions aimed at counteracting the effects of tumor cytokines, altered GI functioning, and cancer-therapy drugs and radiation. Anti-anorectic agents cannot reverse the dramatic catabolism and profound aversion to food in aggressive malignancies like pancreatic cancer. Expectations for "reversal" of weight loss or "return" of appetite should be discussed to set realistic expectations; appetite and dysgeusia can be improved to a much greater extent than weight loss. Corticosteroids offer an immediate but time-limited boost in appetite and ability to tolerate food, but difficult side effects occur both acutely and with longer use. More sustainable long-term agents include megestrol acetate which works by altering metabolic balance and increased fat production, and dronabinol and mirtazapine which work by improving the sensations of taste, smell, and interest in food. All three can lead to weight gain, but with some risks and side effects; megestrol carries an increased risk of deep vein thrombosis and may be incompatible with other hormonal therapies. Dronabinol causes dysphoria and drowsiness, while mirtazapine can cause confusion and somnolence in the elderly. Anxiety and depression can independently cause both nausea and anorexia; these symptoms can improve with targeted psychiatric agents.

### *Fatigue*

Reduced endurance for physical activity and cognitive functions of memory, problem solving, concentration, and mood stability are features of cancer-related fatigue. This is a ubiquitous symptom in advanced disease causing isolation, loss of autonomy, and depression when patients become unable to complete their activities of daily living, homebound, or even bedbound. Multiple pathways including cachexia, reduced fluid intake, fatigue, nausea, depression, insomnia, overall tumor burden, and many others leave patients without enough energy to maintain their age-appropriate activity. Effective interventions target the underlying pathophysiology—nutrition, chemotherapy, and normalizing impaired organ functioning—and are the only measures that can bring long-term relief for profound fatigue [14]. Evidence for fatigue symptom relief in cancer supports gentle regular exercise which results in improved perfusion, increased appetite, and endorphin production; promotes a sense of “well-being”; and lessens the sense of “inertia” that ill patients commonly have. Psychostimulants have not shown efficacy in fatigue although they are specifically helpful for opiated-related somnolence and poor concentration.

## Ambulatory Palliative Care

Ambulatory palliative care is a thriving new frontier in palliative medicine that has tremendous promise in improving quality of life for our patients as well as increasing goal concordance, reducing unnecessary and ineffective care, and possibly extending survival. As compared to the long-established inpatient hospital palliative service, ambulatory palliative practice presents the opportunity to develop long-term relationships with patients and to support their coping with illness through all phases [15]. In this setting, there are long periods of stability between episodes of acute illness, and the focus of the visits turns to healthy coping and living well with illness. Particularly in cancer, where patients have frequent visits to their cancer center and access to palliative care providers, ambulatory palliative care is an ideal opportunity to address difficult issues of coping with illness, understanding prognosis, planning for the future, and managing complex symptoms. In the following sections, we present the work of ambulatory palliative care with a focus on cancer patients; first we describe recent work defining the interventions and effects of palliative practice, followed by essential provider skills and knowledge related to communication, coping, and understanding.

A landmark paper by Temel et al., 2010 [16], demonstrated that patients with lung cancer referred early to a palliative care provider, and having an average of 4-monthly palliative care visits before death, showed the anticipated improvements in quality of life and depression scores over the course of their care. A surprise was a statistically significant accompanying survival advantage over patients treated with "usual care," 11.6 months instead of 8.9 months. "Early" in this study meant the point of diagnosis of metastatic non-small cell lung cancer, already an advanced state of disease with a prognosis of less than 1 year. Despite its limitations—single institution, single diagnosis, 151 total patients—the randomized controlled methodology and dramatic results galvanized an effort in palliative care and oncology to explore a somewhat automatic or "triggered" referral process to palliative care for ongoing visits focused on symptom management and improved understanding and coping with illness. The true innovation here is the change from the usual symptom-based referral to a disease stage- or prognosis-based reason for referral. Patients, families, medical societies, advocacy groups, and society at large have taken notice of these results, and the field has focused on creating and studying systems for earlier palliative care interventions, and on delineating the effective processes and methods of ambulatory palliative care practice.

At least nine subsequent studies published between 2012 and 2016 generally confirm the hypothesis that early, intentional, and focused palliative care intervention for patients with cancer results in improved quality of life [17]. The American Society of Clinical Oncology has reviewed these works for evidence of benefit, primarily in improved quality of life and psychological distress scores, and describes the conclusions as evidence based, of moderate quality, and strong in strength [17]. Known limitations are the high prevalence of advanced cancers and solid tumors over hematological malignancies in study populations, the need to define the appropriate starting point or "trigger" to invite palliative care, and the wide variety of interventions studied without information on which specific palliative actions are beneficial. Conclusions from the review have led to the society's position that "Inpatients and outpatients with advanced cancer should receive dedicated palliative care services, early in the disease course, concurrent with active treatment. Referral of patients to interdisciplinary palliative care teams is optimal, and services may complement existing programs. Providers may refer family and friend caregivers of patients with early or advanced cancer to palliative care services."

Two studies included above deserve special mention for the unique interventions applied. Bakitas [18] studied an implementation of the ENABLE intervention [19], an advanced-practice nurse-led project based on the chronic care model used in case management; this entailed an educational approach to encourage patient activation, self-management, and empowerment. Program nurses led four initial in-person group sessions for patients followed by available telephone support, an education manual, and monthly phone "check-ins." Overall distress was measured during phone contact using the National Comprehensive Cancer Network's "Distress Thermometer" tool [20] and patients were guided by the nurse practitioner in a problem-solving approach using an assigned module from their education manual [21]. Zimmerman [22] created a seamless program of palliative care support for cancer patients using defined assessment tools, regular phone follow-up, and a uniform multidisciplinary approach delivered by inpatient, outpatient, and home care teams that addressed physical, psychosocial, social, and spiritual needs. The finely integrated care in this Canadian study demonstrates an aspirational goal possible in a large single-payer program with a common medical record.

There are more than 20 studies in the surgical literature since 1998 reporting interventions aimed at improving various combinations of symptom management, end-of-life communication, and patient decision-making; results are quite heterogeneous regarding selection of surgical disease, palliative interventions applied, and methodologic quality. The approaches used were unique to surgical settings—one-third involved interventions applied to patients and families in the intensive care unit, and the remaining majority applied to interventions applied before and immediately after a surgical procedure. A systemic review describes this current evidence for effectiveness as "sparse" and calls for increased rigor and standardization in the study of palliative care in surgery [23]. The applicability of the longer term medical studies cited earlier is not difficult to accept for surgical patients, particularly in cancer where the disease span is much longer than a single hospitalization or procedure, and care is shared by surgeons, radiation oncologists, medical oncologists, and palliative care providers.

The impressive quality of life gains in the cited studies raise the question of which palliative care practices generate these results. The answer is not known precisely, but many common elements are illustrated in a follow-up analysis [24] of the content of palliative care visits in the 2010 lung cancer study. Records from the visits reveal a defined series of tasks and a usual progression that coincides with disease advancement. There is significant overlap in some of these tasks between the palliative and the medical oncology provider visits; others were "owned" primarily by one or the other. Initial visits began with relationship and rapport building between provider, patient, and family, and then a discussion of the illness, eliciting the patient's preferences for receiving information, a review of current prognostic awareness, and information sharing about the effects of cancer treatment. All visits included assessment and management of symptoms and current coping issues; illness status was reviewed each time, and outreach and engagement of family members were promoted. Final visits focused on decision-making about available cancer treatments and planning for end-of-life caregiving and logistics. The exact trajectory of symptoms, coping, and awareness over time through the progression of illness is unique to the individual but there themes are common enough for the provider to anticipate and prepare the patient for coming challenges and "shepherd" him or her through when they arrive.

**Table 13.5** Conversation supporting adaptive coping [15]

| |
|---|
| • Developing rapport with basic communication techniques of sitting down, asking open-ended questions, listening carefully, and taking time to learn about the patient's life beyond illness |
| • Reassessing the patient's entire spectrum of needs, not just the clinical, on every visit |
| • Anchoring the discussion around the patient's hopes and worries. Titrating discussion according to the patient's coping helps ensure that he or she is not overwhelmed by information |

Originally published in Mary Ann Liebert, Inc., Jacobsen J, Kvale E, Rabow M, Rinaldi S, Cohen S, Weissman, D, Jackson V. Helping Patients with Serious Illness Live Well through the Promotion of Adaptive Coping: A Report from the Improving Outpatient Palliative Care (IPAL-OP) Initiative. J Palliat Med. 2014;17(4):463–468

As we highlighted in the symptom management section, the importance of addressing symptoms (seen above as a component of all visits) cannot be underestimated. Patients' cognition is distracted and diminished by active symptoms, and their thoughts are gloomy and frightening. It is essential to improve symptoms through expert attention and intervention to allow the relationship and communication to develop with the palliative provider and grow to include prognostic understanding and coping (Table 13.5).

When symptoms are controlled, attention turns to promoting the patient's adaptive coping with illness. Conversation at each visit follows three themes as outlined below [15]. This work is part of a larger effort from CAPC [1], the Center to Advance Palliative Care, which includes white papers, courses, and materials to promote the practice of ambulatory palliative care.

Adaptive (or constructive) coping is a term from psychology meaning the conscious process of solving personal and interpersonal problems to reduce psychological stress [25]. Translating to palliative care, adaptive coping is a collection of strategies and skills to cope with the stress of illness. The palliative provider can develop these important traits by discussing specific strategies and counseling the patient on how and when to use them to overcome stress and psychological suffering. Identifying and supporting coping strategies such as distraction, optimism, meditation, and intellectualization, among others, provide the patient with tools that allow them to tolerate unpleasant affect, discouraging thoughts, unwelcome news, and uncertainty about the future [15]. The "difficult conversation" becomes a process over time with much less of the urgency and ultimatums of inpatient crises; the ambulatory relationship provides the opportunity for evolving coping skills in a measured and comfortable way.

Palliative care providers consider prognostic awareness to be a unique and profound understanding of the intersection of disease and the future [26]; such awareness for patients requires cultivation over time with repeated adjustments and reinforcement. In this technique, prognosis is broken into manageable pieces that allow for slow assimilation despite the normal swings and variability in the patient and family's optimism and strength. The abstract and unreal vagary of what is ahead can yield to a much clearer and confident approach when the patient can safely explore the meanings and uncertainties of their future in limited episodes of intense communication, separated by time at home to reflect and filter in solitude and with their loved ones. The work of cultivating prognostic awareness is described in a stepwise process that is accessible to palliative providers, generalists, and specialists in any field (Table 13.6).

As you can see, this approach is a dissection of components of prognosis and a careful assessment of when to deliver difficult news—particularly the challenging step that physicians sometime face, when the patient is going to be surprised and shocked by prognostic information or when he or she must assimilate it quickly for clinical decision-making; this situation is summarized as "naming the dilemma" [26]. The palliative care provider fosters trust and develops the awareness and implications of prognosis for the patient and family—this is not in conflict with the oncologist or other disease specialists, but a specific use of prognosis to craft the "what does this mean for me" understanding that is so important to patient agency and quality of life. A specific technique in bridging this divide is to provide a "dual framework" where a patient can talk about living well AND tolerate the possibility of dying [27]. Appealing to metacognition, the patient can "talk about talking about it" and learn safe ways to contain fear and speculation about worsening disease and death while living well and feeling optimistic.

A growing challenge in presenting cancer prognosis is the impact of immune and genetically targeted therapies such as pembrolizumab (Keytruda) in melanoma and lung cancer and trastuzumab (Herceptin) in breast cancer [28]. Subsets of patients with cancers showing specific genetic features may be eligible for FDA-approved or clinical trial therapies that have the potential to extend prognosis. A minority of these patients will have astounding results: near or complete eradication of disease without serious toxicity, or an extended period of reduced symptoms and disease regression. There are difficult dilemmas faced in these situations regarding repeat tissue sampling, eligibility and payment for therapy, severe complications, and therapy failure, and much is unknown about the duration of disease control, susceptibil-

**Table 13.6** Cultivating prognostic awareness [26]

| |
|---|
| **Step 0:** Prepare—both provider and patient |
| **Step 1:** Assess the patient's prognostic awareness—"what is your sense of how you are doing?" |
| **Step 2:** Inquire whether the patient can imagine a poorer health state. "What would it be like if you got sicker?" |
| **Step 3:** Judge patient readiness and clinical urgency: "Do I need to discuss prognosis now?" |
| **3a:** For a patient who demonstrates readiness (regardless of clinical status): Indicate that you will discuss the information |
| **3b**: For a patient who is ambivalent or resistant and clinically stable: Hold off on giving the information and reassess |
| **3c:** For a patient who is ambivalent or resistant and clinically declining: "Name the dilemma." |
| **Step 4:** Deliver prognostic information tailored to patient readiness and clinical urgency |
| **4a:** For the patient who demonstrates a degree of readiness |
| **4b:** For a patent who is ambivalent or resistant and clinically declining |

Originally published in Mary Ann Liebert, Inc., Jackson VA, Jacobsen J, Greer JA, Pirl WF, Temel JS, Back AL. The Cultivation of Prognostic Awareness Through the Provision of Early Palliative Care in the Ambulatory Setting: A Communication Guide. J Palliat Med. 2013;16(8):894–900

ity to adverse effects, and major long-term adverse effects. Patients, palliative care providers, and oncologists are appropriately hopeful for meaningful response to treatment in late-stage disease; for palliative care providers, a new degree of prognostic uncertainty is introduced which can complicate and delay prognostic awareness and planning for the future.

Prognostic misunderstanding is a common problem that many providers and patients face. Studies show that both groups overestimate prognosis and survival, with patients often not hearing that their disease is incurable even when this is stated directly at earlier visits. There is science to unpacking these situations [29]: a lengthy differential diagnosis for the cause of misunderstanding, and a pendulum-like variation in the patient's perspective ranging from frankly unrealistic to morbidly dire. Solutions include effective communication between providers to reduce ambiguity or conflict in the delivered messages and a consistent coordinated approach to reinforce appropriate understanding through different emotional states, care settings, symptom burdens, and new developments. The collaboration achieved and the visible positive effects on the patient and family's distress are remarkably effective and represent gratifying moments in the care of cancer patients.

Palliative care adds a partner or even a team for the medical oncologist or surgeon to provide several styles of approach to promote patient and family engagement with prognosis; there are differing and complementary answers for questions of "how long will I survive," "what will my death look like," "what will cause me distress and discomfort at the end," and "how will I cope with everything that is going to happen." By providing a guide, confidence, and essential language and structure, the palliative care provider and ambulatory visit sequence allow for a comprehensive, nuanced, and evolving adaptation to these difficult essential questions.

## Communication

Expert communication between patients is a necessary requirement for developing the adaptive coping that leads to enhanced satisfaction and disease outcomes. Such communication is often stressful for everybody, patient, family, and provider, and there is a risk of delay or avoidance altogether due to this difficulty and providers' lack of knowledge and experience. Specific skills are available to allow effective communication, and they can be learned through study, reflection, and practice; three essential techniques are presented here.

### *Ask-Tell-Ask*

The Ask-Tell-Ask sequence [30] is helpful to present new information by building on what the patient already knows about their illness. Ask-Tell-Ask allows the provider to remain aware of the patient's current and evolving understanding, and it guides where to go next in the conversation and when the patient is reaching their fill. Ask-Tell-Ask can be applied to the large topic of prognosis and survival or to a focused event such as the interpretation of a scan. Examples of the Ask-Tell-Ask sequence are illustrated below (Example 13.3).

**Example 13.3** Ask-Tell-Ask

Ask—"What have you heard most recently about what is going on with your illness?"
Tell—"Results from the current scan show your cancer has progressed despite treatment."
Ask—"What is going through your mind right now?"

## *Expanding the Conversation*

Like the second step in the Ask-Tell-Ask sequence, it is necessary to listen to the patient for clues about what is the best next step for conversation. Providers often cannot gauge what is most important to him or her at that moment; it is easy to be swayed by what we as the provider or other contributors think is the primary immediate issue. Short open-ended questions allow the patient to control the direction of the conversation, and they reveal the patient's present state of thinking. Allowing silence after the question, without interruption or clarification by the provider, is very helpful to give patients a feeling of comfort and control. The response following silence often is very rich with meaning and emotion. Common examples are the following:

"How do you feel about what we have discussed today?"
"What are your thoughts about getting through the next few months?"
"How are you coping with your cancer these days?"

## *Surgical Communication Checklist*

An emerging template or "checklist" approach to patient-provider communication involves the Serious Illness Care Project [31], and its recent application to emergency surgical conditions [32]. This technique is tailored to the needs of the surgeon when a critical decision must be made with patient and family under time pressure with significant ramifications for ultimate quality of life and goal-concordant care. The checklist approach provides uniformity and completeness in critical communication and improves the overall quality of information sharing and decision-making (Table 13.7). The authors eloquently reduce the aims and approach to communication and then go on to provide a stepwise progression of the conversation and sample language. Educational offerings and materials specifically for surgeon communication using this paradigm are under development by this research group.

**Table 13.7** Goals of a structured surgical communication framework [32]

| |
|---|
| • Place the patient's acute surgical condition in the context of the patient's underlying illness |
| • Elicit the patient's goals, priorities, and what is acceptable to the patient regarding life-prolonging and comfort-focused care |
| • Describe treatment options—including palliative approaches—in the context of the patient's goals and priorities |
| • Direct treatment to achieve these outcomes and encourage the use of time-limited trials in circumstances of clinical uncertainty |
| • Affirm continued commitment to patient's care |



## *Responding to Emotion*

Strong emotions are natural and should be expected when discussing difficult topics like prognosis or planning for a future with progressing illness. For the provider, strong emotion is challenging and anxiety provoking, but can become easier and more effective with techniques to help the patient feel understood and to allow them to progress the conversation onwards. Illustrated in Table 13.8 is the NURSE model [33], describing a stepwise progression of response to emotion. These can be used in sequence or, for the more experienced provider, individually to provide options for demonstrating empathy and advancing the conversation.

## *Goals-of-Care Discussion*

A goals-of-care discussion is a specific kind of provider-patient conversation that serves several critical functions: clarifying the patient's goals and wishes for the future, demonstrating provider understanding and alignment with the patient's values, and preparing for goal-concordant caregiving. The goals-of-care approach can apply to all important care decisions, and it is not limited to provider-patient-family conflicts or specific resuscitation or POLST issues (physician order for life-sustaining treatment). The goals-of-care style fits every important decision, and it is very important early in the disease course to elicit and define values and demonstrate respect, interest, and alignment. In the ideal situation, discussion takes place between the patient and their trusted long-term provider; themes and choices are captured in the common medical record for others to follow and expand in subsequent hospital or specialist encounters. Organizing these discussions is facilitated by a "talking map" or mental model to increase the consistency and timeliness of the conversation. The REMAP model [33] is illustrated here in Table 13.9.

**Table 13.8** NURSE model of responding to emotion [33]

| | | |
|---|---|---|
| N | Name | Naming a patient's emotion notes what is happening in the encounter, shows the patient that you are attuned to what she is experiencing, and may help the patient herself gain more insight into the situation. For example, "It sounds like you are worried that the cancer may be recurring." To name an emotion may require that physicians read nonverbal clues that patients display. It is important that when using naming, the physician is suggestive, not declarative. "I wonder if you're feeling angry," or "Some people in this situation would be angry," rather than "I can see you're angry about this." People don't like being told what they are feeling |
| U | Understand | The most effective empathic statements link the "I" of the doctor to the "you" of the patient: "I sense how upset you are feeling about the results of the CT scan." It is not necessary to have had the experience to empathize; but it is necessary to put yourself in the patient's position and to communicate that understanding back to the patient. A sensitive appreciation of the patient's predicament or feelings is an important prerequisite for responding in a way that builds the relationship. By making an "understand" statement the physician is telling the patient that they "get" what they are going through and they are aligned with them. This can be very simple such as "It must be hard as you think about the effect your chemotherapy has had on your kids," and serves to validate patient emotions. Paradoxically, saying "I cannot imagine what it is like to (X)" is a good way to show you understand |
| R | Respect | This can be a nonverbal response, involving facial expression, touch, or change in posture, but a verbal response is helpful because it can be more explicit in giving patients the message that their emotions are not only allowable but also important. Acknowledging and respecting a patient's emotions is an important step in showing empathy. In terms of how much to do on this step, consider matching the intensity of your acknowledgment to the patient's expression of emotion—a strong emotion deserves a strong acknowledgment. Praising the person's coping skills is a good way to show respect. "I am very impressed with how well you've cared for your mother during this long illness. You have been a godsend for her." This really makes people feel good about themselves and implies respect |
| S | Support | Several types of supporting statements are possible. Physicians can express concern, articulate their understanding of a patient's situation, express willingness to help, make statements about partnership, and most importantly acknowledge the patient's efforts to cope. Given that many dying patients fear abandonment, making statements—if truthful—that you will be there for the patient is very useful, e.g., "I'll be with you during this illness, no matter what happens." |
| E | Explore | Distressed patients frequently do not share their emotions or what they are thinking directly or clearly. In these situations, the simple statement, "Tell me more," can be extremely effective to open people up more and help them articulate what was, at first, hard to say |

Used with permission from VitalTalk, http://vitaltalk.org/guides/transitionsgoals-of-care/

**Table 13.9** REMAP model for goals-of-care discussion [33]

| | |
|---|---|
| Reframe why the status quo isn't working. | You may need to discuss serious news (e.g., a scan results) first. "Given this news, it seems like a good time to talk about what to do now." "We're in a different place." |
| Expect emotion and empathize. | Use one of the NURSE statements: "It's hard to deal with all this." "I can see you are really concerned about [x]." "Tell me more about that—what are you worried about?" "Is it ok for us to talk about what this means?" |
| Map out the future. | "Given this situation, what's most important for you?" "When you think about the future, are there things you want to do?" "As you think towards the future, what concerns you?" |
| Align with the patient's values. | "As I listen to you, it sounds the most important things are [x, y, z]." |
| Plan medical treatments that match patient values. | "Here's what I can do now that will help you do those important things. What do you think about it?" |

Used with permission from VitalTalk, http://vitaltalk.org/guides/transitionsgoals-of-care/

## *Best Case–Worst Case Scenario in Surgical Communication*

A very useful technique in surgical decision-making with high-risk procedures is the best case–worst case formulation [34], a technique that helps the surgeon, patient, and family go beyond the often-scant numerical data and tie the operative risks to the patient's overall condition and future goals. The surgeon presents surgery and no surgery as two available strategies instead of surgery as the "dominant plan with a secondary alternative" of avoiding surgery. He or she then describes the best and worst outcome of each strategy. The surgeon can provide rich detail of the alternatives from personal experience and use clinical judgment regarding the patient's condition and available data to estimate what is most likely to occur with each strategy (Example 13.4).

**Example 13.4** Best Case–Worst Case in Surgery

A 49-year-old woman has been treated for cervical cancer with chemotherapy and radiation brachytherapy. She has no detectable active disease, but her treatment has resulted in cachexia; incontinence; fistulas between bladder, vagina, and rectum; and chronic infection requiring IV antibiotics and tube drainage. She is unable to leave the hospital because of the complex infection care and total parenteral nutrition. At the patient's and family's request, the surgical oncologist describes a pelvic exenteration as a risky but potentially curative procedure. Best case–worst case presentation of this option might be as follows:

**Surgery—Best Case:** With surgery, your infections would resolve and you can leave the hospital for a rehabilitation center in 1 week, and then return home 2 weeks later without TPN. After 2 months of physical therapy and nutrition, you could eat normally and maintain your weight, and you will be able to drive, walk limited distances at a slowed pace, and tolerate sedentary work on a part-time basis. You would have to manage a urostomy and colostomy indefinitely. You may be able to have further surgery to allow sexual intercourse although it will probably always entail some discomfort.

**Surgery—Likely Outcome:** You will have a rocky 2 weeks after the surgery with increased pain and further drainage procedures required. Ultimately, you can move to a rehabilitation center, but wound care, poor nutrition, and recurrent infections will result in a life lived at rehab with monthly hospitalizations. There will be ongoing pain and very limited mobility and endurance with most of your time spent in bed. Ultimately, an infection will become so severe that we will not be able to control it, and you may die (comfortably) at the rehab or in the hospital within the next 1–2 years.

**Surgery—Worst Case:** The surgery will be initially successful, but will then fail resulting in continued fistulas, infections, incontinence, ongoing dependence on TPN, and more severe pain and increased somnolence from opiates. Similar to your current situation, you will not be able to survive outside of the hospital and you will ultimately die from overwhelming infection in the next few months.

**No Surgery—Best Case:** We will simplify your infectious drainage and antibiotic regimen to allow your return home with hospice care, initially including continued total parenteral nutrition. You will be comfortable and able to ambulate short distances inside initially. Over the next 3 weeks you will become progressively weaker and bed bound, and develop worsening infection. We will stop TPN and increase pain medication, leading to a more rapid decline with increasing drowsiness and coma and death at home 4 to 6 weeks from now. You will have continuous incontinence of urine and stool that can be managed effectively with frequent scheduled changes of diapers and bedding.

**No Surgery—Likely Outcome:** We will stabilize your symptoms for discharge to rehab or home, but your requirements for pain medication and worsening nutrition and hydration status will result in progressing drowsiness, confusion, and unresponsiveness. You will likely die comfortably at rehab or home in the next 10 days.

**No Surgery—Worst Case:** You will continue your current care in the hospital with antibiotics, tube drainage, incontinence, and TPN. Ultimately, an overwhelming infection will result in organ failure and death, likely sometime in the next few months.

This is a heartbreaking case with little chance for a durable and functional recovery, and the presentation here is artificially abbreviated and limited to text. However, the approach presenting the limits of what is possible gives patients and families the ability to contextualize the range of outcomes instead of facing a stark and polarized surgery vs. no surgery fork. This is not a brief conversation, and likely not a single conversation either. The surgeon is unlikely to be able to supervise and orchestrate the care that each outcome requires, but medical oncology, palliative care, and hospice providers will provide much of the downstream attention. This conversation and decision-making process goes well beyond traditional procedural consent and places the surgeon in a central role in negotiating the goal-concordant care that every patient desires.

The communication techniques presented here allow the provider to develop their skills through experimentation with new language and structure for conversations. More formal training through live coursework is readily available and a very enjoyable experiential learning activity in contrast to our usual didactic learning practices. The importance of refining our communication about prognosis, coping with illness, and end of life cannot be overestimated. With practice and new techniques, all providers can significantly improve both their patient's experience of care and their quality of life through illness. We encourage readers to explore the reference material and develop their skills.

## Summary

This chapter has been a tour of the role and methods of ambulatory palliative care. Through effective symptom management, high-quality communication, and cultivation of prognostic awareness and adaptive coping, palliative care offers hope that the experience of illness can be comfortable, peaceful, and meaningful in physical, spiritual, and emotional realms. Although secondary, the significant societal benefits of reduced intensity of medical intervention at the end of life are increasingly important in the efficiency of our healthcare system. Improving this process is the aim of palliative care, particularly the primary palliative work done by surgeons and providers in all capacities. The opportunity for spiritual and emotional growth during illness and at the end of life is possible with attentive, effective, and available palliative care. This essential role of the healer, as provider of comfort and trusted advisor, is a profoundly important and deeply satisfying bulwark of medical practice.

## References

1. https://www.capc.org/about/palliative-care/. Accessed 8 Apr 2016.
2. Quill TE, Abernethy AP. Generalist plus specialist palliative care--creating a more sustainable model. N Engl J Med. 2013;368(13):1173–5.
3. Abrahm J. A physician's guide to pain and symptom management in cancer patients. 3rd ed. Baltimore: Johns Hopkins University Press; 2014.
4. Hanks GW, Cherny NI, Christakis NA, Fallon M, Kaasa S, Portenoy RK. Oxford textbook of palliative care. 5th ed. New York: Oxford University Press; 2015.
5. Kematick BS, Phantomvanit V, Lynch M, Rickerson E, Zhang M, Nabati L, et al. Pain management tables and guidelines. Boston: Dana-Farber Cancer Institute and Brigham and Women's Hospital; 2016. http://pinkbook.dfci.org/. accessed 2 Jun 2017
6. Portenoy RK, Ahmed E. Principles of opioid use in cancer pain. J Clin Oncol. 2014;32(16):1662–70.
7. Webster LR, Webster RM. Predicting aberrant behaviors in opioid-treated patients: preliminary validation of the opioid risk tool. Pain Med. 2005;6(6):432–42.
8. Butler SF, Fernandez K, Benoit C, Budman SH, Jamison RN. Validation of the revised Screener and Opioid Assessment for Patients with Pain (SOAPP-R). J Pain Symptom Management. 2008;9(4):360–72.

9. Dowell D, Haegerich TM, Chou R. CDC guideline for prescribing opioids for chronic pain — United States, 2016. MMWR Recommendations and Reports. 2016;65(1):1–49.
10. ASCO policy statement on opioid therapy: protecting access to treatment for cancer-related pain. http://www.asco.org/sites/new-www.asco.org/files/2016-ASCO-Policy-Statement-Opioid-Therapy.pdf. Accessed 2 Jun 2018.
11. Ahmedzai SH, Boland J. Constipation in people prescribed opioids. Clin Evidence. 2010. http://www.ncbi.nlm.nih.gov/pmc/articles/PMC2907601/pdf/2010-2407.pdf. Accessed 22 May 2017.
12. Ruston T, Hunter K, Cummings G, Lazarescu A. Efficacy and side-effect profiles of lactulose, docusate sodium, and sennosides compared to PEG in opioid-induced constipation: a systematic review. Can Oncol Nurs. 2013;23(4):236–46.
13. Parshall MB, Schwartzstein RM, Adams L, Banzett RB, Manning HL, Bourbeau J, American Thoracic Society Committee on Dyspnea, et al. An official American Thoracic Society statement: update on the mechanisms, assessment, and management of dyspnea. Am J Respir Crit Care Med. 2012;185(4):435–52.
14. Yennurajalingam S, Bruera E. Palliative management of fatigue at the close of life: "it feels like my body is just worn out". JAMA. 2007;297(3):295–304.
15. Jacobsen J, Kvale E, Rabow M, Rinaldi S, Cohen S, Weissman D, Jackson V. Helping patients with serious illness live well through the promotion of adaptive coping: a report from the improving outpatient palliative care (IPAL-OP) initiative. J Palliat Med. 2014;17(4):463–8.
16. Temel JS, Greer JA, Muzikansky A, Gallagher ER, Admane S, Jackson VA, et al. Early palliative care for patients with metastatic non-small-cell lung cancer. N Engl J Med. 2010;363(8):733–42.
17. Ferrell BR, Temel JS, Temin S, Alesi ER, Balboni TA, Basch EM, et al. Integration of palliative care into standard oncology care: American Society of Clinical Oncology clinical practice guideline update. J Clin Oncol. 2017;35(1):96–112.
18. Bakitas MA, Tosteson TD, Li Z, et al. Early versus delayed initiation of concurrent palliative oncology care: patient outcomes in the ENABLE III randomized controlled trial. J Clin Oncol. 2015;33(13):1438–45.
19. Bakitas M, Lyons K, Hegel M, et al. Project ENABLE II randomized controlled trial to improve palliative care for rural patients with advanced cancer: baseline findings, methodological challenges, and solutions. Palliat Support Care. 2009;7(1):75–86.
20. https://www.nccn.org/patients/resources/life_with_cancer/pdf/nccn_distress_thermometer.pdf. Accessed 22 May 2017.
21. https://rtips.cancer.gov/rtips/viewProduct.do?viewMode=product&productId=22742367. Accessed 22 May 2017.
22. Zimmermann C, Swami N, Krzyzanowska M, et al. Early palliative care for patients with advanced cancer: a cluster-randomized controlled trial. Lancet. 2014;383:1721–30.
23. Lilley EJ, Khan KT, Johnston FM, Berlin A, Bader AM, Mosenthal AC, Cooper Z. Palliative care interventions for surgical patients: a systematic review. JAMA Surg. 2016;151(2):172–83.
24. Yoong J, Park ER, Greer JA, Jackson VA, Gallagher ER, Pirl WF, et al. Early palliative care in advanced lung cancer: a qualitative study. JAMA Intern Med. 2013;173(4):283–29.
25. Lazarus R. Fifty years of the research and theory of R.S. Lazarus: an analysis of historical and perennial issues. Hove: Psychology Press; 2013. p. 185–8.
26. Jackson VA, Jacobsen J, Greer JA, Pirl WF, Temel JS, Back AL. The cultivation of prognostic awareness through the provision of early palliative care in the ambulatory setting: a communication guide. J Palliat Med. 2013;16(8):894–900.
27. Jacobsen J, Brenner K, Greer J, Jacobo M, Rosenberg L, Nipp R, Jackson V, When a patient just can't talk about it: a dual framework to focus on living and tolerate the possibility of dying. J Palliat Med. 2017.
28. Johnson BE. Divide and conquer to treat lung cancer. N Engl J Med. 2016;375:1892–3.
29. Jacobsen J, Thomas JD, Jackson VA. Misunderstandings about prognosis: an approach for palliative care consultants when the patient does not seem to understand what was said. J Palliat Med. 2013;16(1):91–5.

30. Back AL, Arnold RM, Baile WF, Tulsky JA, Fryer-Edwards K. Approaching difficult communication tasks in oncology. CA Cancer J Clin. 2005;55(3):164–77.
31. Bernacki RE, Block SD. Communication about serious illness care goals: a review and synthesis of best practices. JAMA Intern Med. 2014;174(12):1994–2003.
32. Cooper Z, Koritsanszky L, Cauley C, Frydman JL, Bernacki RE, Mosenthal AC, et al. Recommendations for best communication practices to facilitate goal-concordant care for seriously ill older patients with emergency surgical conditions. Ann Surg. 2016;263(1):1–6.
33. http://vitaltalk.org/guides/transitionsgoals-of-care/. Accessed 20 May 2017.
34. Schwarze ML, Kehler JM, Campbell TC. Navigating high risk procedures with more than just a street map [letter]. J Palliat Med. 2013;16(10):1169–71.

# Chapter 14
# End-of-Life Care and Cancer: Psychosocial Needs of Patients and the Bereaved

**Kailey E. Roberts, Aliza A. Panjwani, Allison Marziliano, Allison J. Applebaum, and Wendy G. Lichtenthal**

## End-of-Life Care and Cancer: Psychosocial Care of Patients and the Bereaved

Attention to end-of-life (EOL) care of both patients with cancer and their families has gained an increasingly important place in policy discussions and medical care recommendations [1]. According to the National Cancer Institute, EOL care is initiated when it is determined that the cancer can no longer be managed with active treatment [2]. EOL care encompasses interdisciplinary care-oriented toward quality of life (QOL), symptom management, relief of suffering, and

K. E. Roberts (✉)
The New School for Social Research, New York, NY, USA

Department of Psychiatry and Behavioral Sciences, Memorial Sloan Kettering Cancer Center, New York, NY, USA
e-mail: robek590@newschool.edu

A. A. Panjwani
Department of Psychology, The Graduate Center, City University of New York, New York, NY, USA
e-mail: apanjwani@gradcenter.cuny.edu

A. Marziliano
Department of Psychiatry and Behavioral Sciences, Memorial Sloan Kettering Cancer Center, New York, NY, USA

A. J. Applebaum
Department of Psychiatry and Behavioral Sciences, Caregivers Clinic, Memorial Sloan Kettering Cancer Center, New York, NY, USA
e-mail: applebaa@mskcc.org

W. G. Lichtenthal
Department of Psychiatry and Behavioral Sciences, Bereavement Clinic, Memorial Sloan Kettering Cancer Center, New York, NY, USA
e-mail: lichtenw@mskcc.org



P. Hopewood, M. J. Milroy (eds.), *Quality Cancer Care*,
https://doi.org/10.1007/978-3-319-78649-0_14

comfort [2]. Care at EOL typically falls under palliative and hospice services, both of which involve an interdisciplinary, holistic approach to addressing the physical, psychological, social, emotional, and spiritual needs of the patient, caregiver(s), and families [3]. Notably, clinical practice guidelines have emphasized how attending to psychosocial needs is integral to patient- and family-centered EOL care [4].

The purpose of this chapter is to provide an overview of EOL cancer care from a psychosocial perspective. The focus primarily is on adult care while including a brief overview of the unique needs of children, adolescents, and young adults and their families. The first section includes an orientation to palliative and hospice care, a description of patient and caregiver psychosocial needs at EOL, and potential assessment and intervention approaches. The subsequent section describes bereavement care needs of family members after a cancer loss. Evidence-based interventions for patients and their families directed at enhancing connection to legacy and meaning are highlighted throughout.

## Overview of Palliative and Hospice Care

### *Concept of a "Good Death"*

Both palliative and hospice services provide care intended to maintain a high QOL and help patients experience a "good death." The Institute of Medicine (IOM) defines a "good death" as "one that is free from avoidable suffering for patients, families and caregivers in general accordance with the patients' and families' wishes; and reasonably consistent with clinical, cultural, and ethical standards" [1]. A number of studies have investigated more specific characteristics of a "good death" from the perspective of providers, patients, and caregivers. For example, a national survey asked patients with life-limiting illness, EOL care providers, and bereaved family members about the most important components of a good death. Pain and symptom management, preparation for death, having a sense of completion, decisions about treatment preferences, and being treated as a "whole person" were identified across groups as central [5]. In their recent review of studies assessing the concept of a "good death," Meier et al. [6] identified several additional important components, including preferences for treatment and dying being met, spiritual/religious needs met, and maintaining emotional well-being, connection with family, and quality of life. Across groups, providers, patients, and caregivers identified preferences for dying met, being pain free, and maintaining emotional well-being as most important [6]. Above all, maintaining a sense of dignity, meaning in life, and identity continuity are considered to be essential elements of a "good death" [7, 8]. In contrast, avoiding unnecessary interventions and being perceived as a burden to others have been identified as characteristic of a "bad death" [9].

## Barriers to Quality End-of-Life Care

Despite recommendations for quality EOL care and how it may facilitate a version of a "good death," a number of barriers to such care exist. A central potential barrier, at least in the United States, is death anxiety and general discomfort with discussing death, even among health professionals [10, 11]. Death anxiety influences the underuse of palliative care and hospice, in part because of stigma associated with the terms "palliative" and "hospice" [12] that imply hopelessness, futility, and imminent death. Not only does stigma impact patients and family members, but it also plays a role in medical providers' approaches to care. In a world where advancements in medicine are ever increasing, cancer-related death can be associated with "giving up" or "losing a battle" for providers and their patients [13]. With that viewpoint comes the danger of not recognizing or admitting when a patient may be declining or imminently dying [14] and a concern that referral to EOL care may eliminate hope in patients and families [13].

Additional barriers to EOL care include sociocultural healthcare disparities and lack of access to appropriate, culturally competent communication about EOL issues [14, 15]. In their systematic review focusing on EOL care and minorities with cancer, LoPresti et al. [16] found that compared to Caucasian-Americans, Hispanic-Americans used hospice at less than or equal rates, followed by African and Asian-Americans, confirming what is already broadly known about healthcare disparities related to race and ethnicity. Factors that could contribute to this difference in hospice use include socioeconomic status, health literacy, language barriers, access barriers, health insurance issues, and lack of cultural competence in providers [16]. Notably, LoPresti et al. [16] found that providers tended to adhere to EOL preferences of Caucasian-American patients more than those of African-American patients.

Lopez-Sierra and Rodriguez-Sanchez [17] emphasize the importance of providers developing cultural competence, specifically with regard to the many influences (e.g., social, spiritual, psychological) on patient needs and preferences at EOL. Approaches to destigmatize EOL care and improve these disparities can include increasing interdisciplinary training in EOL care and tailoring EOL care to specific patient and family member needs or be as simple as changing "palliative" to "supportive" care, a movement that has been occurring at some institutions [17, 18].

## Location of Care

End-of-life (EOL) care is generally coordinated by palliative or hospice services and can take place in inpatient or outpatient settings. Whereas patients become eligible for hospice if they are considered to have a prognosis of 6 months or less to live [3], current guidelines recommend early palliative care intervention for patients with advanced cancer [19]. A component of planning for EOL care and facilitating patient goals is determining the location of this care. While not universal, across many cultures dying at home is commonly considered preferable to dying in a facility or hospital for a variety of reasons, including QOL and access to social support [3, 20, 21]. Hales et al. [22] examined reasons why caregivers may rate quality of death as higher for deaths in the home and suggested that this may be related to better social support and fewer medical complications. Despite evidence that most patients and caregivers prefer home-based care for hospice [23], in the United States, 50% of annual deaths occur in the hospital [24]. However, the quality of care provided may be more important than location, as one study of bereaved family members found that communication with family and emotional and spiritual support were important areas of quality of care, regardless of location [25].

Whether providing care through home-based hospice or in a medical inpatient setting, there are many ways professionals can intervene to support a "good death" and reduce barriers to care. To that end, palliative and hospice care offers services addressing the physical, psychological, and spiritual needs of patients and families, as well as practical assistance with EOL-related decision-making [26]. Palliative care and hospice teams can include physicians, nurses, aides, social workers, clergy, volunteers, physical and occupational therapists, psychiatrists, and psychologists [3]. In addition to palliative care providers, mental health professionals can serve as models for approaches to discussing EOL issues, communicate a sense of calm and normalcy in what can be a highly distressing time [26], and empower patients in their care decisions [27].

## Patient Psychosocial Needs at End of Life

Psychosocial needs at EOL can include maintaining autonomy, QOL, psychological well-being, and strengthening relationships [28]. In order to support patients' psychosocial needs, it is important for providers to consider which mental states and behaviors represent a normative process, as well as what may necessitate more targeted psychological or psychiatric interventions. EOL care professionals should be familiar with common presentations of patients in decline and also maintain an open stance as to what is considered normative for each individual given their personal history, social system, and culture [29]. While they are facing the end of their lives, patients at EOL are still *in life* and efforts should be made to nurture opportunities to engage in life, when possible. Within palliative and hospice teams, mental health professionals in particular can play an important role in facilitating the patients' and families' remaining goals for living by assessing patients for psychological distress and utilizing interventions to reduce distress and increase engagement in life. Mental health professionals can serve as consultants, facilitators of communication between patients, their families and providers, assess and treat psychological distress, as well as provide a consistent source of support [26]. As Neimeyer [30] emphasizes, though, specialized training for mental health providers involved in EOL care is important to manage their personal death anxiety and related existential distress in order to be fully and appropriately present with patients.

## *Psychological Assessment at End of Life*

Assessment of patients' psychological distress at EOL should incorporate theories on normative psychological processes at EOL. Perhaps the best known stage theory of dying was proposed by Kubler-Ross [31] in *On Death and Dying*. Kubler-Ross [31] advanced the notion that individuals experience distinct, linear, universal stages at EOL and eventually should reach a point of acceptance of their impending death. Since its original publication, this theory of dying has been critiqued and evidence suggests that, rather than occurring in a linear fashion, these stages constitute distinct and overlapping psychological experiences during EOL [32]. Other theories such as Corr [32] and Doka [33] focus on tasks of dying and phases, respectively, that fall under the physical, psychological, social, and spiritual.

Not every patient at EOL will experience symptoms consistent with a diagnosable psychological disorder; thus, a proper psychological assessment bears in mind normative processes and individual needs [16]. However, it is important to assess patients for more severe experiences of depression, hopelessness, and other psychiatric symptom presentation as both underdiagnosing and overdiagnosing individuals at EOL can have negative consequences. For example, in some case, patients may underreport symptoms so as to appear "strong," or medical providers may assume that a degree of hopelessness is normal in patients with life-limiting cancer [34]. This may result in patients needlessly suffering emotionally without appropriate intervention. Assessment may be informal as the patient declines or may incorporate brief, well-validated measures such as the Patient Health Questionnaire, a 9-item measure of depression symptoms [35]. When assessing for psychological distress, it is important to consider the intersection of physical and emotional experiences and consider differential diagnoses. For example, physical pain increases the chance of psychological distress and vice versa [36, 37]. Additionally, psychological distress can mimic an underlying medical problem such as cardiac arrest, electrolyte imbalance, and dehydration [38]. While psychological distress in patients at EOL can come in many forms, the most commonly identified presentations include delirium, depression, anxiety, and trauma reactions such as adjustment disorder or post-traumatic stress disorder [39].

### Delirium

Delirium is an organically based disturbance in consciousness involving changes in cognition and/or perception that can fluctuate in duration and intensity [40]. It occurs in 26–44% of advanced cancer patients admitted to acute care and in 80% of patients during their last days of life [41]. Though often associated with being drug induced, delirium has a variety of causes [40]. Delirium can cause significant distress in patients and families [42] as patients appear to be confused, highly distressed, agitated, and potentially combative. While interventions for delirium are primarily pharmacological, mental health professionals involved in EOL care can assist with management by providing education to the family [40]. Additionally, following a delirium episode, patients may be engaged in calming interventions such as diaphragmatic breathing or music therapy to reduce stress in the environment and anxiety [43].

### Depression

Some degree of sadness and dysphoria is common in people with advanced illness but can be differentiated from severe depression [44]. The frequency of severe depressive disorders in patients at EOL has been identified as between 20 and 25% [44]. It is important to assess patients for depression as it can impact QOL, lead patients to refuse visits from professionals and loved ones, and contribute to them avoiding or struggling with important healthcare decisions or making plans for care. Depression at EOL can present as a loss of meaning and purpose, low self-worth, desire for hastened death, or suicidality [45]. Hopelessness has also been identified to be a related but distinct construct from depression at EOL that can be related to not only prognosis but also meaning in life and relationships [44]. It has been found to be an independent predictor of desire for hastened death and, when not addressed, can influence patients refusing treatment or requesting assisted suicide [44, 46]. While in some states assisted suicide is legal (e.g., Oregon and Washington), it is important to determine patients' competence to make such decisions and to differentiate these types of wishes from suicidality. To distinguish depression from a more normative, passing state of sadness related to EOL, clinicians can utilize standardized measures, draw on expertise in working with patients at EOL, and determine the negative impact of the depression symptoms on the patient's QOL.

### Anxiety

As with depression, some degree of anxiety and fearfulness is normative at EOL given that patients may be facing distressing physical, spiritual, and emotional experiences. However, for some patients, anxiety can intensify and become more pervasive, potentially needlessly decreasing their QOL. Careful assessment is also necessary with anxiety as physical symptoms of anxiety may be missed given their overlap with medical illness symptoms. Often in this population, anxiety in the form of jitteriness, hyperactivity, insomnia, and shortness of breath can present more than affective or cognitive symptoms [47].

### Post-Traumatic Stress Disorder

For patients who carry a diagnosis of PTSD related to a prior trauma, there can be an exacerbation of PTSD symptoms at EOL, particularly if the patient is in a potentially stressful environment such as a hospital inpatient unit [48]. Patients with

PTSD may present as depressed or anxious initially but may also experience more severe insomnia, nightmares, flashbacks, confusion, mistrust of providers, and paranoia [49]. Certain populations such as military veterans will be more likely to have preexisting PTSD and providers working in setting serving those populations should integrate regular screening for PTSD into any assessment.

## *Psychotherapeutic Interventions*

Psychotherapy at EOL often looks quite different from traditional outpatient psychotherapy [50]. In many cases, a mental health provider will engage with the patient at bedside, either in a hospital setting or in their home. Family members and/or other providers may be present or coming in and out, thus changing the typical frame and boundaries present in traditional psychotherapy and making the therapeutic relationship more informal. Interventions can involve the general provision of emotional support, or they may be more targeted, such as to reduce physical symptoms of anxiety. For example, anxiety and depressive symptoms can be addressed through acute cancer cognitive therapy (CT) [51]. Acute cancer CT is a modified version of cognitive therapy, a form of short-term psychotherapy oriented toward modifying maladaptive thoughts and behaviors [51]. Given the constraints of medical inpatient units and hospice, acute cancer CT acknowledges truth to certain anxieties and fears while also guiding patients to maintain a sense of "realistic optimism." This version of CT can be done in a single-session format and necessitates therapists having the ability to quickly assess and intervene from a cognitive perspective with the goal of reducing distress [51].

Psychotherapy at EOL can also focus on legacy-building and meaning-making. Research with advanced cancer patients has highlighted the importance of the patient's legacy, which can include how one dies, the desire for something good to come out of the death, and being remembered [52]. As patients reach the end of their lives, there may be a sense of urgency to identify and build upon their legacy [53]. Patients may feel a sense of grief over not having enough time to create legacy in the way one would ideally want. Psychotherapeutic interventions can address this through direct exploration of the legacy patients have created throughout their lives as well as identifying opportunities to address unfinished business. Examples of legacy- and meaning-oriented interventions that have demonstrated benefits at EOL include Meaning-Centered Psychotherapy (MCP), therapeutic life review [54], and Dignity Therapy [55].

MCP is an existential approach, based on Viktor Frankl's [56] logotherapy, developed by Breitbart and colleagues. Both 8-session group [57] and 7-session individual [58] formats have demonstrated efficacy in enhancing advanced cancer patients' spiritual well-being, QOL, and physical symptom distress. The group format in particular has been demonstrated to be effective in reducing depression, hopelessness, and desire for hastened death [58]. MCP focuses on connecting patients to sources of meaning in their past and present (e.g., lessons learned, childhood experiences) that may already exist or to sources of meaning they are just beginning to discover (e.g., new priorities) and highlighting the choices they have in how they respond to any suffering they are experiencing. Each session focuses on a different source of meaning and utilizes didactics as well as experiential exercises during session and as homework. The concept of legacy is woven throughout the therapy and patients are given opportunities to reflect on the legacy they were given as well as how they continue to create legacy in the present (e.g., how they are facing death or interacting with loved ones) and future. In addition to engaging in this reflection with the therapist, patients are invited to create a "legacy project" that reflects their sources of meaning or addresses unfinished business. These projects are highly individualized and have ranged from memoirs to artwork and to simply having a long-awaited conversation with a loved one. The therapy concludes with reflections on the sources of meaning as well as the patient's experience having the therapist "bear witness" to their legacy through the therapy. MCP, has been adapted for various populations, in many cases based on feedback given by patients, and includes a modified, shortened version for hospice care [59]. Guidance on administering MCP and its adaptations can be found in a recently published textbook [60].

Dignity therapy is a brief intervention developed by Chochinov [8] and focuses on areas of psychosocial and existential distress in patients with the goal of reconnecting patients with a sense of meaning and dignity. Rather than simply a life review, dignity therapy involves focusing on thoughts, ideas, and events that are most meaningful. Often, patients will be offered the opportunity to audio-record the brief session so that it can later be transcribed and given back to the patient (and their family if they so choose) [55]. Dignity therapy has demonstrated efficacy in increasing sense of dignity, purpose, and meaning, as well as reducing depressive symptoms [55].

Pharmacotherapy should also be utilized when appropriate such as in cases of agitation, intractable depression, and insomnia [26]. As mentioned, careful assessment of the presenting symptoms should be done to determine the most effective medication to use with a given patient, taking into account their physical symptoms and functional status. Additionally, patients at EOL may be on multiple medications for symptom management so expertise in medications used at EOL and their interactions with psychotropic medications is important. A number of useful resources on this topic exist and can be referred to for further information [61–64].

## *Spiritual Care*

Though it is often the realm of chaplaincy and pastoral care, spiritual care at EOL can become important when providing psychological assessment and intervention, particularly in meaning-oriented interventions. Even patients who would not otherwise identify with a particular religion can face spiritually oriented questions at EOL that may either result in distress or be a source of comfort [65]. Spiritual care can focus on helping patients process their general sense of meaning in life or more specifically be related to their beliefs in a higher power or doctrine [66]. Though spirituality can be highly important in coping, there is evidence that the presence of these beliefs does not necessarily reduce depression and anxiety in individuals with advanced cancer [67]. Thus, spirituality should be considered in the context of the whole presentation of the patient, psychologically, physically, and emotionally.

## Family Member Needs at End of Life

### *Caregiver Distress*

Continuity of care has been highlighted as just as important for caregivers as for patients [1]. Caregivers may suffer from physical and mental health problems [68], and intervention provided at EOL can be an essential stepping stone for families receiving bereavement care and making an initial connection to a mental health provider [69]. Caregiving at the EOL has been shown to result in emotional and psychological distress that can extend into bereavement [70]. In their nationwide cohort study of caregivers of patients with a life-limiting illness, Nielsen et al. [70] found that 15% reported severe anticipatory grief symptoms, 16.1% depression symptoms, and 12% a high degree of caregiver burden. They further noted that high levels of anticipatory grief and lack of preparedness in cancer caregivers were related to bereavement-related mental health challenges after the death [70]. Nevertheless, caregiving has also been associated with positive consequences such as sense of mastery, appreciation of others, meaning in life, and new priorities in life [71]. These benefits of caregiving can be nurtured in caregivers in order to reduce distress and make challenges not only bearable but also meaningful.

Caregiver distress has been associated with a number of factors, including anticipatory grief and distress of the patient. Ratkowski et al. [72] surveyed caregivers and found that across illnesses (e.g., cancer and cardiopulmonary) caregivers rated psychological symptoms in the patient as the most distressing as opposed to physical symptoms, suggesting the importance of psychosocial support. Similarly, in another study, family members identified psychosocial problems such as confusion, agitation, and communication issues as the most distressing [14]. However, physical symptoms in patients such as shortness of breath, pain [73], fatigue, and nausea [14] can also be distressing to caregivers. Family members who perceive the patient as experiencing unmanaged physical symptoms such as pain are at greater risk for bereavement-related mental health challenges [74]. Emotional burdens related to decision-making, supporting the patient, and coping with anticipatory grief can also be highly burdensome to caregivers. In particular, Wijnhoven et al. [75] found that caregivers felt more of a responsibility and burden at the transition from active to supportive treatment, suggesting the importance of attending to caregiver psychosocial needs at this transition in care.

### *Support for Families*

Hudson et al. [76] developed guidelines for the psychosocial support of caregivers at EOL based on a systematic review. These include establishing the role of the caregiver and caregiver support, offering appropriate information about the patient's EOL care plan, assessing caregiver needs and creating a plan for care, preparing the caregiver for death by providing information on dying process, assisting with planning and offering support options, and providing bereavement support options [76]. This group found that a brief psychoeducation intervention to provide support with symptom management reduced caregiver distress at EOL [77]. Similarly, another study illustrated that earlier EOL decision-making resulted in reduced stress in caregivers [78], suggesting the importance of psychoeducational intervention early in the process. Some interventions used with patients at EOL can be and have been adapted to support caregivers such as Meaning-Centered Psychotherapy for Cancer Caregivers, an existential intervention designed to be delivered in a web-based format in order to increase accessibility to caregivers and reduce burden [79]. Other interventions target the family as a unit beginning during palliative care through bereavement. Family-focused grief therapy (FFGT) is a brief, time-limited intervention designed to identify concerns specific to a family and, subsequently, devise a tailored plan to address issues around cohesion, communication, and conflict [80]. FFGT has been shown to be most effective in reducing distress and depression in families with mild-to-intermediate dysfunction [80]. By addressing caregiver support needs pre-loss through psychotherapeutic interventions and guidance on advance care planning, quality of death for the patient may be improved and risk for bereavement-related mental health challenges may be reduced [81].

## End-of-Life Care for Children, Adolescents, and Young Adults with Cancer

EOL care for children with cancer presents unique psychosocial issues for both the young patients and their parents. While the child's involvement in decision-making of their own care is ideal, young children may not be cognizant of the myriad options or consequences of said decisions, and thus parents often are responsible for the majority of decisions [82]. The decision-making process can become all the more complicated when the child is an adolescent or a young adult (AYA), though research on the psychosocial needs of these patients and their families is more limited [83]. Parents of children at EOL have a number of unmet needs, chiefly around communication with the healthcare team and their child, as well as managing emotional distress and support needs [84–86].

## *Communication Between Parents and the Healthcare Team*

During and after EOL discussions with the healthcare team, parents are left with the formidable challenge of assimilating and understanding key information [82, 87] while managing accompanying emotional distress [84]. EOL decisions (e.g., withholding resuscitation or withdrawing life support) are cited as the most difficult among all the decisions made throughout their child's cancer [88] and parents may require significant support around coming to terms with their child's prognosis and the appropriate time to transition to EOL [89]. Parent accounts suggest that one of their primary EOL care goals is easing suffering and symptoms such as pain and fatigue [90].

The quality and level of communication at EOL are important for providers to attend to, particularly given differing needs of parents and patients depending on the age of the patient. Studies on EOL communication and pediatrics have demonstrated inadequacies in the amount of information provided [85] and the clarity [86]. Other studies have highlighted parents' perception of providers being inaccessible [91] and uncertainty about which questions were critical or appropriate to ask [85]. Evidence suggests that parents prefer information to be communicated honestly and directly with simplified language [86], as long as the delivery is compassionate and sensitive [87]. In addition to accessibility to the healthcare team, parents appreciate being included in the decision-making process and having their opinions heard by the physicians [86]. At a time when parents feel powerless in the face of their child's suffering [92], this kind of inclusivity can provide some control [93], equip parents to make difficult decisions [94], result in higher satisfaction with medical care [95], and build trust in health professionals [85].

## *Communication with Children at the End of Life*

An important aspect of psychosocial care for parents of child with cancer may be providing support in communicating about EOL with their child. In attempting to maintain their child's sense of hope and protect them from further psychological distress, parents can be reluctant to disclose information about death or EOL care [95]. For example, in one study, most parents (98%) felt that their child should be aware of a cancer diagnosis while fewer parents (68%) felt that their child should be informed if the cancer was no longer treatable [96]. However, research has demonstrated that when children or younger adolescents feel like active participants in their care, not only do they feel less isolated [97], but also less anxious and fearful [90]. Further, studies suggest that avoidance of EOL discussions with children and adolescents or young adults (AYAs) can result in an increased sense of distance from their child [98] and feelings of regret during bereavement [99]. Honest and open communication during EOL has been associated with better quality of remaining life [100]. However, at times such discussions can occur too close to time of death to allow the patient enough time to mentally and emotionally prepare [101].

Though interventions and support designed to help parents communicate with their ill child are limited, there are a number of recommendations to consider. The care team can play a critical role in guiding parents through the process of disclosing EOL information to their children [102]. Psychoeducation around children's needs can be provided, specifically noting the benefits of children being involved in their own care such as reduced anxiety and isolation [90]. Bearing in mind the child's age and developmental level, parents can also consider involving the child in making decisions [103]. Simply asking what is important to the child can help them feel more empowered. For AYAs, the use of an advanced care planning tool such as the Five Wishes [104] or Voicing My Choices [105] may be a way to honor their priorities as well as keep lines of communication open between the patient, care team, and family [106].

## *Managing Family Distress*

Parents experience a range of difficult emotions like sadness, powerlessness, worry, guilt, and anticipatory grief, about their child's suffering and impending passing [107]. With respect to EOL decisions and ensuing emotional turmoil, parents report a need for providers to utilize gentle guidance to help parents move from the "preservation mode" into "letting go" [84]. Even the delivery of information can influence parents' experiences at EOL. One study showed that when the healthcare professional delivering troubling information expressed kindness and compassion, parents felt validated, empathized with and bonded over a shared experience of sorrow [108]. The way the care team treats the family can have an influential impact and may even affect how parents grieve after the loss of their child [109].

Often parents come to rely heavily on their immediate care team and having reduced contact with the team after death of the child can be experienced as additional loss (78). Therefore, it is important to help parents connect with a variety of support services prior to the loss such as pastoral care, funeral planning, psychological services, and community support [110]. Peer support from other parents with similar experiences may also help parents to feel more emotionally prepared to cope with EOL and bereavement [111]. Though these services can help alleviate some of the distress or assist the parent in processing information, many parents remain unaware of services available to them [112]. It is recommended that pediatric care teams apply a standard of at least one outreach call to parents following the loss of a child [113].

Following the death of a child, parents may struggle with decisions related to their child's cancer treatment and EOL experiences [114], which can add to their emotional distress (e.g., feelings of regret) and potentially complicate grief. Parents' engagement in open and informed communication with their healthcare team as well as the ill child when possible can mitigate some of this distress [115]. Continuity of care for parents is important and at a minimum should be provided through an outreach phone call. When possible, other support services such as bereavement groups should be offered [113, 116].

## Bereavement Care for the Family

For both caregivers of adults and those of children, care should not end with the death of the patient. Continuity of care through bereavement may have benefits for both family members and providers [113]. When it is offered, bereavement care should include assessment of the psychological, physical, and social state of the bereaved [117].

Although bereaved family members often express a desire for bereavement care [117], services are often underutilized [69, 118]. For example, in a study of 86 bereaved caregivers of patients with advanced cancer, the authors found that less than half of the sample (44%) discussed emotional health concerns with a professional after the patient's death and even fewer (40%) reported mental health service use following the patient's death [69]. A variety of factors contribute to this underutilization, including family members not wanting to return to the hospital where care was provided, stigma associated with mental health, and family members becoming disconnected from medical providers after the death due to lack of follow-up [119].

This lack of follow-up is related to numerous systemic barriers to providing high-quality, consistent care to families during palliative care and bereavement [76]. Particularly in cases where there is not a staff position dedicated to following up with families, one such barrier is the absence of standard procedures for outreach to bereaved family members. The frequency with which oncologists and other providers reach out to bereaved family members varies by and within hospitals, and even from family member to family member [120]. For example, in one study evaluating the frequency and nature of provider bereavement practices of telephoning the family, sending a card, or attending the funeral among oncologists and palliative care physicians, the authors found that only 33.3% reported usually or always engaging in the practice [121]. Providers indicated that they were most likely to place a telephone call to the bereaved rather than sending a card or attending a funeral service [121].

### *Identifying Family Members in Need of Bereavement Support*

Given the inconsistency in outreach and underutilization of services, it is important to be able to identify family members in most need of more targeted intervention. While the grieving process can be intensely painful and characterized by acute distress, deep sadness, and anxiety symptoms, many individuals are able to adapt and resume functioning within the first 1–2 years post-loss [122]. However, some individuals may continue to experience more impairing and prolonged bereavement-related mental health challenges following their loss [123, 124]. These can come in the form of a variety of psychological disorders, including prolonged grief disorder (PGD), major depressive disorder (MDD), and post-traumatic stress disorder (PTSD), and affect a relatively small but important subset of bereaved family members [125].

### Prolonged Grief Disorder

A substantial minority of bereaved individuals, estimated at approximately 10%, experience a persistent and impairing set of symptoms related to grief, referred to as Prolonged Grief Disorder (PGD) [37, 124]. Symptoms of PGD include difficulty accepting the reality of the death, feeling as if part of oneself is lost, anger over the death, guilt regarding the death, or difficulty with social situations. For a diagnosis of PGD to be warranted, these symptoms must remain apparent beyond a period considered normal within an individual's culture (i.e., often 6 months or greater post-loss), interfere with functioning, and be severe beyond what is expected based on social/cultural norms [37].

### Major Depressive Disorder

Substantial numbers of bereaved individuals experience major depressive disorder (MDD) following their loss, with one study finding that 9% of bereaved individuals met the criteria for MDD at 4 months post-loss [126]. The Diagnostic and Statistical Manual of Mental Disorders [127] indicates that a bereaved individual may be diagnosed with MDD as early as 2 weeks post-loss, though careful assessment should be done before assigning a diagnosis as some symptoms of MDD can mimic normative and/or acute grief [128]. Symptoms of MDD include sadness, hopelessness, anhedonia, guilt, negative cognitions about oneself, suicidal ideation, and chances in sleep or appetite. Clinically, bereaved individuals with MDD may be less likely to look for opportunities for treatment than non-bereaved individuals [128]. Therefore, the development of a method to identify those at risk for MDD pre-loss is critical in order to connect this population with mental health services post-loss.

### Post-Traumatic Stress Disorder

Although generally associated with violent deaths, individuals can develop post-traumatic stress disorder (PTSD) related to an illness death, particularly if the death was perceived as a traumatic experience [129–131] or if tumultuous experiences occurred during caregiving, such as life/routine disruption, lack of self-care, and chronic negative affect [132]. Symptoms of PTSD include reexperiencing the traumatic event through intrusive thoughts, flashbacks, and nightmares, avoiding places or people that serve as reminders of the trauma, and increased feelings of arousal.

## Bereavement Risk Screening

Bereavement risk screening as part of a standard of care can be useful in allowing individuals to be identified and offered information about support services prior to the death of a family member to cancer or shortly afterward so that they are less likely to "fall through the cracks" if they experience bereavement-related mental health challenges. Particularly important in busy settings lacking the resources to conduct formal assessments with all family members, risk screening may act as an initial point of contact for caregivers to connect with clinical staff. This could also facilitate later mental health referrals through a "warm handoff" and potentially decreasing underutilization of bereavement services due to stigma [133].

Studies have identified numerous risk factors for the development of bereavement-related mental health challenges [134, 135] that can be categorized as background risk factors, illness/death related factors, and bereavement-related factors. Background characteristics of the bereaved individual that can be risk factors include older age [136], prior mental health problems, low socioeconomic status, less education [137], female gender [138], high levels of worry [139], insecure attachment [140], and lack of acceptance and denial or self-blame [141].

Illness and death-related factors such as the type of death, circumstances, and difficult caregiving experiences may put family members at higher risk for challenges in bereavement. Deaths that are violent are more likely to lead to PGD and PTSD than nonviolent, expected deaths [130–132, 137, 142]. In the case of illness deaths, the perception of the quality of death may contribute to the caregivers' post-loss adjustment as illustrated in the *Coping with Cancer* study findings demonstrating that caregivers who perceived their loved one's quality of life at end of life to be poor were at greater risk for suicidal ideation post-loss [143]. Factors surrounding the post-loss experience also increase the risk of developing negative mental health outcomes. Difficulty with making sense of their loss and inability to identify benefits associated with the loss are positively related to more severe grief [144]. Further, feelings of regret, guilt, shame, or self-blame place individuals at greater risk [145, 146].

Finally, the bereaved individual's relationships, both with the deceased and with others [147], can be considered risk factors. Research shows that insecure attachment styles [148, 149] or excessively dependent personality [150] can increase risk for mental health challenges. The quality of the relationship the bereaved individual had with the deceased, such as having a great deal of conflict [151] or being dependent on the person [152], can impact their grief trajectory. Additionally, the death of a child or spouse/partner can lead to increased risk of family members developing negative mental health outcomes as compared to other types of losses [153, 154].

Bereavement risk screening tools have been developed but many require significant resources, do not address the most salient risk factors for these types of challenges, and have not been systematically validated [155]. In light of the need for bereavement follow-up care, members of our research team have developed the Bereavement Risk Inventory and Screening Questionnaire (BRISQ), based on the latest literature on risk factors, bereavement expert input [134], and family member feedback. The BRISQ [134] is a brief, self-report screening tool that can be used to identify those at risk for various bereavement-related mental health challenges either pre- or post-loss and to track these family members in order to efficiently provide high-quality bereavement care to those most in need.

## *Bereavement Support Services*

Despite the lack of a standard of care and follow-up in bereavement, many settings make concerted efforts to develop high-quality bereavement services within the confines of their available resources. Research suggests that there is no one-size-fits-all approach to bereavement services, and tailored interventions may be necessary to accommodate the wide range of life experiences, situations, and needs of the bereaved. Bereavement care can range from targeted psychotherapy [156] to simply sending a condolence card to family [157]. While an ideal standard of care should involve the provision of services, at least a phone call is advised [113]. Other research has suggested the importance of providers acknowledging the patient's death, the provision of information about what to expect in terms of grief, and visits with the bereaved to assess their coping [158]. According to a nationwide survey of 501 bereaved family members of cancer patients, receiving bereavement care was positively significantly related to the bereaved feeling a sense of mastery, appreciation for others, meaning in life, and reordering of priorities about one's life [71].

In some instances, relatively formal bereavement programs have been implemented and systematically evaluated [159]. For example, a bereavement program specifically designed for bereaved family members of veterans with cancer involved calling the bereaved, sending letters and "what to expect" sheets, and referrals for support services. An evaluation of this program 1 year post-intervention demonstrated the benefit of letters and "what to expect" sheets, as well as the overall benefit the program conferred on the majority of participants [160]. Bereavement programs with available resources may consider offering targeted grief counseling approaches when possible. Options for grief-specific therapy range from FFGT [80], complicated grief treatment [161], and narrative therapy [162] to creative approaches such as those described in "Techniques of Grief Therapy" [163].

In sum, as with EOL care for patients, bereavement care for families should incorporate assessment of not only distress, but also risk for mental health challenges. Bereavement services can not only aid family members in adapting to loss but also improve the center or hospital's reputation by offering care in an area that is highly desired. For this reason, it is recommended that when possible, hospitals and cancer centers incorporate bereavement care that includes assessment and intervention. When resources are limited, an outreach phone call with referrals for community resources as part of a standard of care should be implemented [113].

## *Supporting Bereaved Parents*

Parents who have lost a child to cancer experience unique bereavement needs [164]. Similar to bereaved individuals who have lost an adult in their life, bereaved parents report a desire for bereavement care following the death of their child and benefit from continued interactions with their child's oncology team [113, 165]. Bereavement experts suggest that the standard of care in pediatrics should consist of at least one meaningful contact between the oncology team and bereaved parents to both assess risk and provide referral [113]. Nevertheless, an empirically validated psychosocial standard of care for bereavement follow-up with parents does not exist, despite research to suggest that bereaved parents need and want bereavement services [166]. As a result, outreach to parents varies. According to an web-based survey completed by pediatric oncologists, most (82%) of the sample stated that they "at least sometimes" call the bereaved family members, send a condolence card, attend the memorial service or other family meeting, or provide a counseling referral [167]. Indeed, the vast majority of the sample (96%) reported that bereavement care is part of good clinical practice, whereas 8% deemed it not to be their responsibility [167].

Although the desire for services is present, and there is evidence that the majority of clinicians believe bereavement care to be part of their duty, other barriers prevent optimal delivery and utilization of services [116]. On the delivery end, providers, even those in mental health, may hesitate to initiate bereavement care out of fear of saying the "wrong" words to comfort the bereaved, becoming themselves too emotional, or because of their own unresolved grief issues [168], particularly in the case of the death of a child. Other commonly cited barriers are lack of time on both the parts of the parents and the oncology team, as well as the oncology team lacking the resources to reach out to all bereaved parents [167]. In another study assessing 120 parents bereaved by cancer between 6 months and 6 years following the loss, 40% of parents who were not receiving bereavement services reported interest in such services, citing barriers to engagement such as the pain associated with speaking about the loss being too great (64%) and difficulty with locating bereavement help (60%) [166].

Where they do exist, several components of bereavement programs for parents who lost a child to cancer confer benefit. Bereavement follow-up has the potential to show empathy and provide validation of feelings, offer respect for the child's memory, provide an avenue to access further support, and incorporate practical suggestions [164]. A systematic review of bereavement services offered in pediatric hospital settings concluded that family members receiving such services reported that they felt cared for, supported by staff, less isolated, and greater growth and coping [116].

As with adult loss, bereavement care for parents also can include the provision of grief counseling and more targeted support when indicated. Our group has developed Meaning-Centered Grief Therapy (MCGT), a 16-session grief intervention that incorporates principles of MCP for advanced cancer patients as well as meaning reconstruction [169], cognitive-behavioral [137, 170], and attachment principles [147]. MCGT is designed to reduce prolonged, intense grief symptoms by paradoxically assisting the bereaved to coexist with their grief through connection to sources of meaning and meaningful narration of their and the deceased's story [156]. Our initial efforts to evaluate this intervention have focused on parents who have lost a child to cancer, assisting them with connecting to sources of meaning in their lives, as well as the meaning of their child's life [156]. As is done in MCP, a core principle highlighted in MCGT is that even when faced with out-of-control circumstances like the tragic loss of a child, individuals can decide how they face their suffering. That is, they are able to choose their attitude in the face of suffering [170]. They are also able to choose how they tell their own and their deceased loved one's story. MCGT additionally focuses on strengthening and connection between parents and their child in meaningful ways. Parents are encouraged to honor this connection and transform their caregiving role through a Living Legacy Project that reflects identified sources of meaning and their continuing bond with their child. Efforts to evaluate the efficacy of MCGT are currently under way.

## Conclusion

As this chapter has illustrated, quality EOL care in cancer consists of many intering elements such as physical, emotional, psychological, and spiritual needs and, thus, an interdisciplinary team is optimal. The field has responded to policy recommendations for compassionate, high-quality EOL care and bereavement support [1], but more can be done. For example, continuity of care for families bereaved by cancer can be strengthened through bereavement risk screening [134]. In addition, the role of strong communication between providers, patients, and family members from EOL and through bereavement cannot be overstated. Psychosocial care through thoughtful assessment and flexible interventions for patients and families at EOL can be integral to helping families to maintain a sense of meaning amidst many potentially overwhelming experiences. Mental health providers can utilize specific evidence-based interventions that focus on enhancing meaning, legacy, and dignity in EOL and bereavement settings [55, 60]. Meaning-centered approaches can also help minimize burnout and existential distress among health-care providers, which is critical to providing quality EOL care [171]. Despite the many systemic, institutional, and personal challenges in providing quality EOL care, both formal and informal care providers have a unique opportunity to engage with patients and families at a profound time of life that most will eventually experience themselves and can model the process of maintaining meaning in the face of these challenges [79, 172].

**Acknowledgments** The writing of this chapter and research by our team was generously supported by National Cancer Institute grants T32 CA009461, F31 CA192447, R03 CA139944, K07 CA172216, R01 CA128134, and P30 CA008748.

# References

1. Institute of Medicine. Committee on care at the end of life, Division of Health Care Services. In: Field MJ, Cassel CK, editors. Dying in America: improving quality and honoring individual preferences near the end of life. Washington D.C.: National Academy Press; 2014.
2. National Cancer Institute. End-of-Life Care. National Cancer Institute; 2012.
3. National Hospice and Palliative Care Organization. NHPCO's Facts and Figures, Hospice care in America; 2015.
4. Qaseem A, Snow V, Shekelle P, Casey DE, Cross T, Owens DK. Evidence-based interventions to improve the palliative care of pain, dyspnea, and depression at the end of life: a clinical practice guidelines from the American College of Physicians. Ann Intern Med. 2008;148:141–6.
5. Steinhauser K, Christakis N, Clipp E, McNeilly M, McIntyre L, Tulsky J. Factors considered important at the end of life by patients, family, physicians, and other care providers. JAMA. 2000;284(19):2476–82.
6. Meier EA, Gallegos JV, Thomas LP, Depp CA, Irwin SA, Jeste DV. Defining a good death (successful dying): literature review and a call for research and public dialogue. Am J Geriatr Psychiatry. 2016;24(4):261–71.
7. Block S. Psychological considerations, growth, and transcendence at the end of life: the art of the possible. JAMA. 2001;285(22):2898–905.
8. Chochinov HM. Dignity-conserving care—a new model for palliative care: helping the patient feel valued. JAMA. 2002;287(17):2253–60.
9. De Jong JD, Clarke LE. What is a good death? Stories from palliative care. J Palliat Care. 2009;25(1):61–7.
10. Becker E. The denial of death. New York: Free Press; 1973.
11. Neimeyer R, Fortner B. Death attitudes in contemporary perspective. In: Strack S, editor. Death and the quest for meaning: essays in honor of Herman Feifel. New Jersey: Jason Aronson Inc.; 1997.
12. Hui D, Kim SH, Kwon JH, Tanco KC, Zhang T, Kang JH, et al. Access to palliative care among patients treated at a comprehensive cancer center. Oncologist. 2012;1(17):1574–80.
13. McPhee SJ, Rabow MW, Pantilat SZ, Markowitz AJ, Winker MA. Finding our way—perspectives on care at the close of life. JAMA. 2000;284:2512–3.
14. Clark K. Care at the very end-of-life: dying cancer patients and their chosen family's needs. Cancers. 2017;9(2):11.
15. Heyland D, Dodek P, Rocker G, Groll D, Gafni A, Pichora D, et al. What matters most in end-of-life care: perceptions of seriously ill patients and their family members. CMAJ. 2006;174(5):627–33.
16. Lo Presti M, Dement F, Gold H. End-of-life care for people with cancer from ethnic minority groups: a systematic review. Am J Hosp Palliat Care. 2016;33(3):291–305.
17. Lopez-Sierra HE, Rodriguez-Sanchez J. The supportive roles of religion and spirituality in end-of-life and palliative care of patients with cancer in a culturally diverse context: a literature review. Curr Opin Support Palliat Care. 2015;9(1):87–95.
18. Maciasz RM, Arnold RM, Chu E, Park Y, White DB, Vater LB, et al. Does it matter what you call it? A randomized trial of language used to describe palliative care services. Support Care Cancer. 2013;21(12):3411–9.
19. Smith T, Temin S, Alesi E, Abernethy A, Balboni T, Basch E, et al. American Society of Clinical Oncology provisional clinical opinion: the integration of palliative care into standard oncology care. J Clin Oncol. 2012;6(30):880–7.

20. Gomes B, Calanzani N, Koffman J, Higginson I. Is dying in hospital better than home in incurable cancer and what factors influence this? A population-based study. BMC Med. 2015;13(1):235.
21. Higgins PC, Garrido MM, Prigerson HG. Factors predicting bereaved caregiver perception of quality of care in the final week of life: implications for health care providers. J Palliat Med. 2015;18(10):849–57.
22. Hales S, Chiu A, Husain A, Braun M, Rydall A, Gagliese L, et al. The quality of dying and death in cancer and its relationship to palliative care and place of death. J Pain Symptom Manag. 2014;48(5):839–51.
23. Agar M, Currow D, Shelby-James T, Plummer J, Sanderson C, AP A. Preference for place of care and place of death in palliative care: are these different questions? Palliat Med. 2008;22(7):787–95.
24. Grunier A, Mor V, Weitzen S, Truchil R, Teno J, Roy J. Where people die: a multilevel approach to understanding influences on site of death in America. Med Care Res Rev. 2007;64(4):351–78.
25. Burge F, Lawson B, Johnston G, Asada Y, McIntyre PF, Grunfeld E, et al. Bereaved family member perceptions of patient-focused family-centred care during the last 30 days of life using a mortality follow-back survey: does location matter? BMC Palliat Care. 2014;13:25.
26. Breitbart W, Alici Y. Psychosocial palliative care. Oxford: Oxford University Press; 2014.
27. Prigerson H, Vaughan S, Lichtenthal W. The hidden dangers of a cancer diagnosis. BMJ. 2016;354:4446.
28. Singer P, Martin D, Kelner M. Quality end-of-life care: patients' perspectives. JAMA. 1999;281(2):163–8.
29. Corr C, Corr D. Culture, socialization and dying. In: Meagher D, Balk D, editors. Handbook of thanatology: the essential body of knowledge of death, dying and bereavement. New York: Routledge; 2013.
30. Neimeyer R. From death anxiety to meaning making at the end of life: recommendations for psychological assessment. Clin Psychol Sci Pract. 2005;12:354–7.
31. Kubler-Ross E. On death and dying. New York: Scribner; 1969.
32. Corr C. A task-based approach to coping with dying. Omega. 1992;24:81–92.
33. Doka K. Living with life-threatening illness: a guide for patients, families, and caregivers. Lexington, MA: Lexington Books; 1993.
34. Passik S, Dugan W, McDonald M, Rosenfeld B, Theobald D, Edgerton S. Oncologists' recognition of depression in their patients with cancer. J Clin Oncol. 1998;16(4):1594–600.
35. Kroenke K, Spitzer R, Williams J. The PHQ-9: validity of a brief depression severity measure. J Gen Intern Med. 2001;16(9):606–13.
36. Gibson C, Breitbart W, Tomarken A, Kosinski A, Nelson C. Mental health issues near the end of life. In: Werth J, Blevins D, editors. Psychosocial issues near the end of life: a resource for professional care providers. Washington DC: American Psychological Association; 2006. p. 137–62.
37. Lichtenthal WG, Nilsson M, Zhang B, Trice ED, Kissane DW, Breitbart W, et al. Do rates of mental disorders and existential distress among advanced stage cancer patients increase as death approaches? Psychooncology. 2009;18(1):50–61.
38. Strain J, Liebowitz M, Klein D. Anxiety and panic attacks in the medically ill. Psychiatr Clin N Am. 1981;4(2):333–50.
39. Miovic M, Block S. Psychiatric disorders in advanced cancer. Cancer. 2007;110(8):1665–76.
40. Bush S, Bruera E. The assessment and management of delirium in cancer patients. Oncologist. 2009;14:1039–49.
41. Centeno C, Sanz A, Bruera E. Delirium in advanced cancer patients. Palliat Med. 2004;18:184–94.
42. Breitbart W, Gibson C, Tremblay A. The delirium experience: delirium recall and delirium-related distress in hospitalized patients with cancer, their spouses/caregivers, and their nurses. Psychosomatics. 2002;43:183–94.
43. Meagher D. Delirium: optimising management. Br Med J. 2001;322:144–9.

44. Breitbart W, Rosenfeld B, Pessin H, Kaim M, Funesti-Esch J, Galietta M, et al. Depression, hopelessness, and desire for hastened death in terminally ill patients with cancer. JAMA. 2000;284(22):2907–11.
45. Robinson S, Kissane DW, Brooker J, Burney S. A review of the construct of demoralization: history, definitions, and future directions for palliative care. Am J Hosp Palliat Care. 2016;33(1):93–101.
46. Chochinov H, Wilson K, Enns M, Lander S. Depression, hopelessness, and suicidal ideation in the terminally ill. Psychosomatics. 1998;39(4):366–70.
47. Holland J. Anxiety and cancer: the patient and the family. J Clin Psychiatry. 1989;50:20–5.
48. Alici Y, Smith D, Lu H, Bailey A, Shreve S, Rosenfeld K, et al. Families' perceptions of veterans' distress due to post-traumatic stress disorder-related symptoms at the end of life. J Pain Symptom Manag. 2010;39(3):507–14.
49. Feldman D, Sorocco K, Bratkovich K. Treatment of post traumatic stress disorder at the end-of-life: application of the stepwise psychosocial palliative care model. Palliat Support Care. 2014;12(3):233–43.
50. Connor S, Lycan J, Schumacher D. Involvement of psychologists in psychosocial aspects of hospice and end-of-life care. In: Werth J, Blevins D, editors. Psychosocial issues near the end of life: a resource for professional care givers. Washington DC: American Psychological Association; 2006. p. 203–17.
51. Levin T, Applebaum A. Acute cancer cognitive therapy. Cogn Behav Pract. 2014;21(4):404–15.
52. Coyle N. The hard work of living in the face of death. J Pain Symptom Manag. 2006;32(3):266–74.
53. Breitbart W. The existential framework of meaning-centered psychotherapy. In: Breitbart W, editors. New York: Oxford; 2017.
54. Keall R, Clayton J, Butow P. Therapeutic life review in palliative care: a systematic review of quantitative evaluations. J Pain Symptom Manag. 2015;49(4):747–61.
55. Chochinov H, Hack T, Hassard T, Kristjanson L, McClement S, Harlos M. Dignity therapy: a novel psychotherapeutic intervention for patients near end of life. J Clin Oncol. 2005;23(24):5520–5.
56. Frankl VE. Man's search for meaning : the classic tribute to hope from the Holocaust: Rider; 2011.
57. Breitbart W, Rosenfeld B, Pessin H, Applebaum A, Kulikowski J, Lichtenthal W. Meaning-centered group psychotherapy: an effective intervention for improving psychological well-being in patients with advanced cancer. Palliat Support Care. 2015;33(7):749–54.
58. Breitbart W, Poppito S, Rosenfeld B, Vickers A, Li Y, Abbey J, et al. Pilot randomized controlled trial of individual meaning-centered psychotherapy for patients with advanced cancer. J Clin Oncol. 2012;30(12):1304–9.
59. Masterson M, Rosenfeld B, Pessin H, Fenn N. Adapting meaning-centered psychotherapy in the palliative care setting: meaning-centered psychotherapy-palliative care. In: Breitbart W, editor. Meaning-centered psychotherapy in the cancer setting: finding hope and meaning in the face of suffering. New York: Oxford; 2017.
60. Breitbart W, editor. Meaning-centered psychotherapy in the cancer setting New York. New York: Oxford University Press; 2017.
61. Garcia C, Lynn R, Breitbart W. Psychotropic medications in palliative care. Prim Psychiatry. 2009;16(5):25–32.
62. O'Mahony D, O'Connor MN. Pharmacotherapy at end of life. Age Aging. 2011;40(4):419–22.
63. Grassi L, Riba M. Psychopharmacology in oncology and palliative care: a practical manual. Berlin: Springer; 2014.
64. Thekdi SM, Trinidad A, Roth A. Psychopharamacology in cancer. Curr Psychiatry Rep. 2015;17(1):529.
65. Delgado-Guay MO. Spirituality and religiosity in supportive and palliative care. Curr Opin Support Palliat Care. 2014;8(3):308–13.
66. Sulmasy D. A biopsychosocial-spiritual model for the care of patients at the end of life. Gerontology. 2002;42(suppl 3):24–33.

67. King M, Llewellyn H, Leurent B, Owen F, Leavey G, Tookman A, et al. Spiritual beliefs near the end of life: a prospective cohort study of people with cancer receiving palliative care. Psychooncology. 2013;22(11):2505–12.
68. Kapari M, Addington J, Hotopf M. Risk factors for common mental disorder in caregiving and bereavement. J Pain Symptom Manag. 2010;40(6):844–56.
69. Lichtenthal WG, Nilsson M, Kissane DW, Breitbart W, Kacel E, Jones EC, et al. Underutilization of mental health services among bereaved caregivers with prolonged grief disorder. Psychiatr Serv. 2011;62(10):1225–9.
70. Nielsen MK, Neergaard MA, Jensen AB, Bro F, Guldin MB. Psychological distress, health, and socio-economic factors in caregivers of terminally ill patients: a nationwide population-based cohort study. Support Care Cancer. 2016;24(7):3057–67.
71. Kang J, Shin DW, Choi JE, Sanjo M, Yoon SJ, Kim HK, et al. Factors associated with positive consequences of serving as a family caregiver for a terminal cancer patient. Psychooncology. 2013;22(3):564–71.
72. Ratkowski KL, Washington KT, Craig KW, Albright DL. The stress of sadness: the most stressful symptoms for hospice family caregivers. Am J Hosp Palliat Care. 2015;32(7):745–9.
73. Kehl KA, Kowalkowski JA. A systematic review of the prevalence of signs of impending death and symptoms in the last 2 weeks of life. Am J Hosp Palliat Med. 2013;30(6):601–16.
74. Pitceathly C, Maguire P. The psychological impact of cancer on patients' partners and other key relatives: a review. Eur J Cancer. 2003;39(11):1517–24.
75. Wijnhoven MN, Terpstra WE, van Rossem R, Haazer C, Gunnink-Boonstra N, Sonke GS, et al. Bereaved relatives' experiences during the incurable phase of cancer: a qualitative interview study. BMJ Open. 2015;5(11):e009009.
76. Hudson P, Remedios C, Zordan R, Thomas K, Clifton D, Crewdson M, et al. Guidelines for the psychosocial and bereavement support of family caregivers of palliative care patients. J Palliat Med. 2012;15(6):696–702.
77. Hudson P, Trauer T, Kelly B, O'Connor M, Thomas K, Zordan R, et al. Reducing the psychological distress of family caregivers of home based palliative care patients: longer term effects from a randomised controlled trial. Psychooncology. 2015;24(1):19–24.
78. Yamamoto S, Arao H, Masutani E, Aoki M, Kishino M, Morita T, et al. Decision making regarding the place of end-of-life cancer care: the burden on bereaved families and related factors. J Pain Symptom Manag. 2017;53(5):862–70.
79. Applebaum AJ, Buda KA, Farberov M, Teitelbaum ND, Evans K, Cowens-Alvarado R, et al. Care for the cancer caregiver: A web-based intervention to address caregiver burden. 14th Annual Conference of the American Psychosocial Oncology Society; Orlando, FL; 2017.
80. Kissane DW, McKenzie M, Bloch S, Moskowitz C, McKenzie DP, O'Neill I. Family focused grief therapy: a randomized, controlled trial in palliative care and bereavement. Am J Psychiatry. 2006;163(7):1208–18.
81. Garrido MM, Prigerson HG. The end-of-life experience: modifiable predictors of caregivers' bereavement adjustment. Cancer. 2014;120(6):918–25.
82. Dokken DL. In their own voices: families discuss end-of-life decision making--part 1. Pediatr Nurs. 2006;32(2):173–5.
83. Rogers CH, Floyd FJ, Seltzer MM, Greenberg J, Hong J. Long-term effects of the death of a child on parents' adjustment in midlife. J Fam Psychol. 2008;22(2):203–11.
84. Kars MC, Grypdonck MHF, van Delden JJM. Being a parent of a child with cancer throughout the end-of-life course. Oncol Nurs Forum. 2011;38(4):E260–E71.
85. Davies B, Connaughty S. Pediatric end-of-life care: lessons learned from parents. J Nurs Adm. 2002;32(1):5–6.
86. Contro N, Larson J, Scofield S, Sourkes B, Cohen H. Family perspectives on the quality of pediatric palliative care. Arch Pediatr Adolesc Med. 2002;156(1):14.
87. Meert KL, Eggly S, Pollack M, Anand KJS, Zimmerman J, Carcillo J, et al. Parents' perspectives on physician-parent communication near the time of a child's death in the pediatric intensive care unit. Pediatr Crit Care Med. 2008;9(1):2–7.

88. Bluebond-Langner M, Belasco JB, Goldman A, Belasco C. Understanding parents' approaches to care and treatment of children with cancer when standard therapy has failed. J Clin Oncol. 2007;25(17):2414–9.
89. Matsuoka M, Narama M. Parents' thoughts and perceptions on hearing that their child has incurable cancer. J Palliat Med. 2012;15(3):340–6.
90. Wolfe J, Grier HE, Klar N, Levin SB, Ellenbogen JM, Salem-Schatz S, et al. Symptoms and suffering at the end of life in children with cancer. N Engl J Med. 2000;342(5):326–33.
91. Widger K, Picot C. Parents' perceptions of the quality of pediatric and perinatal end-of-life care. Pediatr Nurs. 2008;34(1):53–8.
92. Farrell MF, Frost C. The most important needs of parents of critically ill children: parents' perceptions. Intensive Crit Care Nurs. 1992;8(3):130–9.
93. Branchett K, Stretton J. Neonatal palliative and end of life care: what parents want from professionals. J Neonatal Nurs. 2012;18(2):40–4.
94. Rini A, Loriz L. Anticipatory mourning in parents with a child who dies while hospitalized. J Pediatr Nurs. 2007;22(4):272–82.
95. Zimmermann K, Cignacco E, Eskola K, Engberg S, Ramelet AS, Von der Weid N, et al. Development and initial validation of the parental PELICAN questionnaire (PaPEQu)--an instrument to assess parental experiences and needs during their child's end-of-life care. J Adv Nurs. 2015;71(12):3006–17.
96. Ellis R, Leventhal B. Information needs and decision-making preferences of children with cancer. Psycho-Oncology. 1993;2(4):277–84.
97. Beale EA, Baile WF, Aaron J. Silence is not golden: communicating with children dying from cancer. J Clin Oncol. 2005;23(15):3629–31.
98. Wiener L, Zadeh S, Wexler LH, Pao M. When silence is not golden: engaging adolescents and young adults in discussions around end-of-life care choices. Pediatr Blood Cancer. 2013;60(5):715–8.
99. Kreicbergs U, Valdimarsdóttir U, Onelöv E, Henter J, Steineck G. Talking about death with children who have severe malignant disease. N Engl J Med. 2004;351(12):1175–86.
100. Hurwitz CA, Duncan J, Wolfe J. Caring for the child with cancer at the close of life. JAMA. 2004;292(17):2141.
101. Bell CJ, Skiles J, Pradhan K, Champion VL. End-of-life experiences in adolescents dying with cancer. Support Care Cancer. 2010;18(7):827–35.
102. Stevens MM, Jones P, O'Riordan E. Family responses when a child with cancer is in palliative care. J Palliat Care. 1996;12(3):51–5.
103. Anderzén-Carlsson A, Kihlgren M, Svantesson M, Sorlie V. Parental handling of fear in children with cancer; caring in the best interests of the child. J Pediatr Nurs. 2010;25(5):317–26.
104. Wiener L, Ballard E, Brennan T, Battles H, Martinez P, Pao M. How i wish to be remembered: the use of an advance care planning document in adolescent and young adult populations. J Palliat Med. 2008;11(10):1309–13.
105. Zadeh S, Pao M, Wiener L. Oening end-of-life discussions: how to introduce voicing my CHOiCES™, an advance care planning guide for adolescents and young adults. Palliat Support Care. 2015;13(03):591–9.
106. Wiener L, Zadeh S, Battles H, Baird K, Ballard E, Osherow J, et al. Allowing adolescents and young adults to plan their end-of-life care. Pediatrics. 2012;130(5):897–905.
107. Dighe M, Jadhav S, Muckaden M, Sovani A. Parental concerns in children requiring palliative care. Ind J Palliat Care. 2008;14(1):16.
108. Meyer EC, Ritholz MD, Burns JP, Truog RD. Improving the quality of end-of-life care in the pediatric intensive care unit: parents' priorities and recommendations. Pediatrics. 2006;117(3):649–57.
109. Hooyman NR, Kramer BJ. Living through loss. New York: Columbia University Press; 2008. p. 452.
110. Michelson KN, Steinhorn DM. Pediatric end-of-life issues and palliative care. Clin Pediatr Emerg Med. 2007;8(3):212–9.

111. Tan JS, Docherty SL, Barfield R, Brandon DH. Addressing parental bereavement support needs at the end of life for infants with complex chronic conditions. J Palliat Med. 2012;15(5):579–84.
112. Davies B, Contro N, Larson J, Widger K. Culturally-sensitive information-sharing in pediatric palliative care. Pediatrics. 2010;125(4):e859–e65.
113. Lichtenthal WG, Sweeney CR, Roberts KE, Corner GW, Donovan LA, Prigerson HG, et al. Bereavement follow-up after the death of a child as a standard of care in pediatric oncology. Pediatr Blood Cancer. 2015;62(Suppl 5):S834–69.
114. Hinds P, Oakes L, Furman W, Quargnenti A, Olson M, Foppiano P, et al. End-of-life decision making by adolescents, parents, and healthcare providers in pediatric oncology: research to evidence-based practice guidelines. Cancer Nurs. 2001;24(2):122–34.
115. Hendricks-Ferguson VL, Pradhan K, Shih C-S, Gauvain KM, Kane JR, Liu J, et al. Pilot evaluation of a palliative and end-of-life communication intervention for parents of children with a brain tumor. J Pediatr Oncol Nurs. 2017;34(3):203–13.
116. Donovan LA, Wakefield CE, Russell V, Cohn RJ. Hospital-based bereavement services following the death of a child: a mixed study review. Palliat Med. 2015;29(3):193–210.
117. Chan HY, Lee LH, Chan CW. The perceptions and experiences of nurses and bereaved families towards bereavement care in an oncology unit. Support Care Cancer. 2013;21(6):1551–6.
118. Ghesquiere A, Thomas J, Bruce M. Utilization of hospice bereavement support by at-risk family members. Am J Hosp Palliat Med. 2016;33(2):124–9.
119. Cherlin EJ, Barry CL, Prigerson HG, Green DS, Johnson-Hrzeler R, Kasi SV, et al. Bereavement services for family caregivers: how often used, why, and why not. J Palliat Med. 2007;10:148–58.
120. Seamark D, Blake S, Brearley SG, Milligan C, Thomas C, Turner M, et al. Dying at home: a qualitative study of family carers' views of support provided by GPs community staff. Br J Gen Pract. 2014;64(629):e796–803.
121. Chau NG, Zimmermann C, Ma C, Taback N, Krzyzanowska MK. Bereavement practices of physicians in oncology and palliative care. Arch Intern Med. 2009;169(10):963–71.
122. Bonanno GA, Kaltman S. The varieties of grief experience. Clin Psychol Rev. 2001;21:705–34.
123. Aoun S, Breen LJ, Howting D, Rumbold B, McNamara B, Hegney D. Who needs bereavement support? A population based survey of bereavement risk and support need. PLoS One. 2015;10(3):e0121101.
124. Prigerson HG, Frank E, Kasl SV, Reynolds CF 3rd, Anderson B, Zubenko GS, et al. Complicated grief and bereavement-related depression as distinct disorders: preliminary empirical validation in elderly bereaved spouses. Am J Psychiatry. 1995;152(1):22–30.
125. Lichtenthal WG, Prigerson HG, Kissane DW. Bereavement: a special issue in oncology. In: Holland J, editor. Psycho-oncology. 2nd ed. New York: Oxford University Press; 2010.
126. Barry L, Kasl S, Prigerson HG. Psychiatric disorders among bereaved persons: the role of perceived circumstances of death and preparedness for death. Am J Geriatr Psychiatry. 2002;10:447–57.
127. American Psychiatric Association, American Psychiatric Association. DSM-5 task force. Diagnostic and statistical manual of mental disorders, DSM-5. Washington, D.C.: Am Psychiatr Assoc; 2013. http://BN7ZQ5YK2C.search.serialssolutions.com/?V=1.0&L=BN7ZQ5YK2C&S=JCs&C=TC0000893411&T=marc&tab=BOOKS
128. Auster T, Moutier C, Lanouette N, Zisook S. Bereavement and depression: implications for diagnosis and treatmen. Psychiatr Ann. 2008;38(10):655–61.
129. Azoulay E, Pochard F, Kentish-Barnes N, Chevret S, Aboab J, Adrie C, et al. Risk of post-traumatic stress symptoms in family members of intensive care unit patients. Am J Resp Crit Care Med. 2005;171:987–94.
130. Sanderson C, Lobb EA, Mowll J, Butow PN, McGowan N, Price MA. Signs of post-traumatic stress disorder in caregivers following an expected death: a qualitative study. Palliat Med. 2013;27(7):625–31.
131. Zisook S, Chentsova-Dutton Y, Shuchter SR. PTSD following bereavement. Ann Clin Psychiatry. 1998;10(4):157–68.

132. Kristensen P, Weisaeth L, Heir T. Bereavement and mental health after sudden and violent losses: a review. Psychiatry. 2012;75(1):76–97.
133. Downar J, Barua R, Sinuff T. The desirability of an Intensive Care Unit (ICU) clinician-led bereavement screening and support program for family members of ICU decedents (ICU Bereave). J Crit Care. 2014;29(2):311.e9–e16.
134. Roberts K, Holland J, Prigerson HG, Sweeney C, Corner G, Breitbart W, et al. Development of the Bereavement Risk Inventory and Screening Questionnaire (BRISQ): item generation and expert panel feedback. Palliat Support Care. 2017;15(1):57–66.
135. Burke LA, Neimeyer RA, editors. Prospective risk factors for complicated grief. New York: Routledge; 2012.
136. Lundorff M, Holmgren H, Zachariae R, Farver-Vestergaard I, O'Connor M. Prevalence of prolonged grief disorder in adult bereavement: a systematic review and meta-analysis. J Affect Disord. 2017;212:138–49.
137. Boelen PA. Improving the understanding and treatment of complex grief: an important issue for psychotraumatology. Eur J Psychotraumatol. 2016;7:32609.
138. Lai C, Luciani M, Galli F, Morelli E, Cappelluti R, Penco I, et al. Attachment style dimensions can affect prolonged grief risk in caregivers of terminally ill patients with cancer. Am J Hosp Palliat Care. 2015;32(8):855–60.
139. Eisma MC, Boelen PA, Schut HA, Stroebe MS. Does worry affect adjustment to bereavement? A longitudinal investigation. Anxiety Stress Coping. 2017;30(3):243–52.
140. Field NP, Gao B, Paderna L. Continuing bonds in bereavement: an attachment theory based perspective. Death Stud. 2005;29(4):277–99.
141. Elvira de la Morena MJ, Cruzado JA. Caregivers of patients with disorders of consciousness: coping and prolonged grief. Acta Neurol Scand. 2013;127(6):413–8.
142. Currier JM, Holland JM, Neimeyer RA. Sense-making, grief, and the experience of violent loss: toward a mediational model. Death Stud. 2006;30(5):403–28.
143. Abbott CH, Prigerson HG, Maciejewski PK. The influence of patients' quality of life at the end of life on bereaved caregivers' suicidal ideation. J Pain Symptom Manag. 2014;48(3):459–64.
144. Lichtenthal WG, Currier JM, Neimeyer RA, Keesee NJ. Sense and significance: a mixed methods examination of meaning making after the loss of one's child. J Clin Psychol. 2010;66(7):791–812.
145. Rozenzweig A, Prigerson H, Miller MD, Reynolds CF 3rd. Bereavement and late-life depression: grief and its complications in the elderly. Annu Rev Med. 1997;48:421–8.
146. Kelly B, Edwards P, Synott R, Neil C, Baillie R, Battistutta D. Predictors of bereavement outcome for family carers of cancer patients. Psychooncology. 1999;8(3):237–49.
147. Bowlby J. Attachment and loss: retrospect and prospect. Am J Orthopsychiatry. 1982;52(4):664–78.
148. Johnson JG, Zhang B, Greer JA, Prigerson HG. Parental control, partner dependency, and complicated grief among widowed adults in the community. J Nerv Ment Dis. 2007;195(1):26–30.
149. van Doorn C, Kasl SV, Beery LC, Jacobs SC, Prigerson HG. The influence of marital quality and attachment styles on traumatic grief and depressive symptoms. J Nerv Ment Dis. 1998;186(9):566–73.
150. Prigerson HG, Shear MK, Bierhals AJ, Zonarich DL, Reynolds CF 3rd. Childhood adversity, attachment and personality styles as predictors of anxiety among elderly caregivers. Anxiety. 1996;2(5):234–41.
151. Heeke C, Stammel N, Heinrich M, Knaevelsrud C. Conflict-related trauma and bereavement: exploring differential symptom profiles of prolonged grief and posttraumatic stress disorder. BMC Psychiatry. 2017;17(1):118.
152. Coelho AM, Delalibera MA, Barbosa A. Palliative care caregivers' grief mediators: a prospective study. Am J Hosp Palliat Care. 2016;33(4):346–53.
153. Bonanno GA, Wortman CB, Lehman DR, Tweed R, Haring M, Sonnega J, et al. Resilience to loss and chronic grief: a prospective study from pre-loss to 18-months post-loss. J Pers Soc Psychol. 2002;83:1150–64.

154. Kersting A, Brahler E, Glaesmer H, Wagner B. Prevalence of complicated grief in a representative population-based sample. J Affect Disord. 2011;131(1–3):339–43.
155. Sealey M, Breen LJ, O'Connor M, Aoun SM. A scoping review of bereavement risk assessment measures: implications for palliative care. Palliat Med. 2015;29(7):577–89.
156. Lichtenthal W, Napolitano S, Roberts K, Sweeney C, Slivjak E. Meaning-centered grief therapy. In: Breitbart W, editor. Meaning-centered psychotherapy in the cancer setting: finding hope and meaning in the face of suffering. New York: Oxford; 2017.
157. Muta R, Sanjo M, Miyashita M, Wakabayashi R, Ando E, Morita T, et al. What bereavement follow-up does family members request in Japanese palliative care units? A qualitative study. Am J Hosp Palliat Care. 2014;31(5):485–94.
158. Morris SE, Block SD. Adding value to palliative care services: the development of an institutional bereavement program. J Palliat Med. 2015;18(11):915–22.
159. Goldstein J, Alter CL, Axelrod R. A psychoeducational bereavement-support group for families provided in an outpatient cancer center. J Cancer Educ. 1996;11(4):233–7.
160. Abrahm JL, Cooley M, Ricacho L. Efficacy of an educational bereavement program for families of veterans with cancer. J Cancer Educ. 1995;10(4):207–12.
161. Shear MK, Frank E, Houck PR. Treatment of complicated grief: a randomized controlled trial. JAMA. 2005;293(21):2601–8.
162. Neimeyer R. Narrative strategies in grief therapy. J Constr Psychol. 1999;12:65–85.
163. Neimeyer R, editor. Techniques of grief therapy. New York: Routledge; 2012.
164. Welch JG, Mannix MM, Boergers J, Jelalian E, Barbosa F, Fujii-Rios H, et al. Parental interest in a bereavement support visit when a child dies from cancer. Omega. 2012;65(4):335–46.
165. Snaman JM, Kaye EC, Levine DR, Cochran B, Wilcox R, Sparrow CK, et al. Empowering bereaved parents through the development of a comprehensive bereavement program. J Pain Symptom Manag. 2017;53(4):767–75.
166. Lichtenthal WG, Corner GW, Sweeney CR, Wiener L, Roberts KE, Baser RE, et al. Mental health services for parents who lost a child to cancer: if we build them, will they come? J Clin Oncol. 2015;33(20):2246–53.
167. Jensen J, Weng C, Spraker-Perlman HL. A provider-based survey to assess bereavement care knowledge, attitudes, and practices in pediatric oncologists. J Palliat Med. 2017;20(3):266–72.
168. Ruden BM. Bereavement follow-up: an opportunity to extend nursing care. J Pediatr Oncol Nurs. 1996;13(4):219–25.
169. Neimeyer RA. Reauthoring life narratives: grief therapy as meaning reconstruction. Isr J Psychiatry Relat Sci. 2001;38(3–4):171–83.
170. Lichtenthal W, Neimeyer R. Directed journaling to facilitate meaning-making. In: Neimeyer R, editor. Techniques of grief therapy. New York: Routledge; 2012. p. 165–8.
171. Fillion L, Duval S, Dumont S, Gagnon P, Tremblay I, Bairati I, et al. Impact of a meaning-centered intervention on job satisfaction and on quality of life among palliative care nurses. Psycho-Oncology. 2009;18(12):1300–10.
172. Pessin H, Fenn N, Hendriksen E, DeRosa A, Applebaum A. Existential distress among health care providers caring for patients at the end of life. Curr Opin Support Palliat Care. 2015;9(1):77–86.

# Chapter 15
# Physician Leadership

**Carl E. Heltne and James G. Brueggemann**

## Overview

Today's healthcare leaders face unprecedented pressure. They are tasked with transformation of the organization or units thereof, meeting the growing demands for high-quality, accessible, and cost-effective care. These goals have been articulated as the "triple aim," which is the simultaneous presence of improved patient experience (including quality and satisfaction), improved health of the population, and reduced per capita cost of health care [1]. The physician leader is also challenged with improving the work life of all healthcare providers: physicians, clinicians, and staff.

For patients to receive care and for care delivery to be sustainable within our society, all four of these aims, care, cost, health, and meaning in work, must be pursued. This has been referred to as the quadruple aim [2]. For this to be a sustainable reality, physicians must assume leadership roles. Stoller et al. in the *Harvard Business Review* further supports this premise by presenting information which demonstrates higher quality of care in those hospital systems led by physicians, relating that not only in medicine but also in other fields, domain experts lead to better organizational performance [3]. Although the article by Stoller et al. refers to "hospital systems," the systems that are referenced are integrated health systems; we believe that the evidence provided is applicable to health systems and clinical practices in general.

Specific areas where health systems can benefit from physician leadership skills and engagement relate most strongly to physician culture and clinical quality. Physicians tend to relate more specifically to proposals for changes in practice

C. E. Heltne (✉) · J. G. Brueggemann
Emeritus Physician,
Essentia Health, Duluth, MN, USA



P. Hopewood, M. J. Milroy (eds.), *Quality Cancer Care*,
https://doi.org/10.1007/978-3-319-78649-0_15

methods if these are brought to them by another physician, perceived as knowledgeable in their field of practice. This is most obvious in peer review, but extends to planning treatment protocols, championing clinical innovation, developing strategies to improve clinical process and outcome quality, and helping to develop methods of managing clinical risk. Physician leader involvement in organization strategic planning and resource allocation helps to engage other physicians in improving care delivery models.

## What Is Physician Leadership?

Within this chapter we reflect on what is leadership, what physician leaders actually do, how leadership differs from management, and the foundational components within the discipline of leadership. Within those components, we examine the necessary skills, structures, processes, and capabilities physician leaders must cultivate to be successful.

This is a focused reflection. The goal is to stimulate you to think with intentionality about the physician leader's role and to take advantage of resources which can enable you to be an effective, influential, and confident physician leader. Leadership is akin to the practice of medicine; to be successful in each of these endeavors one must study, practice, reflect, study, and practice.

This proposition begs for a definition of leadership. Warren Bennis states that "leadership is the capacity to translate vision into reality" [4]. Bill Gates defines leaders as those who empower others [4]. Peter Drucker opines that "the only definition of leadership is someone that has followers" [4]. All of these definitions point toward the work of leadership and are valid definitions. A definition providing additional guidance for this chapter's discussion is one by Terri McCarthy M.D., a former cohort member of the University of St. Thomas's Physician Leadership College, who defines the work of physician leadership as "cultivating and employing our knowledge and skills to facilitate and support our values for our patients" [5].

It is accepted by most that the quality of leadership drives an organization's long-term performance. In health care, high-quality physician leadership fosters higher patient, staff, clinician, and physician engagement which translates into high-quality, safer care and strong financial performance. Leadership is not management. Management is important, but it is about arranging, telling, and a disciplined approach to carry out the needed processes and tasks. Leadership is about putting first things first. It fosters a sense of being part of something greater than ourselves for a greater good. Leadership stems from "social influence," not authority, power, or title. It is a result of relationships. Leadership requires others. It is not simply "direct reports."

Physician autonomy is naturally cherished by physicians. In the traditional independent practice model, this autonomy is usually linked to practice ownership. As more and more physicians become employees of hospitals and health systems, the independent model shifts toward a new model of physician autonomy, one in which physicians' unique skills are leveraged toward leadership of clinical teams, demonstrable professional productivity, and enhanced clinical service value [6].

## Three Interwoven Foundational Components of Effective Leadership

### *Leadership of Self*

There are many paths to effective leadership. Leaders have various personal traits and attributes but the key element, the foundational component of effective leadership, is for one to know oneself, to understand one's values, to be true and authentic to these values, and thus to possess integrity. This work is then *leadership of self*. It is the inner work of leadership, defining the physician leader's mindset. This is the lens through which you see your work, your relationships, and the world, allowing you to accurately see yourself, and the impact you have on others and they on you.

To be an effective leader one must develop an understanding of self. Bill George, in his excellent book *True North: Discover Your Authentic Leadership*, speaks to knowing your authentic self [7]. The inner work of leadership is an ongoing process. We live in a complex world. We are constantly exposed to various perspectives, experiences, and other stimuli which lead us to evolve as we find our place in this world. Without self-awareness it is impossible to know your role, to understand your sources of seduction, and to know what may ring your chimes. It is difficult to be responsive rather than reactive, to accept ourselves, and to be vulnerable. It is also important to realize that vulnerability is a much hidden source of strength for effective leadership. It is important that one articulates which values are important and which we consider inviolable. From the exercise leading to self-awareness arise principles upon which we base our leadership actions. It is of utmost importance to develop a clear sense of our values before we enter into making difficult decisions or face difficult dilemmas. Integrity in our work and actions becomes a reality when this is in place. Integrity leads to trust. Trust is a tangible, intentional act in which one cedes power to another. Trustworthiness is the foundation of both personal and professional success. When what one thinks and feels is in alignment with what one says and does, one is authentic: secure yet vulnerable, in control without being controlling. This leads to effective leadership.

There can be decisions that are truly paradoxes, such as which services to provide and where or how to expend resources, both of which impact our patients and our organizations. Knowing your values makes these difficult calls not easier but understandable. Understanding your values also comes into play in decision-making when one deals with unacceptable clinical care or unprofessional behavior of a colleague. Knowing who you are and what your role calls from you, bringing your inner self into the process, leads to more effective leadership.

It is a common misunderstanding that the key elements of leadership are the technical ones such as finance, strategy development, and many other vital components. The real foundational element determining one's effectiveness is one's understanding of oneself.

## *Leading Others*

Just as it is imperative that as a leader you know yourself, that you are authentic and lead with integrity, it is also true that the effective leader knows the organization. This is the *work of leading others.* The totems that reveal the organization's identity are articulated in its collective statements of vision, mission, and values. These statements guide the organization. If they do not, then the issue of integrity becomes an organizational reality that the leader must address.

The vision statement is a declaration of what is possible, the picture of the future that you want to create for those that benefit from your group's impact. The mission statement flows from the vision. It reflects the work to be done to carry out the vision. The values statement articulates how you do the work, how you walk the talk. This is foundational. Any discussion which focuses on "what is more important, this or that" is a values discussion. It is therefore best to have these statements articulated before the questions arise.

Vision, mission, and values statements are practical tools that also guide and measure your planning and actions. One helpful exercise is to start your meetings by reviewing and discussing these statements so they become part of the fabric of your organization. An interesting question that can lead to the same effect is to occasionally start the meeting by asking those at your table, "Why are we here today?"

This helps to clarify what you are really there for, what future you are trying to create and for whom, and upon what you base your decision-making. The outcome of these three statements (vision, mission, and values), their interpretation and resulting action, is the culture of the organization. Schein, in his book *Humble Inquiry*, states that culture is the sum total of what a group has learned and now takes for granted as the way to deal with the external environment and its internal integration [8]. In simplified terms, culture can be defined as the way we do things around here. This is a learned reality. It does not result from someone announcing it. It is the leader's responsibility not only to understand the culture, but also to view it critically in the context of the tacit assumptions of vision, mission, and values. One then both affirms and nurtures the culture or one transforms it, thus transforming the organization. Culture is not immutable.

The key to the process of cultural transformation is to understand the task, the phases of change, and how to engage others in true dialogue. William Bridges in his text *Managing Transition* helps us understand the aspects of this process [9]. He begins by reminding us of the difference between change and transition: change is situational whereas transition is psychological. Transition is a process that people go through as they come to appreciate the reality of the new situation produced by change. If change occurs without individuals going through transition, the way things are done will never be truly different. The process of transition starts with an ending of the old ways and finishes with a beginning, a new "way things are done here."

To implement this transition, one needs to move from task accomplishment to relationship building. The responsibility of leadership as suggested by Heifetz in his book *Leadership Without Easy Answers* is to help people face reality and mobilize them to change [10]. To be effective, leadership requires building and utilizing highly functional relationships. Relationships are the key to good communication. Good communication is the key to successful transformation. Relationships that yield trust in turn create an environment where people are more confident, proactive, and helpful. We then have a virtuous circle where the chains of actions reinforce themselves through a feedback loop. It is also important to be transparent. There should be a reality where there is no hidden information and that the input of each member is needed and valued.

An example of the need for effective communication occurs in moving from an existing care model to another perceived by the physician leader and others as potentially able to deliver improved clinical care or service quality. If physicians and their care teams are enabled to clearly see the cost (to patients, physician, and other caregivers and/or the health system) of maintaining the status quo, compared with the benefit of moving to a new care model, some will readily make the switch. Others, however, will be more hesitant, focusing on the personal cost of change and risk of failure. If the physician leader can build a trusting relationship with these individuals, recognizing their concerns as valid rather than obstructionist, working with them to involve them personally in the transition, their receptivity to the new care model is likely to be greater.

Communication is also the key to good relationships. There are two aspects of communication: content, what we talk about, and the process, how we engage with one another. It is helpful to engage in dialogue which has the objective of increasing the overall knowledge and wisdom of the participants. This form of interaction is characterized by honesty, curiosity, and a willingness to learn, and very importantly the willingness to learn in public. Successful dialogue requires from the leader personal vulnerability. A simple helpful start is to make the statement "help me understand." The key practices to successful communication are to be truly present; to listen with curiosity; and to notice and suspend your judgments and assumptions, yet speak your truth with honesty. In all aspects of leading others, we come back to the essentials discussed in leading oneself. It is important to be self-aware. It is important to act with integrity and thus engender trust. It is important for you as a leader to understand that anytime you interact with others to accomplish something, culture changes. Your actions in large part determine if these changes are positive or negative.

Focusing on "leading others" more narrowly, let us consider the organizational unit described as teams. In your sphere of responsibility as a physician leader, this may be a cancer committee. Teams are a special collection of people. A team is defined by Katzenbach and Smith in their book *The Wisdom of Teams* as "a small number of people with complementary skills who are committed to a common purpose for which they hold themselves mutually accountable" [11]. Team members need to have the right skills, contribute time and ideas, challenge assumptions, and sign on to complete the task.

The leader's role is not that of "chief problem solver." The leader creates the environment for the work to be done and sets the direction. An analogy can be made to an orchestra conductor. The conductor brings knowledge of the message conveyed by the score, gathers the right people with the right skills, and brings the best out of them. The conductor, in addition to bringing the best out of each individual performer, brings together the various components so that together they make even more beautiful music than they can as an individual. The conductor does not play the music but enables the performance. The leader of the team or an organization gives the work to the team. Some years ago, one of the authors as the Chief Medical Officer and a cardiologist by training and practice was given the charge to develop a system-wide primary care model. This was done by fulfilling the leaders' responsibility of first establishing the expectations, knowing the message of the score. The charge given was to "provide a care model for our patients that resulted in high quality, accessible care in a manner sustainable for the organization." The second responsibility was to assemble the right individuals who had the requisite knowledge, experience, and perspectives (in this case those included were primary care physicians and dyad leadership, organizational content experts, and decision makers such as finance, payor relations, and human resource personal and most importantly patients). This is, as with the conductor of the orchestra, gathering the right people with the right skills and asking for the best effort of each individual and giving the time and resource to work collaboratively to build something better than each one alone or the leader would have developed. The leaders' role was then to champion the outcome and bring it through the organization in a manner that allowed resources to be allocated and the model to be operational.

Such an approach is articulated by Heifetz and Linsky; in their text "*Leadership on the Line,*" they speak to the leader's responsibility as giving the work to the people and very importantly creating a holding environment that is productive [12]. The phrase "holding environment" was brought from psychoanalysis to the leadership literature by Heifetz and Linsky where it refers to a supportive but not tension-free environment where one is neither stressed out to the point where one can no longer function well nor so stress free that one can avoid doing the needed work. It is important for the leaders to be observing the working of the team and to be mindful of their own role. Heifetz and Linsky use the metaphor of getting up on the balcony observing and being on the dance floor in the mix of the activity. With this perspective one can then see what is in play and attempt to create a workable holding environment, returning the work to the people, not simply empowering them but giving the work to those who are most impacted. This in turn leads to fruitful engagement of team members in a most productive manner.

Dov Seidman articulates an additional concept in his book "*how*" [13]. He postulates that one motivates by either coercion, by using promise of reward, or threats of repercussion or the leader can inspire, thus connecting others in a manner that encourages their productive action. The ability to inspire people, to give them an opportunity to be part of something greater than self, is fundamental to leading others.

Daniel Pink in his book "*Drive*" would also suggest that the most successful and sustainable means to motivate is to inspire individuals to be part of something greater than themselves, believing in them to accomplish the task [14]. He cautions us to avoid carrots and sticks, i.e., extrinsic motivators. Such a posture suggests that the task at hand is undesirable and can only be accomplished by punishment or rewards.

Pink suggests that if one is to use rewards they should be unexpected and maybe even whimsical [14]. It has been our practice to send a handwritten note to the individual who has stepped up to the challenge. This note expresses appreciation for the specific actions taken and the specific results witnessed and it is opened in that person's home to be shared with family. We would encourage you to try something similar to reward those you lead.

The majority of the science to date cited by Pink tells us to rely on the intrinsic motivators, which are presence of a purpose; the freedom to accomplish the task in a manner of one's choosing, i.e., autonomy; and the sense of mastery. This echoes the work of Heifetz and Linsky and of Dov Seidman. The message for the leader is that to be effective, one must provide the purpose, give the space for the work to be done, and allow individuals to show their mastery. It is not to be the chief problem solver.

In leading others, there is always the reality of conflict and the need for negotiation. These realities merit further discussion, for there are approaches that can change conflict into opportunity. Conbere and Heorhiadi in their lectures at the University of St. Thomas Physician Leadership College relate that "conflict occurs when there are different opinions about an issue and this difference really matters to one or more members of the group" [15]. Conflict is often presented to the leader as a story. Such stories usually follow a fundamental prototype described by Cloke and Goldsmith in their book, *Resolving Personal and Organizational Conflict* [16]. They reference the classic conflict triangle where there is the princess, prince, and the dragon. The princess is the one afflicted by the problem, the dragon is the source of the problem, and the prince is the one responsible for the solution. It is important for the leader to understand these roles and importantly not to assume the role of the prince. Here again the constructs explained by Heifetz suggest that the leader should not solve the problem but establish a holding space and give the work back to those in conflict. One encourages all within the conflict to be vulnerable and thus aid those involved to move from a posture of positions to one of interests and thus hopefully to resolution. This act of moving from positions to interests lays the foundation for successful negotiation. Negotiation should be true dialogue where the intention is to reach a mutually beneficial outcome for the parties involved. For the leader, it is important when involved in negotiation to separate the problem from the person, to separate the position from the issue, to work with the participants on developing options, and to prepare in advance, so that one fully understands what will be either the minimum result of negotiation or the best alternative, should negotiation fail, that one can and will accept.

To lead others, one must understand how to function collectively, excel at teamwork, have the ability to listen, and possess a high degree of emotional intelligence. Your knowledge and technical competency are the tickets that allow you to become an "accidental" leader [17]. Emotional intelligence is what allows you to be a successful and authentic leader. This was touched on in the discussion of *"leading oneself"* but merits repeating as it is so very important.

Daniel Goleman defines emotional intelligence as "the capacity for recognizing our own feelings and those of others, and for managing emotions well in ourselves and in our relationships" [18]. It is important for you to know your feelings and know how your feelings impact those around you. You must keep your disruptive emotions from being the message. The reality is that as a leader you will be challenged and that will at times feel very personal; it will ring your chimes. You do not have the freedom to act out. We talk about taking a moment to pause. When challenged, it is helpful to tune into your feelings, recognize your triggers, beware of the story you have made in your mind, then pause, and proceed by either reframing the issue or continuing, but most importantly to respond and not react. To not take this pause can lead to destroyed relationships and inappropriate decisions.

In this situation, it is useful to remember that those challenging you as a physician leader are usually challenging the news you bring, the change you represent, or the strategy you are suggesting. Not internalizing these comments may help you to respond appropriately.

## *Leadership of the Organization*

The leader must also be able to lead the organization. (In this discussion we use the word organization to include structures such as medical divisions, sections, departments of the organization, committees, and teams.) This aspect of leadership focuses on its more technical aspects, disciplines such as finance, human resources, legal and regulatory matters, payer relationships, and operations, all critical for the functioning of an organization. *Leadership of the organization* requires access to data and ability to transform data into information. One must have the ability to see within health care all the dimensions that need to work in concert. Each of these dimensions—clinical, operational, and financial—has different content experts and lexicons. One must translate the various languages and effectively coordinate these for the betterment of patient care. Without the investment in leading oneself and leading others, the investment in learning the intricacies of these components will not yield the potential that is needed to lead effectively.

As a physician leader, it is helpful to consider the perspectives espoused by C.J. Peek in his lectures [19]. In those presentations he postulates that healthcare organizations operate simultaneously in three worlds: the clinical world, the operational world, and the financial world. It is important for the physician leader to recognize and understand that for the organization to be successful and sustainable, it must have a structure and processes that satisfy the demands of all three of these worlds so that they harmonize and do not clash. Each of these worlds has its goal. In the clinical world, the goals are caring and quality. In the operational world, the goals are efficiency and effectiveness. In the financial world, the goal is to obtain the right price and ensure good value for the resources allocated.

To successfully lead as a physician, one does not need to be a content expert in operations or finance. One needs to understand the language of each of these worlds and be able to translate them in an effective manner. A most effective way of accomplishing this is to work in a dyad relationship. As Peek relates that this is defined as "a working pair (physician and non-physician) characterized by a singular mission, shared accountability and equal stature but contrasting perspective, knowledge and skills" [19]. Such a relationship is based on trust built on communication and thus on all the ingredients we have mentioned in the discussions of leading self and leading others.

The physician leader in a dyad builds the physician culture, manages physician clinical quality and physician behavior, champions clinical innovation, and forms relationships with referring physicians. The administrative leader manages clinical operations and staffing, revenue and expenses, and reporting of clinical and patient experience outcomes [20]. Each dyad pair will find the correct balance in roles and responsibility. There is no set definition of roles and responsibilities, but there is the need to effectively and completely communicate with each other and thus share the responsibility for decisions and results.

In practical terms the dyads cannot act as though they are fused at the hip. Each member has areas where they act independently. The physician leader may deal with mentoring or coaching a new physician where the administrative partner may have a greater focus on facilities. There are also times when coordination is of importance. The standard example would be the development of a clinical protocol which is led by the physician and the subsequent embedding into the electronic medical record and staff education would be the responsibility of the administrative partner.

As suggested above, a united front on the part of dyad partners is also a posture that is required. If there are significant changes for example in the practice model, the dyad must be unified. There can be no selling out by one or the other. Such action leads to a failure of trust in leadership and the negative consequences that arise from such dysfunction.

Simple acts of respect and civility are important to assure that a productive personal relationship is in place. Through a good working relationship, the art of using each other's style and personalities becomes second nature and effective. The dyad pair must act as partners in front of others. To be successful, they must respectfully deal with differences in private. This working model allows the dyad to become more than the sum of its parts. It brings forth in a productive manner the needed skills and wisdom of the participants in a manner that truly benefits patient care.

In addition to an effective dyad relationship, the physician leader needs to develop collaborative working and learning relations with individuals in areas such as finance, human resources, legal, payer relations, and other disciplines that are of importance in this complex world of health care. Such relations enhance the knowledge of the physician and each person who is part of the interaction. It allows the physician to gain more knowledge, to be able to translate the language from one world to the other, and also to make the work more enjoyable for all.

A separate yet related matter is the understanding of "how things get done." Each organization has policies and procedures that lead to strategic planning and resource allocation. One must understand these policies and procedures and most importantly the pathways within the organization that enable one to execute on needed programs or be successful with capital requests.

In health systems with a cancer program, physician leadership positions may be health system-appointed positions with a written job description, clear accountability, and, if the time required is significant, pay for the time expended in the job. These position descriptions add value for the health system in its quest to improve quality, efficiency, and effectiveness of care. They also clarify for physician leaders their specific responsibility, authority, and accountability. For these reasons, health systems may intentionally groom physicians for leadership, knowing that future success depends on having the right physicians in the right leadership places. What can be achieved for patient care by physicians actively engaged in leadership is valued by everyone in the organization.

## How Do Physician Leaders Succeed?

Leadership is not a title but an attitude based on core values which express one's highest aspirations and fundamental belief. It is an attitude that moves from the position of "Tell and Do" to the diagnostic framework of inquiry which builds trust and allows one to enlist and share with others the opportunity to successfully pursue a vision that is greater than any one individual.

For a physician assuming a leadership role, it is important to remember that to lead is not to command. Curiosity about the many philosophies and theories of leadership, a desire to serve others, and willingness to listen intentionally to others and to give work to others in an environment at a rate that allows them to be successful are critical to leadership success. Leaders engage others in the desire to become part of something greater, whether in a large organization or one of its many vital components.

Physician leaders need to be relentlessly focused on clinical quality and thus the care delivered to those who entrust them with that awesome responsibility. Without this championing role, the teams they lead, whether a disease management program, a committee, or some other unit of the health system, lose heart. With this focus, physicians can engage members of the team, physician and nonphysician alike, in selecting appropriate quality metrics and developing strategies and tactics to meet them.

It is useful for physician leaders to be actively engaged, if possible, in the management of clinical risk. Often this is left to a risk manager working with the legal department, but it is more effective if physicians see both the welfare of their patients and the quality of their team's work at risk from defective processes or systems of care, participating in developing strategies to minimize risk and sharing an open, proactive mind-set toward using clinical risk information to improve clinical quality.

Throughout this discussion we have mentioned the importance of values and integrity in leadership. Trust is a matter of credibility, reliability, and authenticity over self-interest. When trust is present, the work gets done and leadership is manifested. We have then served an interest greater than ourselves, serving our patients.

To be successful, one must be a student of leadership just as one is a student of medicine. Committee members and staff such as those from administration, finance, nursing, and others must be versed and experienced in the discipline of leadership. However, the role of the physician leader is unique both by position and profession and for bodies such as a cancer committee to be effective it is of utmost importance for the physician leader to seek out and obtain the needed education. Being a physician is not enough. Leadership is a discipline that requires education and practice. An understanding of useful basic concepts of physician leadership is of importance and can be acquired through courses offered by a variety of healthcare leadership education organizations and universities, often with online options.

In addition, developing a collegial relationship with others, be it physicians in leadership positions or leaders outside of medicine, is always useful as a mentoring opportunity. As alluded to above, positions such as Cancer Committee Chair are often viewed by organizations as a stepping stone to roles of increasing responsibility. Therefore, if one is interested in such opportunities, it is prudent to seek out educational opportunities.

## Final Thoughts

Lastly, as a physician leader one must develop capacity and resilience. Heifetz and Linsky discuss this in their book "Leadership on the Line" [12]. As you practice leadership it is inevitable that you may at times feel personally challenged or may, for a variety of reasons, see your efforts fall short of your goals. You may feel hurt or disillusioned. It is impossible to experience the joy of leadership without the pain. Heifetz and Linsky say, "the difficult work of leadership involves learning to experience the distress without becoming numb" [12]. We have found that the antidote for this is basically to embrace vulnerability; to work on deeper relationships; to engage in dialogue, not debate; and to focus on the positives of possibilities and choices rather than what is wrong.

We have found the rewards in leadership to be multiple. By taking on this role, you are actively validating the trust that patients have placed in you and your organizations. We wish you the best as a physician leader.

## References


1. Berwick DM, Nolon TW, Whittington J. The triple aim: care, health, and cost. Health Aff. 2008;27(3):759–69.
2. Sikkal R, Moreth J, Leape L. The quadruple aim: care, health, cost and meaning in work. BMJ Qual Saf. 2015;24(10):608–10.
3. Stoller J, Goodall A, Baker A. Why the best hospitals are managed by doctors. Harvard Business Review; 2016. https://hbr.org/2016/12/why-the-best-hospitals-are-managed-by-doctors.
4. Kruse K. What is leadership? Forbes; 2013. https://www.forbes.com/sites/kevinkruse/2013/04/09/what-is-leadership/#341517425b90.
5. McCarthy T. Capstone presentation. Lecture Presented at 2013; University of St. Thomas Physician Leadership College.
6. Brueggemann J, Zismer D. Physician autonomy in integrated health systems. Group Pract J. 2008;57(9):39–43.
7. George B. True north: discover your authentic leadership. San Francisco, CA: Jossey-Bass; 2007.
8. Schein E. Humble inquiry. Oakland, CA: Berrett-Koehler; 2013.
9. Bridges W. Managing transitions. Philadelphia, PA: Da Capo Press; 2009.
10. Heifetz R. Leadership without easy answers. Cambridge, MA: The Belknap Press of Harvard University Press; 1994.
11. Katzenbach J, Smith K. The wisdom of teams: creating the high performance organization. Brighton MA: Harvard Business School Press; 1993.
12. Heifetz R, Linsky M. Leadership on the line. Brighton, MA: Harvard Business Review Press; 2002.
13. Seidman D. How: why how we do anything means everything. Hoboken, NJ: John Wiley & Sons; 2011.
14. Pink D. The surprising truth about what motivates us. New York NY: Penguin Publishing Group; 2009.
15. Conbere J, Heorhiadi A. Negotiation and conflict management. Lecture Presented at 2017; University of St Thomas Physician Leadership College.
16. Cloke K, Goldsmith J. Resolving personal and organizational conflict. San Francisco, CA: Jossey-Bass; 2000.
17. Robbins H, Finley M. The accidental leader: what to do when you are suddenly in charge. San Francisco, CA: Jossey-Bass; 2004.
18. Goleman D. Emotional intelligence: why it can matter more than IQ. New York NY: Bantam Dell; 1995.
19. Peek C. Dyad leadership. Lecture Presented at 2015; University of St Thomas Physician Leadership College.
20. Zismer D, Brueggemann J. Examining the "Dyad" as a management model in integrated health systems. Physician Exec. 2010:14–19.

# Index





P. Hopewood, M. J. Milroy (eds.), *Quality Cancer Care*,
https://doi.org/10.1007/978-3-319-78649-0

**Q**



**R**

MIX
Papier aus verantwortungsvollen Quellen
Paper from responsible sources
FSC® C105338

If you have any concerns about our products,
you can contact us on
**ProductSafety@springernature.com**

In case Publisher is established outside the EU,
the EU authorized representative is:
**Springer Nature Customer Service Center GmbH**
**Europaplatz 3, 69115 Heidelberg, Germany**

Printed by Libri Plureos GmbH
in Hamburg, Germany